# Imaging in GLAUCOMA

# Imaging in GLAUCOMA

**Joel S. Schuman, MD**

Director, Glaucoma Service
Director, Residency Training
Associate Professor
New England Eye Center
Tufts University School of Medicine
Boston, Massachusetts

SLACK Incorporated • 6900 Grove Road • Thorofare, NJ 08086-9447

Chapter 2: Supported in part by the Massachusetts Lions Eye Research Fund and Research to Prevent Blindness. The author acknowledges expert photographic assistance by Audrey C. Melanson.
Chapters 4 and 6: Supported in part by NEI EY11008, NEI EY11158, Foundation for Eye Research, and an unrestricted grant from Research to Prevent Blindness Inc.
Chapter 7: Supported by NIH 1-R29-EY11006-01, NIH 9-RO1-EY11289, MFEL N00014-94-1-0717, and Research to Prevent Blindness, Inc., New York, NY.

Publisher: John H. Bond
Editorial Director: Amy E. Drummond
Associate Editor: Jennifer J. Cahill
Art Director: Linda Baker
Cover Art: Laurel C. Lhowe

Copyright © 1997 by SLACK Incorporated



Imaging in glaucoma/[edited by] Joel S. Schuman.
     p. cm.
   Includes bibliographical references and index.
   ISBN 1-55642-319-5
   1. Glaucoma--Imaging. I. Schuman, Joel S.
   [DNLM: 1. Glaucoma--diagnosis. 2. Diagnostic Imaging. 3. Eye--radiography. WW 290 I31
     1996]
   RE871.I52 1996
   617.7'41--dc20
   DNLM/DLC                                96-42146
   for Library of Congress

Printed in the United States of America
Published by:    SLACK Incorporated
               6900 Grove Road
               Thorofare, NJ 08086-9447 USA
               Telephone: 609-848-1000
               Fax: 609-853-5991

Contact SLACK Incorporated for more information about other books in this field or about the availability of our books from distributors outside the United States.



Last digit is print number: 10  9  8  7  6  5  4  3  2  1

# Dedication

*To my parents, who taught me the value of knowledge.*

*To my teachers, especially W. Morton Grant and David L. Epstein, who taught me to question.*

*To Carmen A. Puliafito, who allowed me free rein of his laser laboratory to probe ophthalmic technology.*

*To my wife, Carole, and children, Alexandra, Eric, and Ari, for their support and love, and for their understanding, which permits me the time to explore.*

# CONTENTS

# CONTRIBUTING AUTHORS


**Louis Cantor, MD**
*Director, Glaucoma Service*
*Indiana University Medical Center*
*Associate Professor of Ophthalmology*
*Indiana University School of Medicine*
*Indianapolis, Indiana*

**David S. Greenfield, MD**
*The New York Eye and Ear Infirmary*
*New York, New York*
*Clinical Assistant Professor of*
*Ophthalmology and Neurology*
*New York Medical College*
*Valhalla, New York*

**Alon Harris, PhD**
*Director, Glaucoma Research and Diagnostic Center*
*Associate Professor of Ophthalmology,*
*Physiology, and Biophysics*
*Indiana University School of Medicine*
*Indianapolis, Indiana*

**Raymond Iezzi, MD**
*The New York Eye and Ear Infirmary*
*New York, New York*

**Larry Kagemann, MS**
*Assistant Director*
*Glaucoma Research and Diagnostic Center*
*Indiana University School of Medicine*
*Indianapolis, Indiana*

**Sara Krupsky, MD**
*The Sam Rothberg Glaucoma Center*
*Goldschleger Eye Institute*
*Tel-Hashomer, Israel*

**Philip Lempert, MD**
*Visiting Fellow in the Department of Physiology*
*College of Vetrinary Medicine*
*Cornell University*
*Ithaca, New York*

**Jeffrey Liebmann, MD**
*Associate Director, Glaucoma Service*
*Clinical Associate Professor of Ophthalmology*
*The New York Eye and Ear Infirmary*
*New York, New York*

**Marcia de Souza Lima, MD**
*Research Fellow in Glaucoma*
*Glaucoma Center and Research Laboratories*
*University of California—San Diego*
*La Jolla, California*

**Cynthia Mattox, MD**
*Assistant Professor of Ophthalmology*
*New England Eye Center*
*Tufts University School of Medicine*
*Boston, Massachusetts*

**Shlomo Melamed, MD**
*Director, The Sam Rothberg Glaucoma Center*
*Goldschleger Eye Institute*
*Tel-Hashomer, Israel*
*Associate Professor of Ophthalmology*
*Sackler School of Medicine*
*Tel-Aviv University*
*Tel-Aviv, Israel*

**Peter A. Netland, MD, PhD**
*Associate Director of Glaucoma*
*King Khaled Eye Specialist Hospital*
*Riyadh, Kingdom of Saudi Arabia*

**Robert Ritch, MD**
*Chief, Glaucoma Service*
*Surgeon Director*
*Professor of Clinical Ophthalmology*
*The New York Eye and Ear Infirmary*
*New York, New York*

**Joel S. Schuman, MD**
*Director, Glaucoma Service*
*Director, Residency Training*
*Associate Professor*
*New England Eye Center*
*Tufts University School of Medicine*
*Boston, Massachusetts*

**Celso Tello, MD**
*The New York Eye and Ear Infirmary*
*New York, New York*

**Giora Treister, MD**
*Director, Goldschleger Eye Institute*
*Tel-Hashomer, Israel*
*Professor of Ophthalmology*
*Sackler School of Medicine*
*Tel-Aviv University*
*Tel-Aviv, Israel*

**Robert N. Weinreb, MD**
*Professor and Vice Chairman*
*Glaucoma Center and Research Laboratories*
*University of California—San Diego*
*La Jolla, California*

**Linda Zangwill, PhD**
*Assistant Professor*
*Glaucoma Center and Research Laboratories*
*University of California—San Diego*
*La Jolla, California*

# Preface

The impetus for this book was a course given in March 1996 at New England Eye Center, Tufts University School of Medicine, called "Imaging in Glaucoma: The Boston Glaucoma Course 1996." This course gathered the world's experts in the various imaging technologies to discuss the techniques and interpretation of optic nerve head, nerve fiber layer, blood flow, and anterior segment imaging. A CD-ROM was produced, also called "Imaging in Glaucoma," providing an interactive audiovisual transcript of the course.

**This text is not a transcript of the "Imaging in Glaucoma" course.** It is written by the speakers at that meeting, but represents a comprehensive evaluation of the current and emerging technologies for clinical assessment of glaucoma. The information in this book is both current and cutting-edge, and also clinically relevant. The authors have designed their chapters with the clinician in mind to present options for ocular imaging in an accessible fashion, and to make available the approaches for interpretation of what is often novel patient information. Tables are often included outlining specialized techniques or comparing competing technologies.

This book is concerned with various means for imaging in glaucoma, including conventional means, such as stereoscopic fundus photography and nerve fiber layer photography, as well as more advanced technologies. Technologies discussed include both anterior and posterior segment imaging methods. The analysis of the optic nerve head with the Glaucoma-Scope and confocal scanning laser ophthalmoscopy are covered. Means for nerve fiber layer analysis, including the Nerve Fiber Analyzer and Optical Coherence Tomography, are reviewed. Color Doppler imaging, as well as confocal scanning laser flowimetry and angiography, are covered with regard to blood flow in glaucoma. In the anterior segment, ultrasound biomicroscopy is discussed.

This book is written for both general ophthalmologists and glaucoma specialists to attempt to answer the following questions:

- Which, if any, technology for optic nerve head or nerve fiber layer analysis should I buy?
- Which devices can I use to determine blood flow in glaucoma, and what do the results mean?
- What tests should I order on my patients, and what can I expect the tests to tell me?

# INTRODUCTION—WHAT DO I NEED IMAGING FOR?

Glaucoma is a disease characterized by loss of neural tissue over time. This damage is irreversible, and even optimal treatment cannot reclaim neurons destroyed by glaucoma. The key then to dealing with this disease is early detection of its presence or progression, with the rapid initiation or advancement of appropriate treatment.

The ophthalmoscope, introduced by Helmholtz in 1851,[1] allowed ophthalmologists to examine the optic nerve head (ONH). This permitted von Graefe in 1855 to describe optic nerve damage in glaucoma, which he characterized as "amaurosis with excavation of the optic nerve."[2] Nerve fiber loss in glaucoma was described by Schnabel,[3] and later work by Fuchs[4] and Elliot[5] illustrated glaucomatous changes in the optic nerve. Fuchs identified the disappearance of anterior glial fibers, which preceded the atrophy of the deeper glial fibers, as well as the backward bowing and thinning of the lamina cribosa in response to elevated intraocular pressure (IOP). Fuchs felt that these structural ONH changes occured prior to visual field loss.[4]

## THE NEED FOR NEW TOOLS

The ONH appearance has been used by clinicians since the time of Helmholtz and von Graefe to assess the status of glaucoma; however, the interpretation of the ONH is subjective, and there is wide variation between observers, and even between examinations by the same observer.[6,7] Although the judgment of the observer is necessary to estimate the degree of glaucomatous optic nerve damage, this parameter, together with IOP and visual field performance, is used to diagnose glaucoma and determine progression. As clinical evaluation of the ONH is subjective and visual field results are both variable and difficult to interpret, and while IOP may or may not be elevated in glaucoma, and even moderately elevated IOP is not diagnostic of glaucoma, it is imperative that objective tools be devised to enable diagnosis of the disease at the outset, and to detect progression at the earliest possible point.

Attempts at the production of such tools have been introduced over the past half century, with possibly the greatest advances achieved during the past 5 to 10 years.

## STEREOSCOPIC OPTIC NERVE HEAD PHOTOGRAPHY

Stereoscopic ONH photography is discussed in the chapter by Greenfield. This is one of the simplest technologies that can be used by the clinician in practice, yet the utility is extremely high. Cost is relatively low, and stereoscopic ONH photographs permit objective recording of the ONH appearance. These photographs enable the clinician to compare ONH appearance in three dimensions between visits, providing a permanent record of change over time.[8]

## OPTIC NERVE HEAD ANALYZERS AND CONFOCAL SCANNING LASER OPHTHALMOSCOPY

Despite the low cost and high value of stereoscopic ONH photography, it does not provide a truly objective system for interpretation of ONH appearance and change over time. Even experts examining stereoscopic ONH photographs are not able to agree in discrimination between normal and glaucomatous ONHs.[6] This is not to diminish the importance of stereoscopic ONH photography; it is certainly better than clinical disc drawings or cup-to-disc ratios. It does not, however, provide an objective interpretation of the ONH.

ONH analyzers preceded the development of the confocal scanning laser ophthalmoscope (CSLO). The ONH analyzers were a necessary first step, but variability and lack of resolution, as well as high cost, eliminated nearly every device of this type. One instrument, the Glaucoma-Scope, produces high quality assessment of the ONH, with reproducibility better than its predecessors and at a relatively low cost. Netland describes the Glaucoma-Scope in his chapter. Lempert demonstrates a technique for "home-made" ONH computer analysis, and includes the necessary programming information in his chapter.

Confocal scanning laser ophthalmoscopy goes beyond ONH analyzers in producing a sequential series of coronal sections progressively deeper through the ONH. These sections are displayed and analyzed by the instrument, and provide a wealth of information regarding the ONH structure. Axial resolution is improved and variability is reduced in the CSLO as compared to ONH analyzers. In addition, since only one spot on the retina is illuminated at any given time with the CSLO, it is a much more comfortable examination for the patient versus ONH photography. The CSLO is the state-of-the-art in ONH assessment, and is described in a chapter by Zangwill, Lima, and Weinreb.

## NERVE FIBER LAYER ANALYSIS

Despite over a century of concentration on the ONH in glaucoma diagnostics, Hoyt and Newman showed nearly 25 years ago that abnormalities in the retinal nerve fiber layer (RNFL) can reveal the earliest signs of glaucoma.[9] To exploit this finding, and because Quigley showed that nearly half of the axons in the eye may be lost before an abnormality is noted by ONH appearance and visual field loss,[10-12] investigators have pursued the development of technologies to evaluate the NFL. According to Quigley, a reduction in NFL thickness of even 10 to 20 microns can be a significant sign of impending visual field loss.[10] NFL defects can precede the appearance of visual field defects.[13,14]

Conventional means of NFL examination provide good information regarding the general appearance of this tissue, as well as indicating the presence or absence of focal damage. Certainly, clinical NFL examination at the slit lamp or the direct ophthalmoscope, and perhaps even NFL photography, as described in the chapter by Mattox, are essential, low cost, highly efficacious means of glaucoma evaluation.

Clinical NFL examination and NFL photography, however, are difficult techniques, require a skilled photographer (in the case of NFL photography), and are subjective and qualitative.[7] In an attempt to increase the utility of an ONH analyzer, Caprioli described a method for mapping peripapillary NFL contour and found depressions in areas of NFL loss that corresponded to cupping and visual field loss.[15,16] Unfortunately, while ingenious, this technique depended on a stable floor from which to measure contour; such a reference plane does not exist.

Two differing technologies are currently employed to perform objective, quantitative NFL measurements. Polarimetry, as described in the chapter by Lima, Zangwill, and Weinreb, utilizes the birefringent properties of the NFL. It shines a polarized light into the eye and measures the change in rotation of this light as it exits the eye.

Optical Coherence Tomography (OCT), as discussed in the chapter by Schuman, uses an interferometer with low coherence light to produce 10-micron resolution, two-dimensional, cross-sectional images of the retina, from which quantitative NFL thickness measurements are made.

These two technologies use different approaches to provide information, not obtainable in any other way, that is both objective and quantitative. This may allow earlier glaucoma diagnosis and detection of change over time.

## OCULAR BLOOD FLOW

Ocular blood flow is critical to maintaining the function of the eye and of the optic nerve. One of the major theories as to glaucoma's pathogenesis relates to decreased blood flow to the optic nerve. An accurate measurement of ocular blood flow, particularly in the region of the optic nerve, would provide critical information relating to tissue health and possibly function. Imaging of blood flow in glaucoma is covered by Harris, Cantor, and Kagemann, as well as by Melamed, Krupsky, and Treister, in their chapters in this section.

Harris, Cantor, and Kagemann discuss color Doppler imaging, as well as blood flow assessments using CSLOs and tomographs. Melamed, Krupsky, and Treister examine the contribution of confocal angiography using exogenous dyes, such as indocyanine green.

## ANTERIOR SEGMENT IMAGING

The sole technology covered in this section, by Ritch, Liebmann, Iezzi, and Tello, is ultrasound biomicroscopy (UBM); however, this chapter is rich with clinical applications for this device.

Although limited by penetration depth to anterior segment imaging, UBM has proved extremely useful in both the clinical diagnosis of glaucoma and the elucidation of mechanisms of glaucomas.

## REFERENCES


1. Helmholtz H. B*eschreiburg eines Augenspiegels zur Untersuchung der Netzhaut in lebenden Augi.* Berlin: A. Forstner; 1851.

2. von Graefe A. Ueber die Wirkug der Iridectomie bei Glaucom. *Arch Ophthalmol.* 1857;3:456.

3. Schnabel I. Die Entwicklungsgeschichte der glaukomatosen Exkavation Z Augenheilkd. 1905;14:1.

4. Fuchs E. Ueber die Lamina cribrosa. *Graefe's Arch Ophthalmol.* 1916;91:435.

5. Elliot RU. *Treatise on Glaucoma.* London: Henry Fraude and Hodder & Stroughton LTD; 1922:195-218.

6. Tielsch JM, Katz J, Quigley HA. Intraobserver and interobserver agreement in measurement of optic disc characteristics. *Ophthalmology.* 1988;95:350.

7. Lichter PR. Variability of expert observers in evaluating the optic disc. *Trans Am Ophthalmol Soc.* 1976;74:532.

8. Drance SM, Fairclugh M, Butler DM, et al. The importance of disc hemorrhage in the prognosis of chronic open angle glaucoma. *Arch Ophthalmol.* 1977;95:226.

9. Hoyt WF, Newman NM. The earliest observable defect in glaucoma? *Lancet.* 1972;1:692-693.

10. Quigley HA, Addicks EM, Green WR. Optic nerve damage in human glaucoma. *Arch Ophthalmol.* 1982;100:135.

11. Quigley HA, Miller NR, George T. Clinical evaluation of nerve fiber layer atrophy as an indicator of glaucomatous optic nerve damage. *Arch Ophthalmol.* 1980;98:1564-1571.

12. Quigley HA, Addicks EM. Quantitative studies of retinal nerve fiber layer defects. *Arch Ophthalmol.* 1982;100:807-814.

13. Sommer A, Miller NR, Pollack I, et al. The nerve fiber layer in the diagnosis of glaucoma. *Arch Ophthalmol.* 1977;95:2149-2156.

14. Sommer A, Katz J, Quigley HA, et al. Clinically detectable nerve fiber atrophy preceded the onset of glaucomatous field loss. *Arch Ophthalmol.* 1991;109:77.

15. Caprioli J, Ortiz-Colberg R, Miller JM, et al. Measurements of peripapillary nerve fiber layer contour in glaucoma. *Am J Ophthalmol.* 1989;108:404.

16. Caprioli J. The contour of the juxtapapillary nerve fiber layer in glaucoma. *Ophthalmology.* 1990;97:358.

# ASSESSING THE STRUCTURE OF THE OPTIC NERVE

# STEREOSCOPIC OPTIC DISC PHOTOGRAPHY

*David S. Greenfield, MD*

## INTRODUCTION

Progressive cupping of the optic nerve head (ONH) is one of the most reliable indicators of inadequate glaucoma control. Therefore, it is of paramount importance that subtle changes in the appearance of the optic disc are accurately recorded during the course of follow-up examinations. A number of technologically advanced modalities have recently become available which may establish objective measurements of optic disc topography and retinal nerve fiber layer (RNFL) thickness. As these digital analysis systems continue to evolve, stereoscopic optic disc photography stands alone as the standard of care in which clinicians document longitudinal changes in the appearance of the ONH. As recommended by the American Academy of Ophthalmology, "Periodic photography of the ONH and stereoscopic photography, if available, will provide a reproducible image and baseline for future comparison."[1]

The evaluation of stereoscopic optic nerve photographs remains a subjective technique. However, stereoscopic optic disc photography represents the modality with which clinicians have had the most experience in documentation of the ONH appearance. In addition, ophthalmic photographers are very familiar with the equipment, and the technique requires only a minimal degree of technical skill to operate. Moreover, fundus cameras represent the most widely available, and perhaps the least expensive, of all available ONH imaging systems.

From a historical perspective, this technique dates back nearly as far as the development of the ophthalmoscope in 1850. In 1889, the development of flexible film coupled with advances in camera technology by George Eastman led to increased interest and popularity in the field of photography. It was only 3 years earlier that Jackman and Webster took the first human fundus photograph.[2]

Fundamentally, there are two ways to obtain stereo images of the ONH: via sequential or simultaneous exposures. Although most ophthalmic photographers create stereoscopic images by taking sequential (consecutive) photographs using a manual shift of the camera joystick, there are a number of advantages associated with simultaneous stereoscopic optic disc photography. This chapter will discuss related background information and principles underlying the production of stereoscopic images of the ONH. The advantages and disadvantages of currently available operating systems will be described.

## HISTORICAL BACKGROUND

Stereoscopic fundus photography has evolved directly through the technological advances independently made in ophthalmoscopy, photographic film, flash, and camera design. Although a plethora of significant contributions have been made over the last century, a number of events are particularly noteworthy and deserve specific mention. A complete historical perspective has been summarized in an earlier review by Hurtes.[3]

Despite the fact that photographs of the human fundus were documented as early as 1886,[2] a number of associated problems were identified shortly thereafter by Howe.[4] These included adequate illumination of the fundus, reflexes from both the light sources and the eye itself, eye movement during film exposure, projection of the image onto a plate of film, and overall poor film sensitivity. Despite these obstacles, Howe was the first individual to successfully create a funduscopic image with sufficient clarity to distinguish discrete funduscopic details.

Over the ensuing years, significant advances in camera design and illumination provided the fundamental basis for what is currently utilized in ophthalmic photography. In 1910, Gullstrand[5] perfected the reflexless ophthalmoscope previously developed by Thorner[6] in 1899. Approximately 15 years later, Nordenson converted a Zeiss fundus camera, essentially a modified Gullstrand ophthalmoscope, to a stereoscopic camera using prisms placed over the objective lens.[7] Although the image quality was poor because of the carbon light source that was utilized for illumination, this camera served as the basis for all subsequent instruments. Shortly thereafter, Bedell published the first English atlas of fundus photography.[8]

The mid-20th century saw a number of technological advances in fundus camera illumination systems. In 1953, Ogle and Rucker[9] were the first to incorporate an electronic flash with a fundus camera. Although their design was modified by a number of individuals, it was eventually perfected by Donaldson in 1964.[10] This design represents the first simultaneous stereoscopic camera to produce truly reliable images using a special flash tube with enhanced illumination. The Donaldson prototype stereoscopic camera was later revised using a single optical axis resulting in significantly enhanced image quality.[11,12] Undisputedly, the Donaldson simultaneous stereoscopic camera has been uniformly regarded as the standard in stereoscopic fundus photography.

Although the Donaldson fundus camera captures very high quality and reproducible stereo images using a simultaneous stereoscopic technique, it is not commercially available. A number of alternative devices are currently available. Some of these modalities are based upon a sequential technique of obtaining a stereo pair of images in a consecutive fashion. Others, based upon the original Donaldson fundus camera, capture stereoscopic images in a simultaneous fashion and are therefore subject to less variability. Each respective modality has inherent advantages and disadvantages, the details of which are summarized herein.

## SEQUENTIAL (CONSECUTIVE) STEREOSCOPIC OPTIC DISC PHOTOGRAPHY

### Allen Stereo Separator

Sequential stereoscopic optic disc photography is a technique that captures stereoscopic images in a consecutive fashion. This technique is often performed using a manual shift of the camera joystick to obtain stereo images through opposite sides of the pupil. Alternatively, an adjunctive device known as an Allen stereo separator may be employed to create stereo disc images.[13]

Developed by Lee Allen in 1964, the original prototype consisted of a special adapter that was designed to fit upon the back of the fundus camera which was equipped with a 2x magnification accessory in place.[14] This would result in 5x print magnification. The unit incorporated a sliding carriage that would house a 4.0- by 5.0-inch film packet. There was a built-in switch that would synchronize the electronic flash

with the Packard-type shutter. Stereoscopic photography was accomplished by sliding the adapter to the right for making the picture to be viewed with the left eye. After this exposure was taken, the sliding carriage would be moved to the left for the picture to be viewed with the right eye.

The stereo separator currently consists of a motorized device that fits over the photographic tube of a standard Zeiss fundus camera. Driven by the camera's power transformer, the unit contains a swiveling glass plate that is suspended over the front camera lens. The alignment of the glass plate primarily is checked manually to ensure adequate exposures. Stereo separation of images, or stereo base, is created by optically directing light toward alternate aspects of the dilated pupil. The degree of arc through which the glass plate swivels may be controlled to standardize the stereo base. Alternate exposures may be obtained in rapid sequence using a motorized foot switch to control the shutter release. In this manner, stereo images may be produced in a relatively reproducible and controlled fashion.

A notable drawback to using this particular technique is the 6-mm minimum pupil diameter required to achieve stereo images. This level of pupillary dilatation is often very difficult to achieve in eyes on chronic miotic therapy. Until recently, the Allen stereo separator could be purchased for approximately $1600 (Humphrey Instruments, San Leandro, Calif). Unfortunately, however, directly obtaining the unit has become increasingly more difficult as the unit is no longer commercially available.

### Manual Shift Technique

The manual shift technique is perhaps the most popular technique utilized to obtain stereoscopic funduscopic images. Although this technique may be performed with any fundus camera, it is typically accomplished using a standard Zeiss fundus camera. For the purposes of this discussion, we will refer to the Zeiss FF-4 fundus camera (Figure 1-1) which is currently available at a cost of approximately $32,000 (Humphrey Instruments, San Leandro, Calif).

The Zeiss FF-4 is a fundus camera that creates stereoscopic images using a sequential technique. As described in Table 1-1, full-frame images are created with a photographic magnification of 2.5x. The viewing magnification is 16x and the minimum pupil diameter is 3 mm. The camera comes equipped for fluorescein angiography with excitation and barrier filters. A green filter is available for performing RNFL (red-free) photography.

In contrast to the Allen stereo separator, which has associated features to augment reproducibility of the stereo base, the manual shift technique may be among the least reproducible of all stereoscopic photographic techniques currently available. One should not infer, however, that this technique

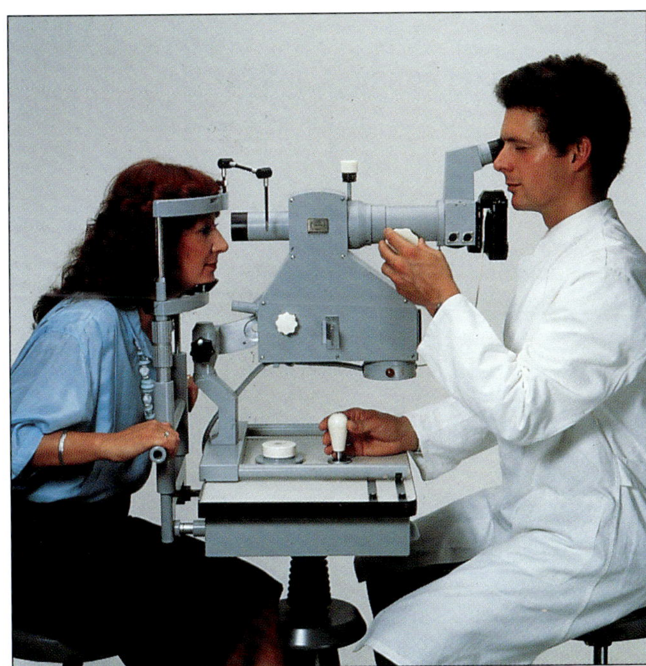

**Figure 1-1.** Photograph of the Zeiss FF-4 fundus camera (Humphrey Instruments, San Leandro, Calif).

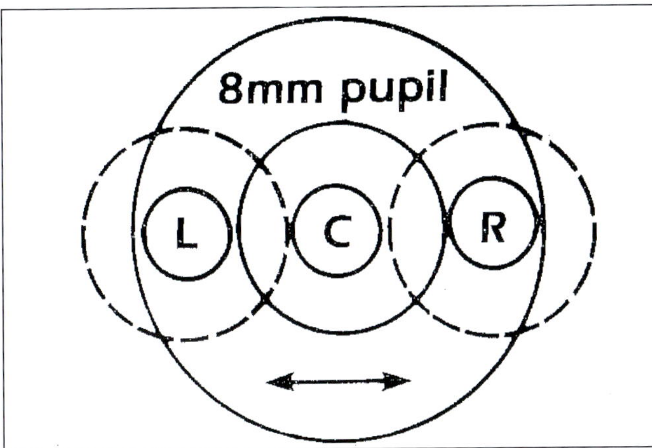



**Figure 1-2.** Schematic of a widely dilated pupil demonstrates the manual shift technique for sequential stereoscopic photography. After an image is captured in the center of the pupil, the joystick is moved to the 9 o'clock position of the pupil capturing the left frame of the stereo pair. The right frame of the stereo pair is then obtained by moving the joystick across the visual axis to the 3 o'clock position of the pupil. Reprinted with permission from Coppinger JM, Maio M, Miller K, eds. *Ophthalmic Photography*. Thorofare, NJ: SLACK Inc; 1988:94-101.

does not afford high quality stereo images to the experienced operator who complies with a standardized technique. In fact, stereo images obtained with this technique are generally of very high stereo quality. Moreover, there are distinct advantages to using this method of stereoscopic photography. For

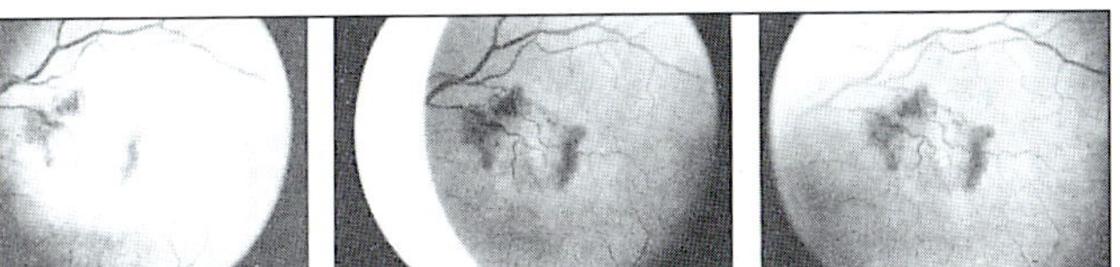

**Figure 1-3.** Fundus photographs demonstrating the camera joystick shift from the center of the visual axis (right image) toward the photographer's left. A crescent-shaped artifact appears (central image) which disappears as the joystick continues to move toward the left (right image). Reprinted with permission from Coppinger JM, Maio M, Miller K, eds. *Ophthalmic Photography*. Thorofare, NJ: SLACK Inc; 1988:94-101.

both the general ophthalmologist and retina specialist, it is perhaps the least expensive technique available since these individuals may already have this camera readily available to them. In addition, the overall longevity of the Zeiss fundus camera compared with newer simultaneous stereoscopic units translates to a higher level of familiarity and experience for the ophthalmic photographer. It is important, however, to emphasize that successful stereo photography using the manual shift technique requires adherence to a standardized technique to enhance image reproducibility.

In short, this technique simply involves manually moving the camera joystick control to the 9 o'clock position of the pupil and capturing the left frame of the stereo pair. The right frame of the stereo pair is then obtained by moving the joystick across the visual axis to the 3 o'clock position of the pupil (Figure 1-2). Adherence to the technique described below may enable the ophthalmic photographer to reduce his or her variability between photographic sessions. These skills have been detailed in an earlier review by Coppinger.[15]

One should obtain maximum pupillary dilation using topical agents such as Neo-Synephrine 2.5% and tropicamide 1%. This may be difficult for patients on chronic miotic therapy. If possible, it may be beneficial to have the patient discontinue miotic therapy approximately 24 hours prior to the expected photographic session. In addition, photographically document the level of pupillary dilatation to help standardize the stereo base between sessions. A uniform stereo base requires a uniform degree of pupillary dilation.

Next, focus on the optic disc in the center of the pupil and obtain a photographic image. Remember to have the patient blink prior to obtaining each image to lubricate the ocular surface and improve the image quality. Move the joystick to the left until a yellow crescent artifact appears (Figure 1-3). Continue to move the joystick toward the left until the artifact disappears. One may need to move the camera body away from the patient if crescent persists. It is important to note that the image will appear noticeably dark-

Table 1-1

**Comparison Between Zeiss, Nidek, and Topcon Fundus Cameras**

| | Nidek 3D$_x$ | Topcon TRC-SS2 | Zeiss FF-4 |
|---|---|---|---|
| **Main Camera Body** | | | |
| Photographic Method | Simultaneous | Simultaneous | Sequential |
| Image Type | | | |
|    35 mm | Split-frame | Split-frame | Full-frame |
|    Polaroid | Optional | N/A | N/A |
|    3D Transparency | Optional | N/A | Optional |
| Picture Angle (diagonal) | 32° | 30° | 30° |
| Magnification (0 D) | | | |
|    Photographic | 2.6x | 2.6x | 1.5x (5x with 2x adaptor) |
|    Viewing | 24.1x | 16.5x | 16x |
|    Polaroid | 7x | N/A | N/A |
| Minimum Pupil Diameter | 4 mm | 5.5 mm | 3 mm |
| Working Distance (obj. cornea) | 54 mm | 45 mm | 37.5 mm |
| Dioptric Compensation (pt.) | -25 to +35 D | -22 to +25 D | -40 to +40 D |
| Pupillary Distance (PD) | 55 to 85 mm | N/A (monocular eyepiece) | N/A (monocular eyepiece) |
| Stereobase | 3 mm | 3 mm | Variable (joystick shift) |
| Grayscale/Color Balance Patch | + | N/A | N/A |
| Internal Fixation Target | 2 fixed LED (L/R) | 1 fixed | 1 moveable |
| Filters | | | |
|    Green (red-free) | + | + | + |
|    Blue | + | + | + |
|    FFA Excitation | Available on 3D$_x$F | + | + |
|    FFA Barrier | Available on 3D$_x$F | + | + |
| Flash | | | |
|    Recycle Time | 1 second | 0.5 to 1 second | 0.5 to 4 seconds |
|    Type | 200 W Xenon lamp | 300 W Xenon lamp | 60 to 720 W Xenon lamp |
| Observational Illumination | 12 V, 50 W | 6 V, 33 W | 110 V, 50 W |
| Cost | $20,000 | $34,900 | $32,000 |
| **Camera Operation** | | | |
| Horizontal Movement | 6 to 10 cm | 8 to 11 cm | 5 cm |
| Vertical Movement | 30 mm | 15 mm | 60 mm |
| Swing Angle | 15° L/R | 30° L/R | 45° L/R |
| Vertical Movement of Chin Rest | 65 mm | 74 mm | 50 mm |
| External Fixation Target | Free-arm | Free-arm | Free-arm |
| **Weight** | Approximately 30 kg | Approximately 34 kg | Approximately 40 kg |
| **Dimensions** | 33 (W) x 56 (D) x 49 (H) cm | 50 (W) x 73 (D) x 67 (H) cm | 45 (W) x 75 (D) x 57 (H) cm |
| **Power Requirements** | 100, 120, 220, 240 V | 100, 120, 220, 240 V | 100, 110, 120, 220, 240 V |
| **Optional Equipment** | | | |
| 2x Objective Sleeve (15° angle) | N/A | N/A | + |
| Allen Stereo Separator | N/A | N/A | + |
| Polaroid Camera Back | + | N/A | N/A |
| Digital Optic Nerve Analysis | + | + | N/A |
|    Cost | Approximately $75,000 | $39,900 | N/A |
|    Optic Disc Topography | + | + | N/A |
|    NFL Measurement | + | + | N/A |
|    Vessel Shift | + | + | N/A |

*N/A=not available*

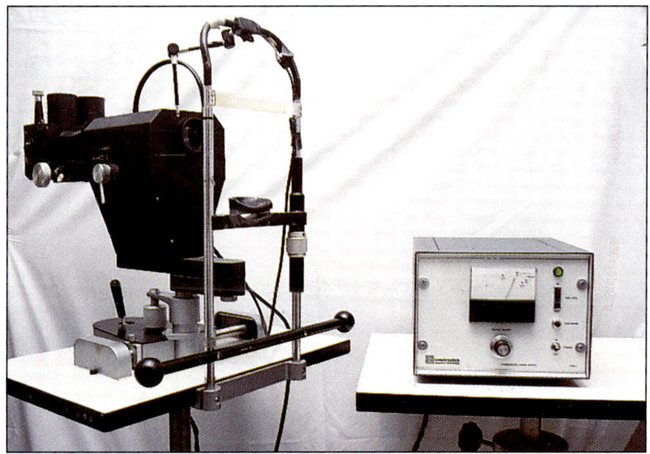

**Figure 1-4.** Photograph of the Donaldson simultaneous stereoscopic fundus camera.

er since a portion of the light entering the eye is obstructed by the edge of the pupil. Obtain an image of the optic disc which will serve as the right frame of the stereo pair.

Move the joystick slightly toward the right across the patient's visual axis. It must be emphasized that the camera axis must remain parallel between images in order to create the stereo base. As outlined above, obtain an image of the optic disc at this side of the dilated pupil after manipulating the joystick to reduce the yellow artifact. This will serve as the left frame of the stereo pair. It is essential to label all images carefully. For purposes of stereo viewing, one should always pair the central image with either the left or right image. One would assume that in order to achieve the greatest stereo base, he or she should pair the left image with the right image. However, in as much as these images are typically the darkest and less clear, the clinician should avoid pairing them during assessments of the optic disc.

To enhance visualization of optic disc detail, one may consider using an auxiliary 2x objective sleeve to provide greater photographic magnification. This device, currently available for approximately $600 (Humphrey Instruments, San Leandro, Calif), reduces the angular field from 30° to 15°. With an increase in photographic magnification from 2.5x to 5x, many clinicians find this adjunctive device essential for accurate and reproducible disc assessments.

## SIMULTANEOUS STEREOSCOPIC OPTIC DISC PHOTOGRAPHY

### Twin Prism Method

In order to help reduce the variability in stereo quality achieved using sequential stereoscopic optic disc photography, Saheb and colleagues designed a device to capture instantaneous stereo images with a single exposure.[16] This device was constructed to fit over the objective lens of a standard Zeiss fundus camera. The design consisted of a pair of 7 diopter prisms mounted apex to apex with a tilt of 15° in the vertical plane.

Saheb and colleagues compared the variability of disc assessments using the twin prism method (simultaneous stereoscopic photography) to that with the Allen stereo separator (sequential stereoscopic photography) using a uniform stereo base of 2.25 mm.[16] The required minimum pupillary diameter was 2 mm larger with the twin prism method (8 mm) compared with the Allen separator (6 mm). Using photogrammetric analysis, simultaneous stereoscopic photography with the twin prism method provided significantly greater reproducibility than with consecutive stereoscopic photography using the Allen separator.

There are notable obstacles to the widespread clinical use of twin prism stereoscopic photography. As previously described, a minimum pupil diameter of 8 mm is required in order to achieve adequate stereoscopic quality. Therefore, patients on chronic miotic therapy would not be acceptable subjects for study. In addition, significant prism-induced distortion is introduced using this method. Although a tilt of 15° in the vertical plane was originally described in order to reduce interfering light reflexes, optical distortion inherent to the prismatic system precludes its use in most clinical settings.

### Donaldson Fundus Camera

A review of the literature reveals that among the earliest camera designs capable of obtaining simultaneous stereoscopic photographs was one reported by Nordenson.[7] This design was based upon the principles of a modified reflex-free Gullstrand ophthalmoscope. In 1953, Norton designed a system attaching a binocular indirect ophthalmoscope to a stereoscopic camera.[17] Four years later, Drews published simultaneous stereoscopic images which, unfortunately, were of poor photographic quality.[18] It was not until 1964, when David Donaldson reported his prototype fundus camera design, that reproducibly satisfactory simultaneous stereoscopic images could be obtained.[10] However, the reflecting surfaces of the rhomboid prisms coupled with the converging paired camera axes produced inherent optical distortion of the images. This distortion was significantly reduced when Donaldson redesigned his fundus camera utilizing a single optical axis.[11,12]

Since its inception, the Donaldson fundus camera has been considered the standard in simultaneous stereoscopic fundus photography (Figure 1-4). The optical principles of the camera are based upon those of binocular indirect ophthalmoscopy. Simply stated, the pupillary space is divided in half vertically so that the illuminating light rays entering the eye are separated from the emerging rays of light leaving the pupil. As

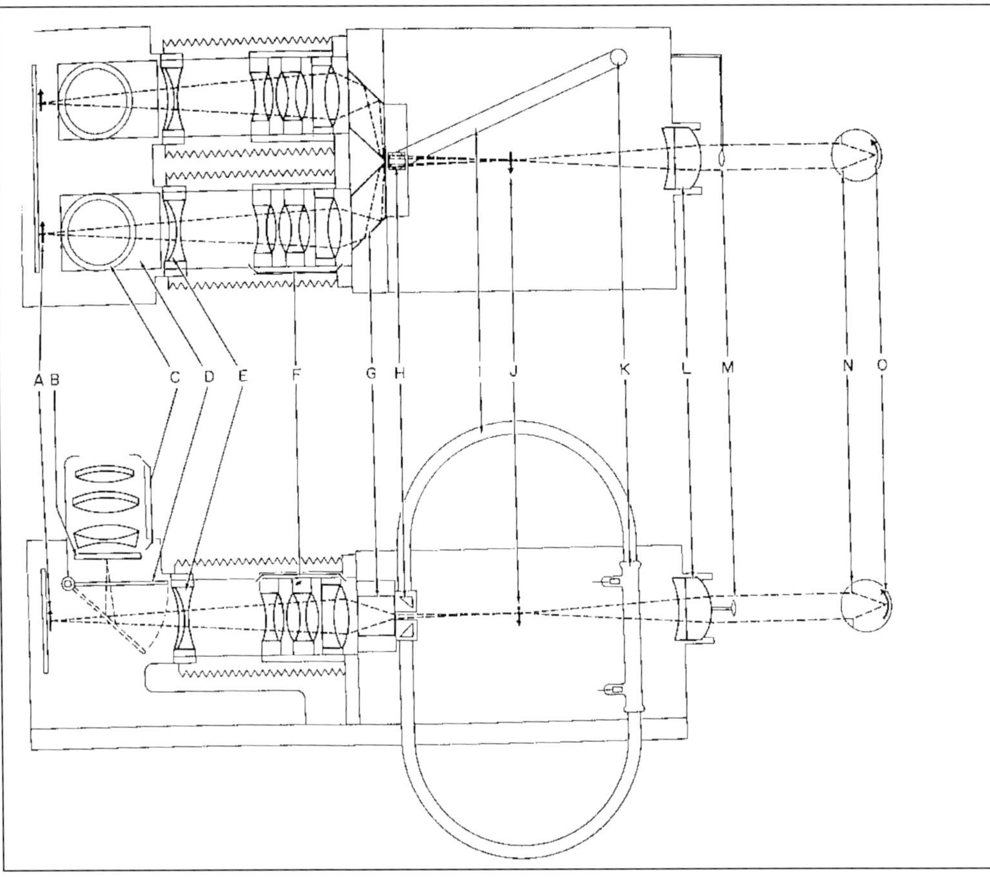

**Figure 1-5.** Optical system of the Donaldson fundus camera. Based upon the principles of binocular indirect ophthalmoscopy, the pupillary space is divided in half allowing the illuminating light rays entering the eye to be separated from the emerging rays leaving the pupil. Reprinted from *International Ophthalmology Clinics*, 119, 1976 by permission of Little, Brown and Company Inc.

demonstrated in Figure 1-5, the optical system of the fundus camera involves capturing images from two distinct vantage points through the 3 and 9 o'clock positions of the pupil. The stereo base depends directly upon the separation of two apertures placed in front of a pair of rhomboid prisms. Light rays from the fundus subsequently pass through a pair of camera lenses and are focused at the film plane after the double reflex mirror system is shifted into a horizontal position. As stated earlier, the illuminating light rays do not pass through the same position of the pupil as the imaging rays returning back to the camera. Light emitted from the electronic flash tube travels through two fiberoptic bundles. A pair of small right-angle prisms then focus the light at the level of the iris plane as two distinct small lights at the 12 and 6 o'clock pupillary positions.

The stereo base may be varied with the use of interchangeable aperture plates placed in front of the rhomboid prisms. Loss of detail and poor image resolution may result if the separation of the apertures is too great. However, the stereoscopic effect will be minimized if the separation is too small. The optimal separation is approximately 5 mm.[11] The minimum pupil diameter recommended to obtain satisfactory images is 4 mm. Photographic magnification of the funduscopic image is 6x and full-frame images are obtained as demonstrated in Figure 1-6. A 30° picture angle of the fundus is captured.[11]

One year after its introduction in 1976, the reproducibility of the single-axis Donaldson fundus camera was compared with that of the Zeiss fundus camera using the Allen stereo separator and the twin prism separator.[19] In this report, Rosenthal and colleagues determined that simultaneous stereoscopic fundus photography using the Donaldson camera provided significantly greater reproducibility of disc assessments than both sequential photography using the Allen separator and simultaneous photography using the twin prism method. These findings were further supported in 1979 by Krohn and colleagues.[20] These investigators found a smaller range of photogrammetric values and a smaller mean percentage error among optic disc measurements from the Donaldson fundus camera than disc measurements from the Zeiss fundus camera.

These reports emphasize the advantages of simultaneous stereoscopic photography. Producing a satisfactory pair of stereoscopic images clearly depends upon a number of variables related to the patient, the camera, and the photographer. Using sequential photography, the patient must maintain a constant head position and fixation, which is often difficult in children, elderly individuals, and patients with poor central vision. Furthermore, maintaining equal focus and illumination between images is difficult, as is maintaining a uniform stereo base between photographic sessions. These variables

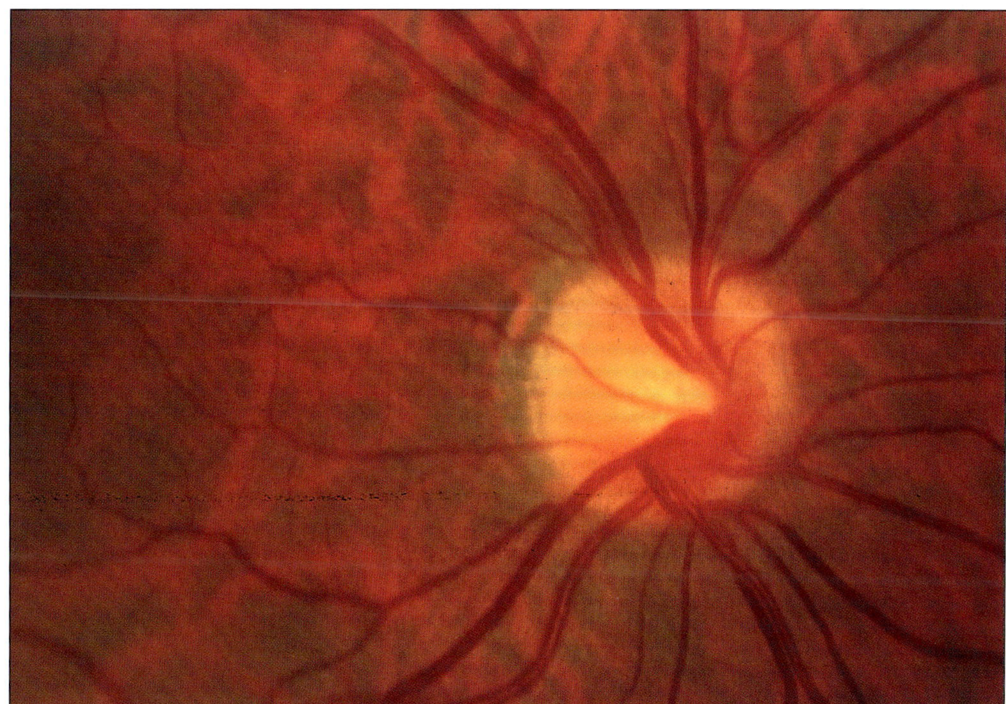

**Figure 1-6.** One of two full-frame images of the ONH obtained with a single exposure using the Donaldson fundus camera.

are reduced using simultaneous stereoscopic photography. Unfortunately, however, the Donaldson fundus camera is not commercially available, precluding its widespread use in the clinical setting. Two simultaneous stereoscopic fundus camera are currently available as described below.

## Nidek 3D$_x$

The prototype of the Nidek 3D$_x$ camera (Nidek Technologies, Inc, Pasadena, Calif) was introduced in 1990 (Figure 1-7). Minckler and colleagues found the camera faster and easier to use than the conventional system of sequential stereoscopic photography with the Zeiss fundus camera.[21] As described in Table 1-1, the Nidek camera captures simultaneous stereoscopic images with a 32° view of the fundus. There is a binocular eyepiece with an adjustable pupillary distance. In comparison to the Donaldson camera, which produces full-frame images, three varieties of images may be obtained with the Nidek unit. Most clinicians document the appearance of the optic nerve using a split-frame image with two adjacent stereoscopic images of the optic nerve that appear on one 35-mm slide (Figure 1-8). These images may be reviewed stereoscopically using a specialized viewing system, such as the Stereoviewer II (Asahi-Pentax Co, Englewood, Colo). Alternatively, one may obtain images in the form of a Polaroid, or by mail as a 3.5- by 5-inch three-dimensional transparency (Lentec Corp, Duluth, Ga). No specialized viewing apparatus is necessary for the latter, which is time-efficient and helpful in demonstrating pathology directly to the patient.

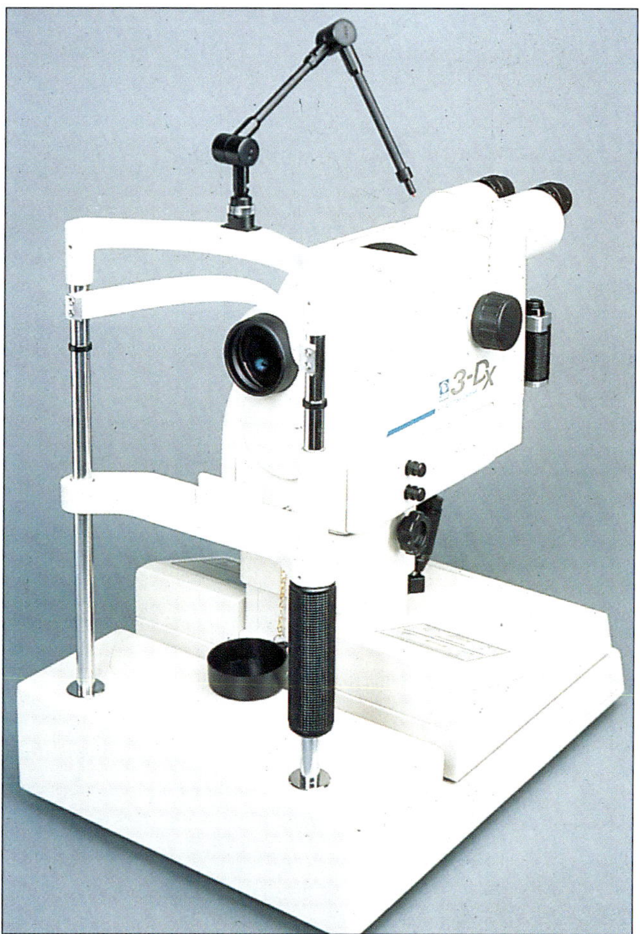

**Figure 1-7.** Photograph of the Nidek 3D$_x$ simultaneous stereoscopic fundus camera (Nidek Technologies, Inc, Pasadena, Calif).

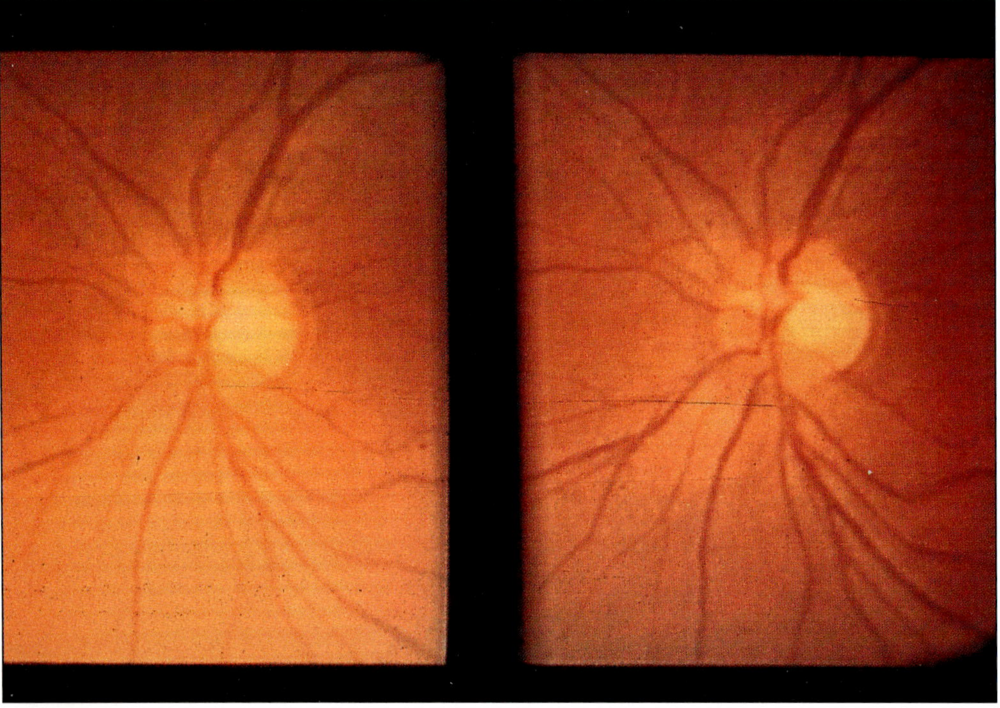

**Figure 1-8.** Split-frame image of the ONH obtained with a single exposure using the Nidek $3D_x$ fundus camera.

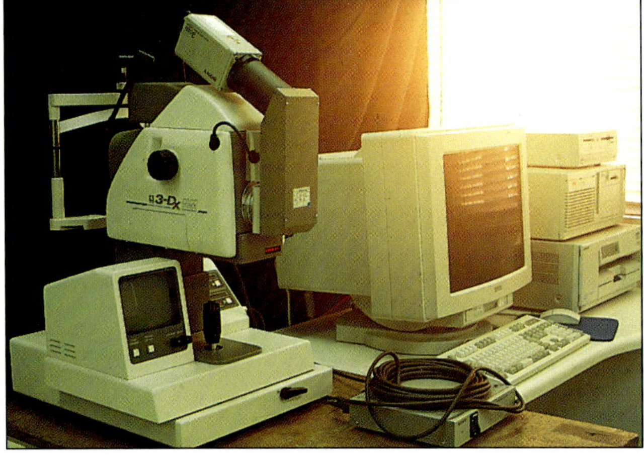

**Figure 1-9.** Photograph of the Nidek Eye Station, an optional digital system capable of analyzing the RNFL and the topography of the ONH.

Photographic magnification is 2.6x with a viewing magnification of 24.1x. A minimum pupil diameter of 4 mm is recommended to obtain satisfactory stereoscopic images with a stereo base of 3 mm. NFL photography may be performed as the Nidek $3D_x$ unit comes equipped with internal green (redfree) and blue filters. Fluorescein angiography may be performed with the $3D_xF$ unit, which contains excitation and barrier filters. Although the camera may be obtained for approximately $20,000, this cost does not include the optional digital ONH analysis system, the Nidek Eye Station, which is commercially available (Nidek Technologies, Inc, Pasadena, Calif) at a cost of approximately $75,000. This technology (Figure 1-

9) has the capacity to digitally display and evaluate the topography of the ONH, to analyze the RNFL, and to detect positional shifts in the major retinal vascular arcades. A digitized wire basket plot of the ONH topography is illustrated in Figure 1-10. It is important to note, however, that to date this system has not been critically evaluated in the scientific literature.

Several studies have compared the Nidek $3D_x$ with other high quality, commercially available fundus cameras. The photographic resolving power of the Nidek fundus camera was reported to be similar to that of the Zeiss, Canon, and Topcon fundus cameras using a high-contrast United States Air Force test target.[22] Boes and colleagues compared the accuracy of relative optic cup depth assessment using Nidek $3D_x$ split-frame images, Lentec transparencies, and Zeiss full-frame slides.[23] These investigators demonstrated that simultaneous stereoscopic slides provide significantly more interobserver consistency for judgments of cup depth, and therefore overall stereoscopic effect, than sequential stereo slides.

Although these investigators reported significantly greater reproducibility of disc assessments using the Nidek camera compared with sequential stereoscopic photography using the Zeiss camera, no comparisons were made with the Donaldson fundus camera, which has traditionally been considered the standard for stereoscopic photography. To this end, Greenfield and colleagues performed a prospective clinical study to compare the stereoscopic quality of images and the reproducibility of disc assessments obtained from the Nidek and Donaldson fundus cameras.[24] Using a custom-designed reticule (Figure 1-11), horizontal and vertical cup

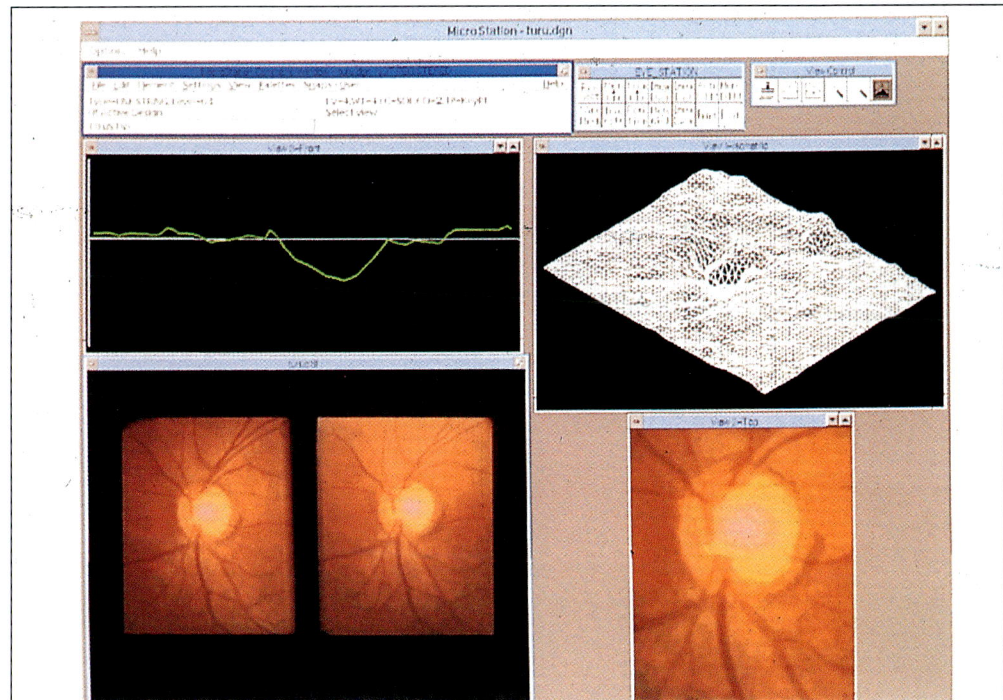

**Figure 1-10.** Digitized wire basket plot of the ONH topography generated using the Nidek Eye Station.

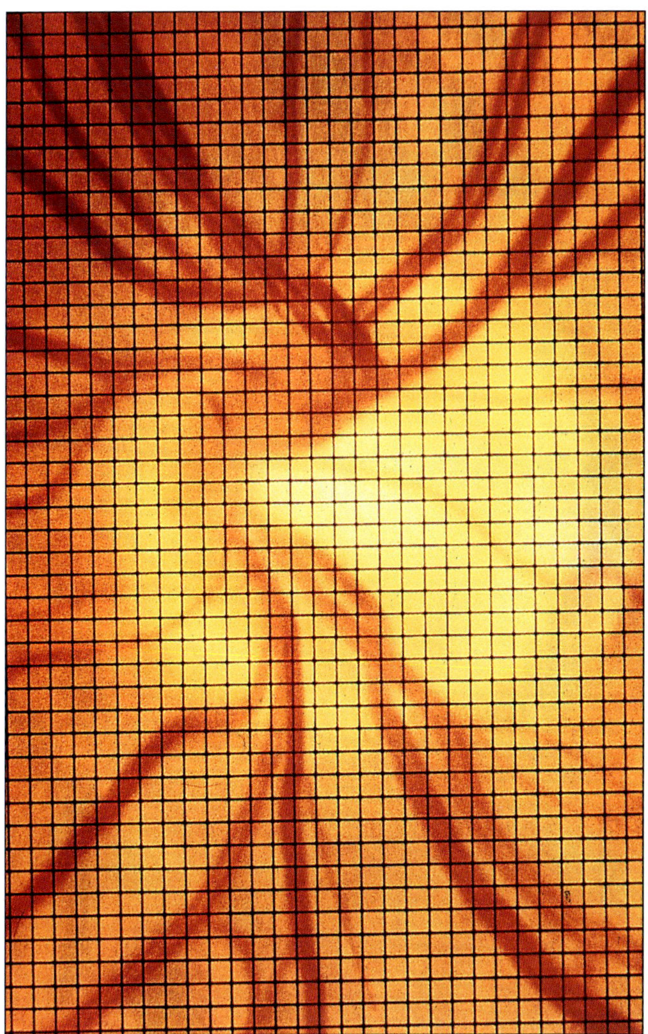

**Figure 1-11.** Reticule utilized to measure horizontal and vertical cup and disc diameters. Reprinted with permission from Greenfield DS, Zacharia P, Schuman JS. Comparison of Nidek 3D$_x$ and Donaldson simultaneous stereoscopic disk photography. *Am J Ophthalmol.* 1993;116:741-747.

and disc diameters were measured. The Nidek fundus camera produced significantly better stereoscopic images than the Donaldson fundus camera. In addition, the Nidek camera produced significantly less variability of disc assessments than the Donaldson. In summary, the Nidek 3D$_x$ fundus camera is capable of providing accurate, high-resolution, reproducible simultaneous stereoscopic images of the ONH.

## Topcon TRC-SS2

The prototype Topcon fundus camera (Figure 1-12) was introduced in the mid-1980s (Topcon Instrument Corporation of America, Paramus, NJ). Similar to the Nidek fundus camera, the Topcon unit produces simultaneous stereoscopic images in the form of a split-frame image (Figure 1-13). However, optional Polaroid and three-dimensional transparencies are not available.

As illustrated in Table 1-1, many similar features are shared by the Topcon and Nidek fundus cameras. Both cameras produce high quality images with a photographic magnification of 2.6x and both are equipped to perform RNFL photography. However, the Topcon unit captures a 30° picture angle of the fundus through a monocular eye piece. The viewing magnification is 16.5x, somewhat reduced compared with the Nidek's 24.1x. In addition, the minimum pupil diameter

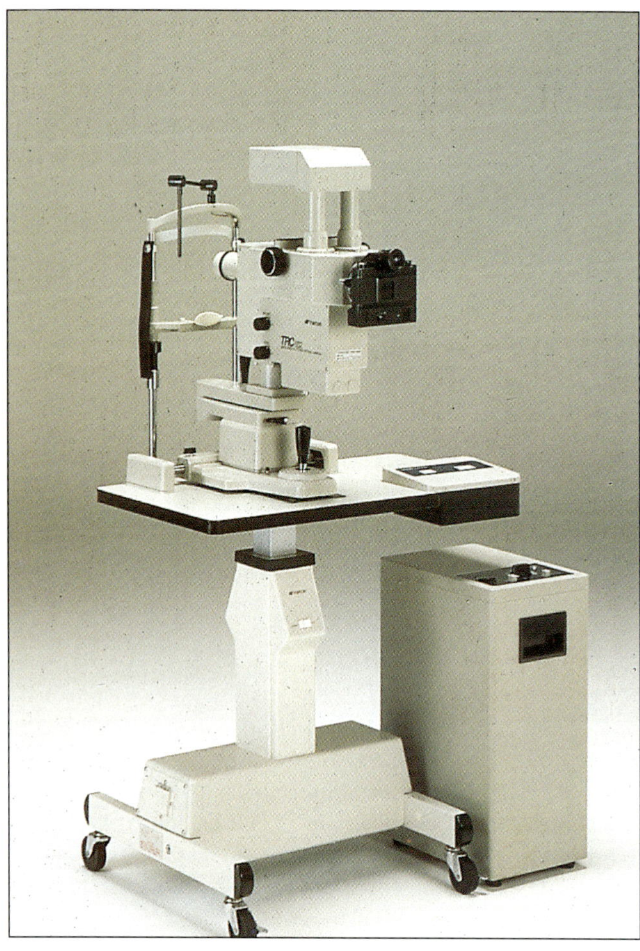

**Figure 1-12.** Photograph of the Topcon TRC-SS2 simultaneous stereoscopic fundus camera (Topcon Instrument Corporation of America, Paramus, NJ).

recommended to obtain satisfactory images is 1.5 mm larger (5.5 mm) than the minimum pupil diameter reported by Nidek (4 mm). It is unclear if this difference is clinically significant.

Similar to the Nidek unit, the Topcon fundus camera is capable of producing accurate, high-resolution, reproducible simultaneous stereoscopic images of the ONH. At a price of $34,900, the Topcon TRC-SS2 fundus camera is 50% more costly than the similar unit produced by Nidek. However, this unit is directly capable of performing fluorescein angiography. In addition, an optional digital ONH analysis system, the Imagenet Stereometric Analysis System, is available at a cost of $39,000 (Figure 1-14). Not only is this price approximately 50% less costly than the Nidek system, but unlike its Nidek counterpart, the Topcon system has been clinically available, scientifically evaluated, and reported in the medical literature over the past 10 years.[25-34] The accuracy, reproducibility, and agreement of this analysis system with optic disc assessments in clinical and experimental glaucoma has been described by many investigators.[26-34] Noteworthy is the fact that this system was found to be two times more sensitive than clinical photographic evaluation alone in detecting vessel shift.[25] In addition, while the overall reproducibility of disc assessments was good, greater variability was seen in optic discs with poorly defined margins, peripapillary atrophy, and poorly defined cup margins with sloping walls.[26,28]

The Imagenet Stereometric Analysis System was developed in 1987, when Topcon acquired the original technology from the PAR Corporation. The system is capable of producing digital analysis of the ONH topography (Figure 1-15) including cup-to-disc ratio, pallor-to-disc ratio, cup volume, and disc peripheral length areas. Overlay sections can be compared using an optic disc change analysis program. Contour wire basket plots, color-coded depth maps, numeri-

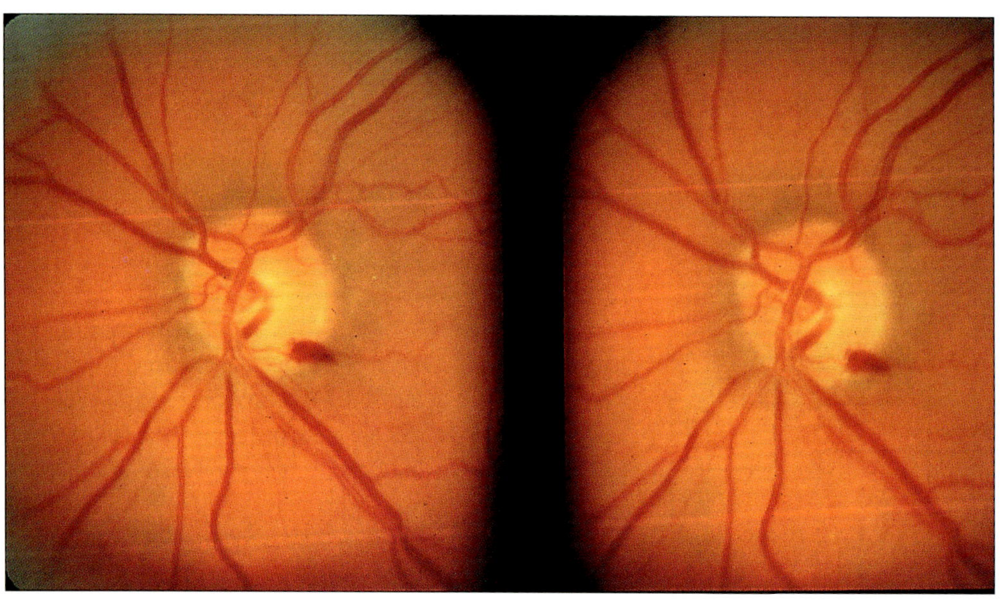

**Figure 1-13.** Split-frame image of the ONH obtained with a single exposure using the Topcon TRC-SS2 fundus camera.

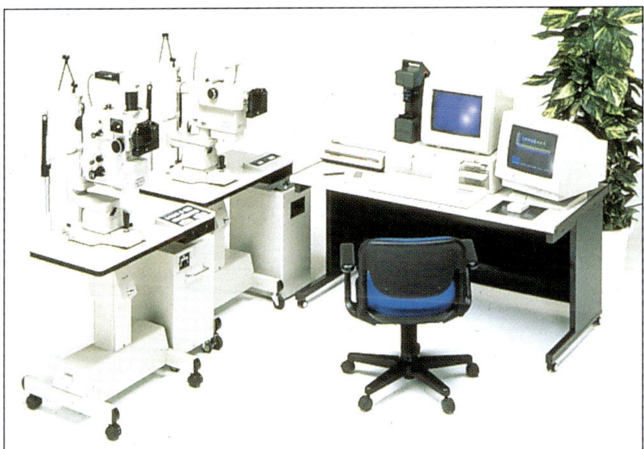

**Figure 1-14.** Photograph of the Topcon Imagenet Stereoanalysis System, an optional digital system capable of analyzing the RNFL and the topography of the ONH.

cal depth maps, and cross-sectional analysis can be performed as well as measurements of the RNFL and analyses of retinal vascular shift. Stereometric analyses and wire basket plots may be generated in approximately 4 to 5 minutes.[35] As new techniques for measuring ONH topography and RNFL thickness evolve, comparative studies will be necessary to determine their clinical roles both in the early detection and progression of glaucomatous optic neuropathy.

## SUMMARY

Stereoscopic photography of the optic nerve provides an excellent means for the objective documentation of change in the appearance of the ONH. This may be accomplished using either sequential or simultaneous photographic techniques. Among these two techniques, the most widely available and utilized modality involves obtaining two consecutive images of the optic nerve using a manual shift of the joystick. These images are then clinically reviewed using a stereoscopic viewing apparatus. The Zeiss fundus camera traditionally has been the standard for obtaining stereoscopic images in a sequential fashion. Alternatively, both images may be captured with a single exposure using a commercially available simultaneous stereoscopic fundus camera, such as the units manufactured by Nidek Technologies, Inc. and Topcon Instrument Corporation of America. The mechanical specifications and optional features of these units are compared herein (see Table 1-1). Noteworthy is that if a clinician is fortunate to have a variety of fundus cameras available for use, maintaining longitudinal follow-up with one uniform fundus camera per patient is recommended. Nicholl and colleagues have reported that the Nidek unit provides significantly smaller estimates of the horizontal cup-to-disc ratio than the Topcon unit.[36] As such, systematic differences may exist between these two simultaneous stereoscopic fundus cameras.

The Zeiss, Nidek, and Topcon fundus cameras have been reported to provide equivalent degrees of image resolution.[22] However, despite the fact that excellent images may be obtained with all three fundus cameras, simultaneous stereoscopic photography has been demonstrated to provide greater reproducibility of disc assessments.[19,20] By corollary, greater reproducibility should translate to more accurate clinical assessments of disease progression.

**Figure 1-15.** Digital plot of the ONH topography generated using the Topcon Imagenet Stereoanalysis System.

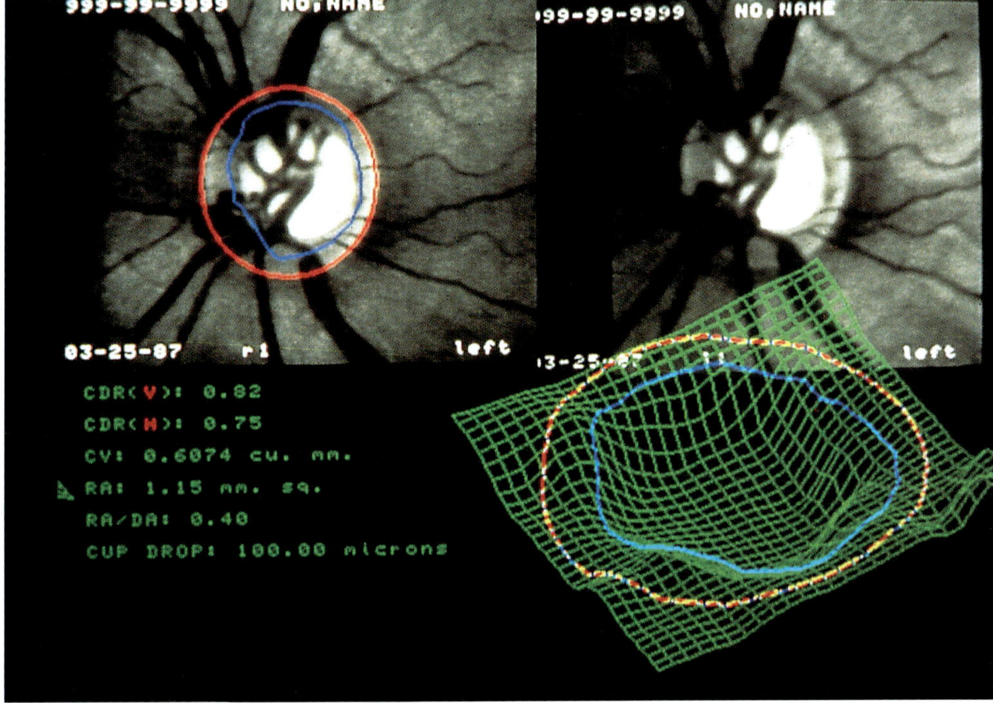

Both the Nidek and Topcon fundus cameras provide optional digital analysis systems to analyze the ONH topography and RNFL. Cost considerations coupled with the emergence and evolution of new ocular imaging devices will further direct the clinical role of each of these technologies. This review emphasizes the clinical significance, both past and present, of stereoscopic ONH photography. Optic nerve photography will unequivocally continue in the future to serve as an invaluable aid in the clinical management of patients with glaucoma. I encourage all clinicians involved in the care of these individuals to use stereoscopic photography to document the appearance of the ONH at regular intervals of time.

## REFERENCES


1. American Academy of Ophthalmology Quality of Care Committee Glaucoma Panel. Primary open angle glaucoma. Preferred practice pattern. American Academy of Ophthalmology, San Francisco, Calif, 1992.
2. Jackman WT, Webster JD. On photographing the retina of the living human eye. *Phil Photographer.* 1886;23:275.
3. Hurtes R. Evolution of ophthalmic photography. In: Justice J Jr., ed. *Int Ophthalmol Clin.* Vol 16. Boston: Little, Brown and Company; 1976:chap 1.
4. Howe L. Photography of the interior of the eye. *Trans Am Ophthalmol Soc.* 1885-7;4:568.
5. Gullstrand A. Neue Methoden der reflexlosen Ophthalmoskopie. *Ber Dtsch Ophthalmol Ges.* 1910;36:75.
6. Thorner W. A new stationary ophthalmoscope without reflexes. Barck C, trans. *Am J Ophthalmol.* 1899;16:330.
7. Nordenson JW. Augenkamera zum stationaren Ophthalmoskop von Gullstrand. *Ber Dtsch Ophthalmol Ges.* 1925;45:278.
8. Bedell AJ. *Photographs of the Fundus Oculi.* Philadelphia, Pa: Davis; 1929.
9. Ogle JN, Rucker CW. Fundus photographs in color using a high-speed flash tube in the Zeiss retinal camera. *Arch Ophthalmol.* 1953;49:435.
10. Donaldson DD. A new camera for stereoscopic fundus photography. *Trans Am Ophthalmol Soc.* 1964;62:429.
11. Donaldson DD. Stereophotographic systems. *Int Ophthalmol Clin.* 1976;16:109-131.
12. Donaldson DD, Prescott R, Kennedy S. Simultaneous stereoscopic fundus camera incorporating a single optical axis. *Invest Ophthalmol Vis Sci.* 1980;19:289-297.
13. Allen L. Ocular fundus photography. *Am J Ophthalmol.* 1964;57:13-28.
14. Allen L. Stereoscopic fundus photography with the new instant positive print films. *Am J Ophthalmol.* 1964;57:539-544.
15. Coppinger JM. Stereo fundus photography. In: Coppinger JM, Maio M, Miller K, eds. *Ophthalmic Photography.* Thorofare, NJ: SLACK Inc; 1988:94-101.
16. Saheb NE, Drance SM, Nelson A. The use of photogrammetry in evaluating the cup of the optic nerve head for a study in chronic simple glaucoma. *Can J Ophthalmol.* 1972;7:466-470.
17. Norton HJ Jr. Absolute three dimensional colored retinal photographs. *Trans Am Acad Ophthalmol.* 1953;57:612-613.
18. Drews RC. Fundus photography by electronic flash. *Am J Ophthalmol.* 1957;44:170-177, 356-359, 522-525, 633-637.
19. Rosenthal AR, Kottler MS, Donaldson DD, Falconer DG. Comparative reproducibility of the digital photogrammetric procedure utilizing three methods of stereoscopic photography. *Invest Ophthalmol Vis Sci.* 1977;16:54.
20. Krohn MA, Keltner JL, Johnson CA. Comparison of photographic techniques and films used in stereophotogrammetry of the optic disk. *Am J Ophthalmol.* 1979;88:859.
21. Minckler DS, Nichols T, Morales RB. Preliminary clinical experience with the Nidek $3D_x$ camera and lenticular stereo disc images. *J Glaucoma.* 1992;1:184-186.
22. Boes DA, Clifton BC, Mills RP. Resolution of Nidek $3D_x$. Zeiss, Canon, and Topcon fundus cameras. *J Glaucoma.* 1994;3:195-200.
23. Boes DA, Spaeth GL, Mills RP, Smith M, Nicholl JE, Clifton BC. Relative optic cup depth assessments using three stereo photograph viewing methods. *J Glaucoma.* 1996;5:9-14.
24. Greenfield DS, Zacharia P, Schuman JS. Comparison of Nidek $3D_x$ and Donaldson simultaneous stereoscopic disk photography. *Am J Ophthalmol.* 1993;116:741-747.
25. Varma R, Spaeth GL, Hanau C, et al. Positional changes in the vasculature of the optic disc in glaucoma. *Am J Ophthalmol.* 1987;104:457.
26. Varma R, Spaeth GL, Steinmann WC, Wilson RP. Variability in digital analysis of optic disc topography. *Graefes Arch Clin Exp Ophthalmol.* 1988;226:435-442.
27. Varma R, Spaeth GL. The PAR is 2000: a new system for retinal digital image analysis. *Ophthalmic Surg.* 1988;19:183-192.
28. Varma R, Spaeth GL, Steinmann WC, Katz LJ. Agreement between clinicians and the image analyzer in estimating cup-to-disc ratios. *Arch Ophthalmol.* 1989;107:526.
29. Burgoyne CF, Varma R, Quigley HA, Vitale S, Pease ME, Lenane PL. Global and regional detection of induced optic disc change by digitized image analysis. *Arch Ophthalmol.* 1994;112:261-268.
30. Varma R, Tielsch JM, Quigley HA, et al. Race-, age-, gender-, and refractive error-related differences in the normal optic disc. *Arch Ophthalmol.* 1994;112:1068-1076.
31. Varma R, Hilton SC, Tielsch JM, Katz J, Quigley HA, Sommer A. Neural rim area declines with increased intraocular pressure in urban Americans. *Arch Ophthalmol.* 1995;113:1001-1005.
32. Burgoyne CF, Quigley HA, Varma R. Comparison of clinician judgment with digitized image analysis in the detection of induced optic disk change in monkey eyes. *Am J Ophthalmol.* 1995;120:176-183.
33. Burgoyne CF, Quigley HA, Thompson HW, Vitale S, Varma R. Early changes in optic disc compliance and surface position in experimental glaucoma. *Ophthalmology.* 1995;102:1800-1809.
34. Burgoyne CF, Quigley HA, Thompson HW, Vitale SV, Varma R. Measurement of optic disc compliance by digitized image analysis in the normal monkey eye. *Ophthalmology.* 1995;102:1790-1799.
35. Varma R, Spaeth GL, Parker KW. *The Optic Nerve in Glaucoma.* Philadelphia, Pa: JB Lippincott Co; 1992.
36. Nicholl JE, Lesk MR, Katz LJ, Spaeth GL, Araujo SV. Comparison of Topcon Imagenet stereometric disc analysis of the Topcon TRC-SS and Nidek $3D_x$ simultaneous stereoscopic fundus cameras. *Invest Ophthalmol Vis Sci.* 1995;36:970.

# THE GLAUCOMA-SCOPE: PRINCIPLE, TECHNIQUES, AND APPLICATIONS

*Peter A. Netland, MD, PhD*

## INTRODUCTION

Optic nerve head (ONH) evaluation is a critical component of glaucoma diagnosis and management. The appearance of the optic nerve has been recorded by clinicians in various ways, including cup-to-disc ratios, drawings, and stereophotographs. These approaches are imprecise and may show considerable variability, even when performed by experienced observers.[1] Because of these limitations, more quantitative, objective, and reproducible methods of ONH analysis have been developed.[2] The Glaucoma-Scope is a computerized ONH analyzer that provides a quantitative assessment of ONH and peripapillary topography.

## PRINCIPLE

The ONH analysis performed by the Glaucoma-Scope is based on a technique of computed raster stereography described by Holm and Krakau[3] and Krakau and Torlegård.[4] A series of equidistant, parallel, straight light lines is projected onto the optic disc at an oblique angle (Figure 2-1). Based on the deflections of the lines, the depth and volume of the papillary excavation (or protrusion) can be calculated. The deflection of the projected lines is proportional to the extent of papillary excavation: small deflections indicate shallow depth, whereas large deflections occur with deep cup excavation.

## TECHNIQUES

The details of the instrument and technique have been reported previously.[5] The Glaucoma-Scope has two major components: the optical head mounted on a joystick for image acquisition and a computer for image analysis (Figure

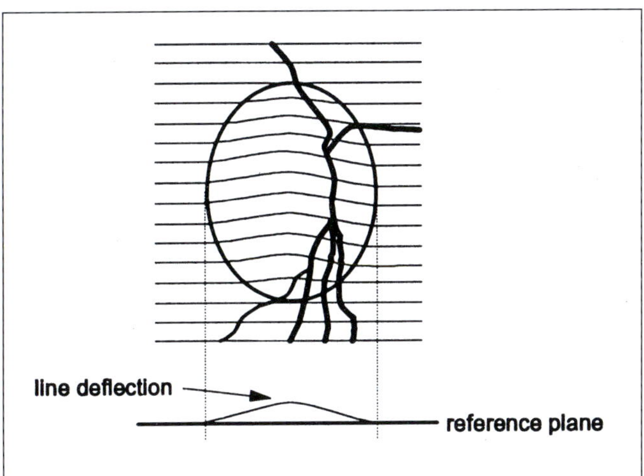


**Figure 2-1.** The Glaucoma-Scope uses a computed raster stereography technique to determine the depth (or height) of the disc. In this technique, parallel lines are projected onto the ONH at an oblique angle. The deflections of the lines relative to a reference plane near the disc are proportional to the depth of the cup.

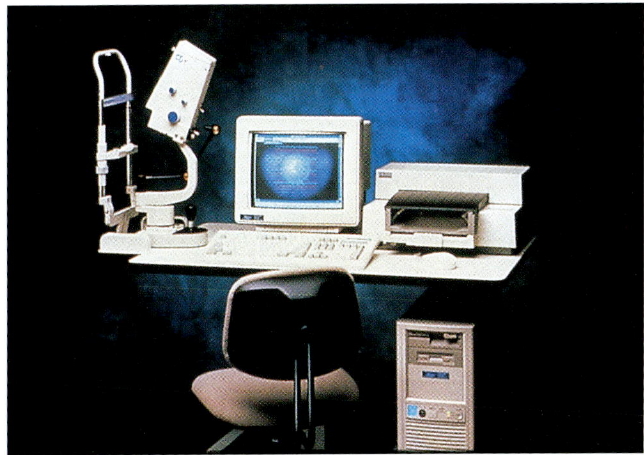

**Figure 2-2.** The Glaucoma-Scope has two major components: an optical head for image acquisition and a computer for image analysis. The optical head (left of the monitor) projects approximately 25 horizontal lines at an angle of 9° to the ONH using near infrared light (750 nm) produced by a halogen lamp illumination system. Courtesy of Christine N. Ritter, Ophthalmic Imaging Systems, Inc, Sacramento, Calif.

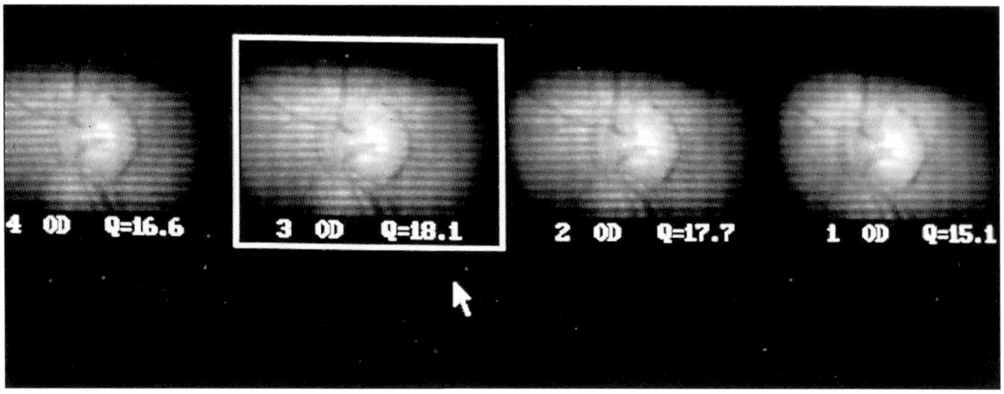

**Figure 2-3.** Glaucoma-Scope images are captured and stored on optical discs. The quality of the images is ranked on a logarithmic scale, which is proportional to horizontal line data in the image. The Glaucoma-Scope automatically selects the image with the highest quality scale (indicated by arrow) for further analysis, although other images may be selected by the operator for analysis.

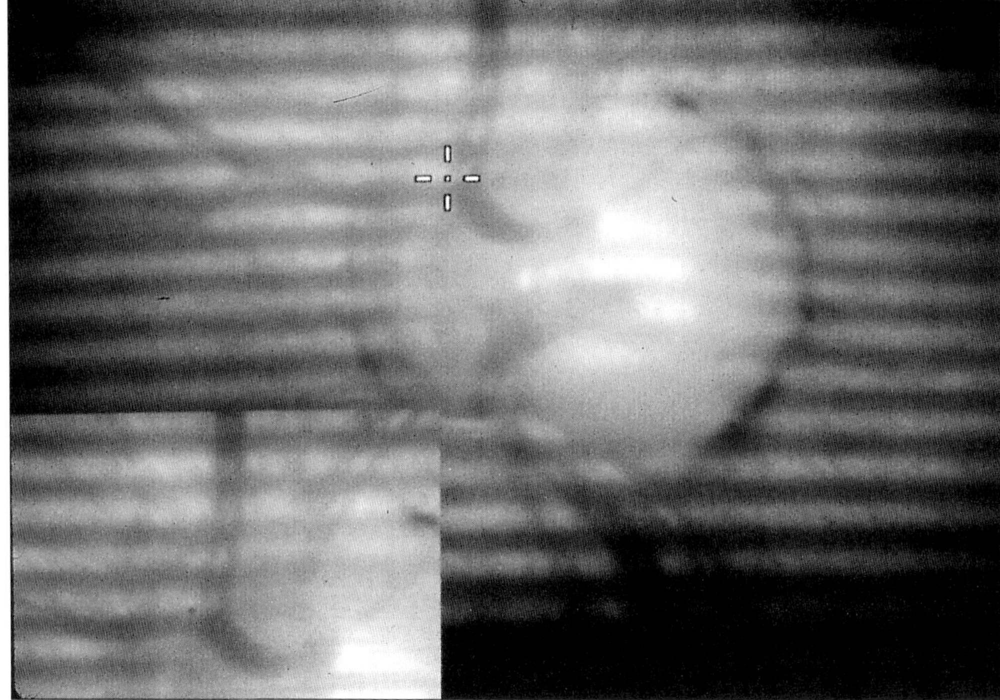

**Figure 2-4.** A reference point is selected by the operator for image registration. Selection of the reference point allows alignment of a 128 by 128 pixel area for comparisons with other images of the same disc. In follow-up examinations, the previously chosen reference point is displayed as shown in the lower left corner of the image. The operator also defines at least eight points on the disc margin and outlines major vessels. The refraction of the eye is entered to correct disc measurements for magnification of the eye.

2-2). A halogen lamp illumination system within the optical head projects a series of about 25 horizontal lines across the ONH. The light lines are projected at an angle of 9° to the ONH using near infrared light (750 nm). A polarizing filter is used to maximize reflection from the anterior surface of the nerve fiber layer (NFL). A video image of the ONH and projected lines is viewed on the monitor, and image quality is optimized by operator control of focus and illumination. Multiple images are captured by pressing a button near the joystick. The captured images are stored in digital form on optical discs.

The quality of the captured images is ranked on a logarithmic scale ranging from zero to infinity (Figure 2-3). This scale is proportional to the ratio of horizontal line data to non-horizontal line data in the image. A secondary feature of the quality scale is an overexposure detector, which sets the quality scale to zero for images that are too bright for analysis. A quality scale of zero indicates that no horizontal lines are present, whereas an image of mostly horizontal lines would produce a large number. Images with a quality scale <4 generate an error message that can be overridden to attempt topographic analysis of the image. In practice, images with a quality scale ≥4 are adequate for image analysis. Images of adequate quality have even illumination and sufficient line contrast. A quality scale of approximately 10 is considered a very good image for analysis, and a scale of ≥15 is an excellent image for analysis.

A reference point is selected for future image registra-

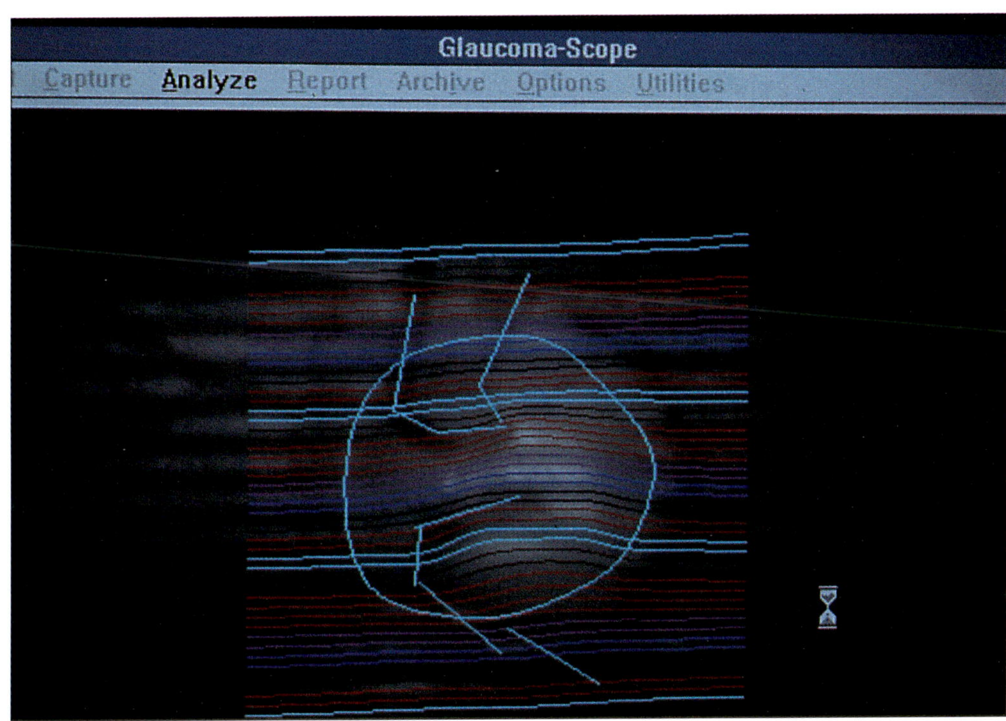



**Figure 2-5.** The Glaucoma-Scope computer algorithm analyzes the line data, then displays this information with the original video image of the disc. The line data are converted into depth values (microns). The reference plane for the depth values is the plane between two 50-micron columns placed 0.3 disc diameters nasal and temporal to the disc. The optic cup is defined as the area of the disc that is $\geq$140 microns below the reference plane.

tion, which denotes the center of a 128 by 128 pixel reference area (Figure 2-4). In subsequent examinations, the previously selected reference point appears in a window in the corner of the image. The operator selects a point on the current image that is near the reference point to allow alignment of the initial and subsequent images. The alignment is the best fit of the 128 by 128 pixel area around the reference point in the initial image compared with the subsequent image. The selected point on the current image must be within the theoretical limit of 64 pixels from the original reference point, but the actual required proximity of these points is determined by the quality of the images. Ideally, the selected point should be within 5 to 10 pixels from the original reference point.

At the initial visit, the operator identifies the disc margin by placing at least eight points around the disc margin and outlines the major vessels. The disc margin and vessel drawings provide landmarks on the report printout but do not affect algorithm calculation of depth values. After analysis of the line data, the line information is displayed with the video image of the disc (Figure 2-5). An algorithm converts the captured horizontal line data from the captured image into corresponding topographic depth values. The reference plane for depth measurements is defined by linear interpolation of data within two 50-micron columns placed 0.3 disc diameters nasal and temporal to the disc margin.

The optic cup area is defined as the area inside the disc margin 140 microns or more below the reference plane. The operator enters the refraction of the eye to allow calculation of the real size of the disc and cup according to the formula described by Bengtsson and Krakau.[6] This formula for telecentric cameras and imaging systems corrects the disc measurements according to an estimate of the magnification of the eye based upon the refraction.

In the ONH analysis, the depths or elevations of over 9100 real data points are determined in an area typically containing 350 by 280 pixels. This corresponds to an area of 2624 by 2624 microns on the retina (6,885,376 microns squared). A total of 98,000 interpolated and real data points are calculated, including the 9100 real data points. The data are reported as a numeric and grayscale printout. Up to 722 numeric depth values appear on the printout in a 19 by 38 number grid, with each value representing the average of approximately 136 data points covering an area of 69 microns vertically by 138 microns horizontally (Figure 2-6). If no line data exist in an area, the depth values are not extrapolated, and an "X" appears on the printout. On subsequent visits, the depth measurements are automatically compared with measurements made at the initial visit, and a change-from-baseline analysis is printed showing any changes in depth values of $\geq$75 microns.

The minimum pupil size is approximately 4 mm, although image capture may be possible in patients with smaller pupils and clear media. Dilation of the pupil is required for most patients. Typical image acquisition requires approximately 1 to 5 minutes. The current algorithm (version 3.17) and microprocessors perform the image analysis in approximately 1 minute. Printing the reports requires approximately 4 minutes, although a batch processing option may

**Figure 2-6.** The Glaucoma-Scope measures approximately 9100 data points, generating a 19 by 38 number grid of up to 722 numeric depth values. If no line data exist in an area, an "X" appears on the printout (arrow).



**Figure 2-7.** On page 1 of the Glaucoma-Scope report, depth information is displayed as a numeric grid and a grayscale (upper left and right, respectively). In the numeric depth information, low confidence numbers appear in lighter type, representing discontinuities in line data. High confidence values are displayed in bold type. In follow-up examinations, the change-from-baseline analysis (lower left and right) shows changes of depth values ≥75 microns.

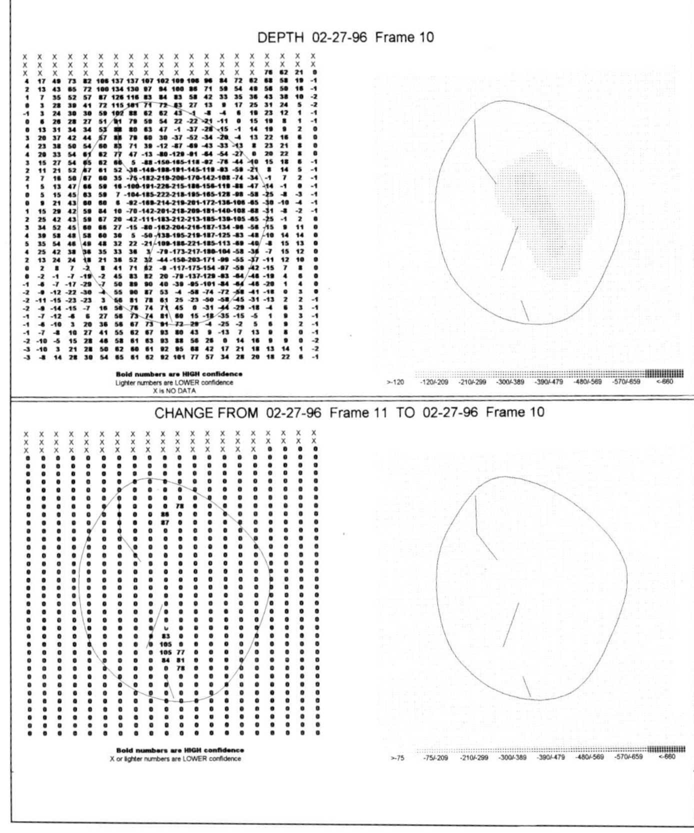

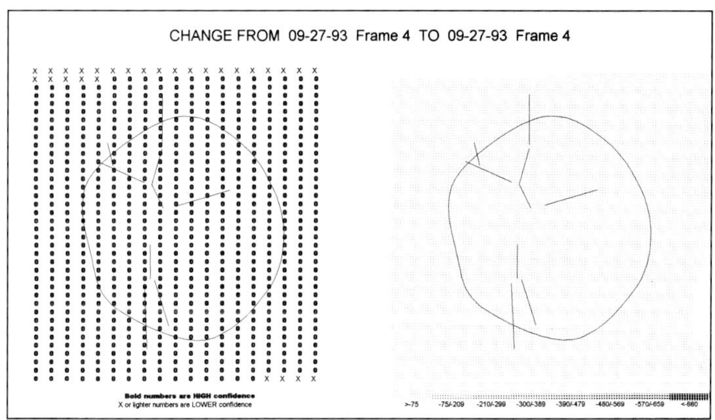


**Figure 2-8.** In the change-from-baseline analysis, variability due to fluctuation of the algorithm is uncommon. The change-from-baseline analysis shown is an image from a patient compared to itself. No points varied in this analysis by ≥75 microns when the line analysis algorithm was run twice on the same image.

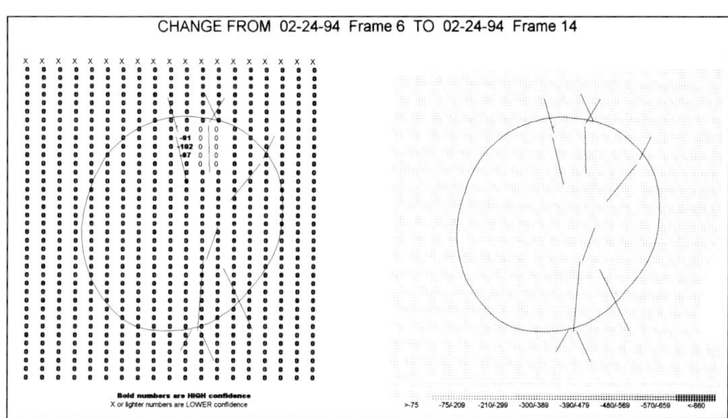


**Figure 2-9.** In the Glaucoma-Scope change-from-baseline analysis, a few points may fluctuate, usually around areas of steep slopes or near blood vessels. In the analysis shown, two different images from the same session in a normal subject were compared to each other, with three points near a blood vessel varying by >75 microns.

be used to print reports at a later, more convenient time. While the reports are printing, another patient image can be captured.

## REPORTS

There are two report pages: page 1 presents depth information as depth numbers (microns) or as a grayscale; page 2 presents color topography maps, profile sections, and common disc parameters. The ONH depth information is presented in a format that is familiar to clinicians.

The numeric depth information is presented on a 19 x 38 number grid (Figure 2-7). Areas where no line data exist are indicated with an "X" on the printout. Numbers defined as low confidence appear as lighter numbers. These low confidence numbers are those numbers with discontinuities in the horizontal line data. These are generally in areas of edges or steep slopes, where horizontal line data are absent. Numbers defined as high confidence are printed in bold type, indicating areas with reliable horizontal line data. The grayscale analysis indicates increasing depth with progressively darker shades of gray, allowing rapid visual assessment of the ONH topography.

In the change-from-baseline analysis, values that have changed by ≥75 microns are shown. These changes may be due to real changes in the topography of the disc or lack of reproducibility. Areas of non-reproducible change may be due to fluctuations of the algorithm (Figure 2-8), or changes due to steep slopes and pulsations around blood vessels (Figure 2-9). Clinically, these areas of artifact may be readily identified by comparing several images captured on the same day to the baseline images (Figure 2-10). Areas of real change are reproducible in comparisons of several images from the same day to the baseline images.

Color topography maps include a three-dimensional map and a two-dimensional disc and cup outline (Figure 2-11). The three-dimensional map is color coded, with shades of blue representing shallow depths, green and yellow indicating intermediate depths, and shades of red showing deeper areas of the cup. The cup outline shows all depth areas greater than 140 microns in red, and shallower areas within the disc margin in yellow.

Profile sections show the cross-sectional depth at the maximum horizontal and vertical cup diameters (Figure 2-12). In these profiles, the disc margins (as indicated by the operator) are shown in bold vertical lines. The depth of the current analysis is represented by a solid red line, whereas the baseline analysis is indicated by a dashed blue line. A "nerve fiber analysis" shows the measurement of the retinal height compared with the reference plane. Areas of peak heights on this analysis usually. represent blood vessels or thicker areas of NFL. The retinal height is shown 200 microns away from the disc margin circumferential to the disc, including temporal (T), superior (S), nasal (N), and inferior (I) areas.

**Figure 2-10.** In the Glaucoma-Scope change-from-baseline analysis, it is often possible to distinguish true changes in disc contour (reproducible changes) from variability (non-reproducible changes) by comparing the baseline image to multiple images from the follow-up session. In the analysis shown, a change-from-baseline analysis of a 36-year-old normal subject showed four points that varied by >75 microns (indicated by squares, upper left) in an area adjacent to blood vessels. This change was non-reproducible when the baseline image was compared to another image from the same session (lower left), indicating that the changes were due to variability rather than a real change of the contour of the disc.

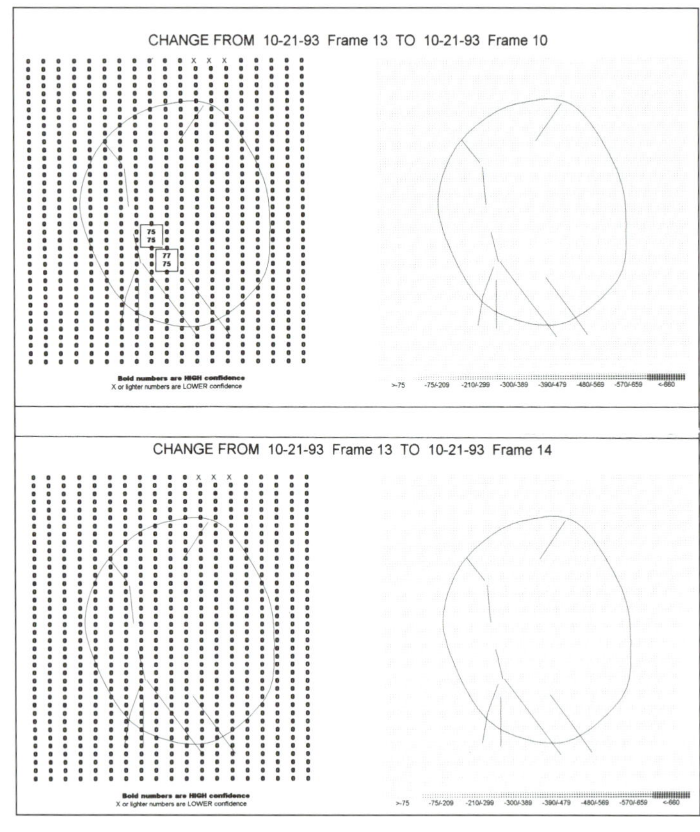

**Figure 2-11.** On page 2 of the Glaucoma-Scope report, color topography maps are shown. A three-dimensional map (left) is color coded according to the depth relative to the reference plane. A two-dimensional disc and cup outline (right) is also displayed, with the cup outline showing the area with depth values $\geq$140 microns.

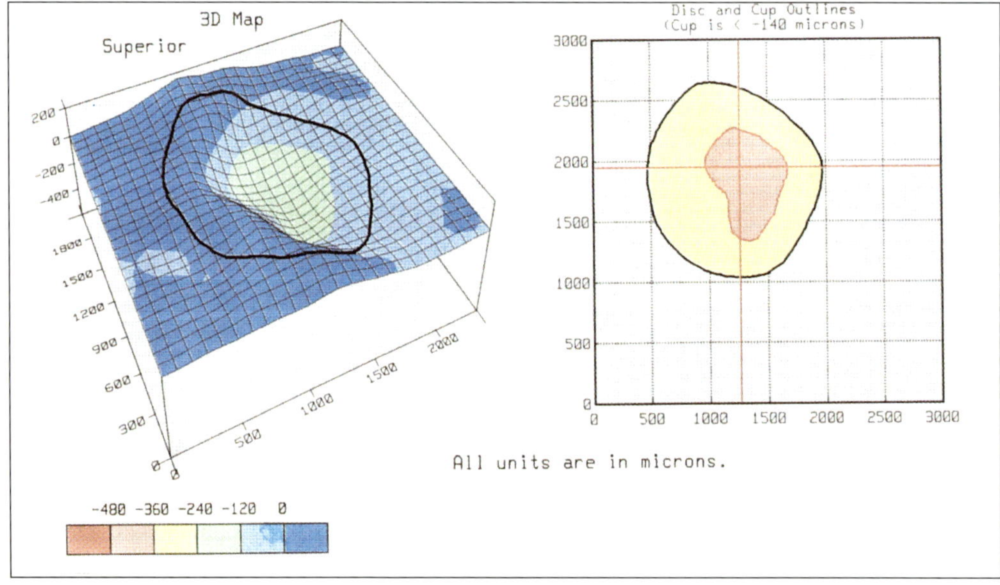

Common disc parameters are also displayed for the current and baseline analyses (Figure 2-13). The cup-to-disc ratio (horizontal and vertical) and the cup-to-disc area ratio are shown. The cup is defined as the area within the disc margin defined by the operator that is at least 140 microns deep. Also displayed are the maximum disc diameter (horizontal and vertical), the disc area, and the cup area, as well as the refraction of the eye. The "MP Disc" is the mean value of the depth numbers inside the disc edge, and the "MP Total Region" is the mean depth of all points measured in the analysis, including points inside and outside the disc.

## REPRODUCIBILITY

Reproducibility is the ability of an instrument to give a consistent result from one measurement to the next in the same individual. With ONH analyzing systems, reproducibil-

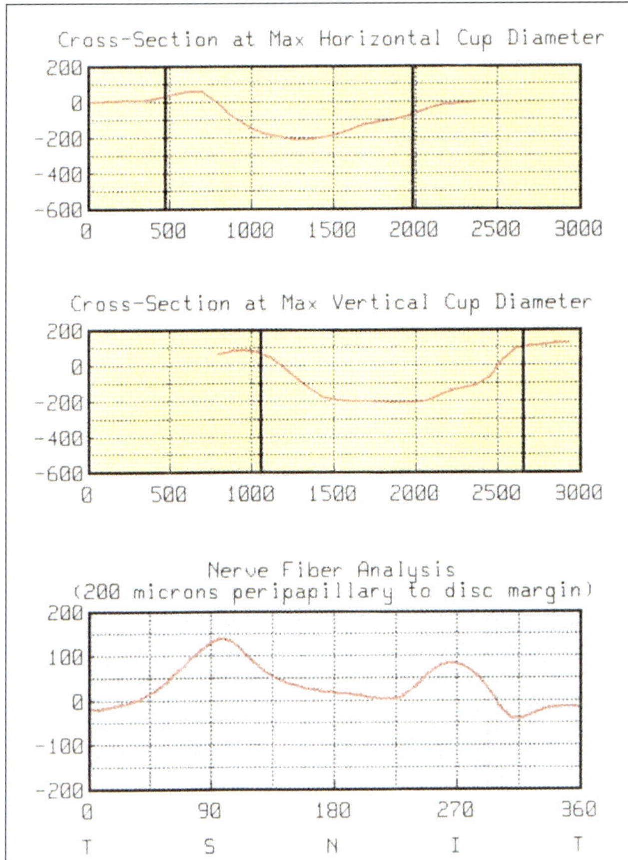

| | CURRENT | PREVIOUS |
|---|---|---|
| Date | 02-27-96 | |
| Analysis | 1 | |
| Frame | 11 | |
| C/D Ratio Vert. | 0.57 | |
| C/D Ratio Horiz. | 0.47 | |
| Cup/Disc Area Ratio | 0.25 | |
| Max Disc Diam Vert | 1,594 | |
| Max Disc Diam Horiz | 1,510 | |
| Disc Area (sq. mm) | 1.836 | |
| Cup Area (sq. mm) | 0.452 | |
| MP Disc | −50.0 | |
| MP Total Region | −6.0 | |
| Rx Sphere | +04.25 | |
| Rx Cylinder | −00.75X180 | |

**Figure 2-13.** Page 2 of the Glaucoma-Scope report shows a table of common disc parameters. The red column shows values from the current analysis, and the blue column shows the values from the previous or baseline analysis. (There was no previous examination in the analysis shown.) Included in the analysis are cup-to-disc ratios, disc diameters, disc and cup areas, the mean position of the disc (MP disc), and the mean position of the total area (MP total region). The MP disc is the mean of depth measurements within the operator-defined disc, whereas the MP total region is the mean of all depth measurements in the analysis. The refraction of the eye, used to correct depth measurements for magnification of the eye, is also shown in this table.

**Figure 2-12.** Profile sections are displayed on page 2 of the Glaucoma-Scope report. The cross-sectional depth at the maximum horizontal (upper) and vertical (middle) cup diameters are shown, with the disc margin as defined by the operator displayed in bold lines. The current analysis is represented by a solid red line, and the baseline analysis (not shown in this analysis) is indicated by a dashed blue line. The "nerve fiber analysis" (bottom) is the retinal height 200 microns away from the disc margin, relative to the reference plane. In the analysis shown, note the double-humped pattern, with the areas of greatest retinal height superior (S) and inferior (I) to the disc.

ity has been expressed in a variety of statistical forms, including coefficient of variation and the standard deviation of a single height measurement.[2] The coefficient of variation is the standard deviation divided by the mean, which measures the variability over an area of several pixel units. The standard deviation of a single height measurement evaluates individual pixels within the images and provides a useful measure of reproducibility of the measurements of an instrument.

Hoskins and associates[5] found that the mean single pixel standard deviation (SD) for the Glaucoma-Scope numerical evaluation was 15.42 microns for the total population, 15.11 microns for healthy discs, and 15.57 microns for glaucomatous discs. Flat areas outside (SD=11.68 microns) and inside (SD=17.91 microns) showed less variability compared with sloped areas within the ONH (SD=20.78 microns) or at the bottom of the cup (SD=32.01 microns). Areas around blood vessels showed the greatest variability (SD=34.76 microns), probably due to vascular pulsations or steep slopes around vessels. Berríos and associates found variability in 5% of the total points displayed within the disc, with most of the variability (75%) found in regions of blood vessels.[7]

Pendergast and Shields[8] evaluated the reproducibility of Glaucoma-Scope measurements by a single observer from one eye of 10 normal subjects and 10 patients with glaucoma on the same day. Reproducibility of depth values was determined in regions of potential clinical interest, including the bottom of the cup, the temporal slope, the nasal disc, and the peripapillary region, as well as 15 randomly selected single points. The mean

**Figure 2-14.** The Glaucoma-Scope change-from-baseline analysis shown compares two different images obtained during the same session from a normal subject, showing reproducible images with no points varying by $\geq 75$ microns. It is common to observe a small proportion of points changing from the baseline image in areas with steep slopes or adjacent to blood vessels.

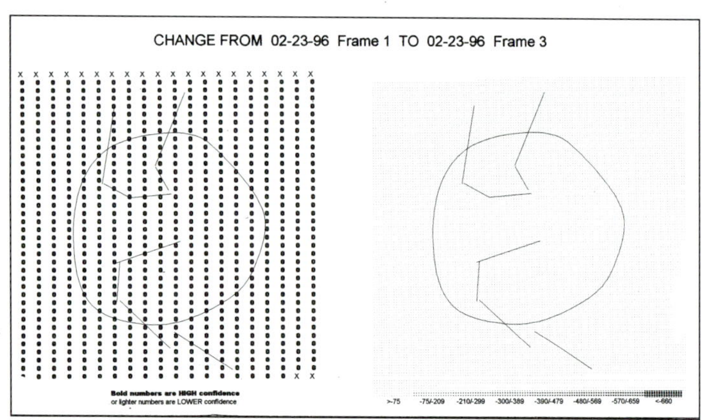


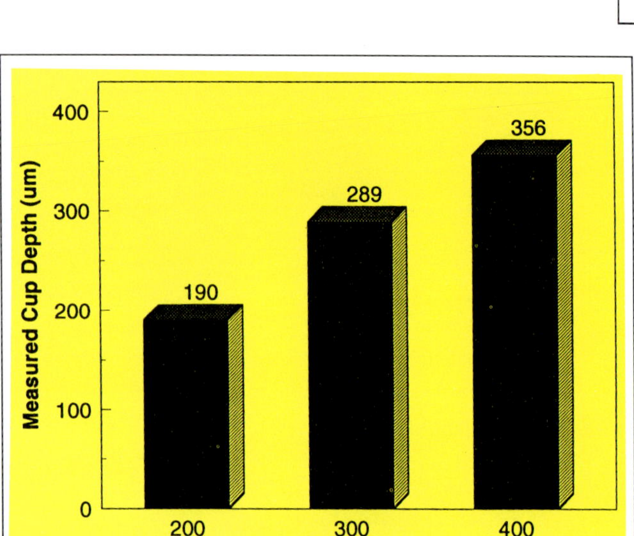


**Figure 2-15.** Accuracy of the Glaucoma-Scope in a model eye. Model eyes with known cup depths of 200, 300, and 400 microns were measured with the Glaucoma-Scope, which found mean±SD cup depths of 190±2, 289±6, and 356±7 microns, respectively. Data provided by P.A. Netland, T. Takamoto, and B. Schwartz.

standard deviations in regions of potential clinical interest among the 20 subjects ranged from 3.98 to 14.09 microns, and the mean coefficient of variation ranged between 4.2% and 8.7%. The 95% confidence intervals for the total population ranged from 9.88 to 34.97 microns for the regions of interest and was 43 microns for the 15 random points. Variability was lowest for the nasal disc and peripapillary retina, which were relatively flat regions, compared with the bottom of the cup and the temporal sloping region. Variability was not statistically significantly different for subjects with and without glaucoma.

The variability of mean position of the disc (MPD) measurements was measured by Quigley and Pease in monkey eyes.[9] The coefficient of variation for MPD measurements was 2.7% in normal monkey eyes. In experimentally induced glaucomatous monkey eyes, the coefficient of variation for MPD measurements was 1.5%, which was not significantly different compared with normal eyes.

Hamzavi, Stewart, and coworkers evaluated the intra- and interobserver variability of depth measurements of the optic disc in cadaver eyes using the Glaucoma-Scope.[10] Intraobserver variation of images was significantly greater with increasing depth of the optic cup (p<0.001). The standard deviation of depth measurements was 9.06 microns over the neural rim, 25.00 microns along the cup wall, and 40.94 microns at the bottom of the optic cup. In this study, the interobserver variability was actually significantly less than intraobserver variability. Depth measurements are objectively determined by the Glaucoma-Scope, which would be expected to minimize interobserver variability.

The Glaucoma-Scope measurements of ONH topography are reproducible (Figure 2-14), with most of the variability occurring in areas around blood vessels or steep slopes. This is probably due to vascular pulsations or differences in algorithm interpretation where line deflections are discontinuous. Patient realignment and algorithm reproducibility contribute little to the variability of the measurements of the Glaucoma-Scope. The reproducibility of the Glaucoma-Scope compares favorably with variability reported for other computerized ONH topography devices.[2,5]

## ACCURACY

Accuracy of ONH analyzers is the ability of these devices to measure the real depth. An instrument with little variability still may not represent the true structure. Accuracy may be difficult to determine in the human eye. Quantitative measurements of the human optic disc must be compared to an accurate "gold standard" and must be corrected for magnification that is dependent upon refractive error, corneal curvature, and axial length. Accuracy determinations also may be directly confirmed with actual sizes and shapes in model eyes (Figure 2-15).

ONH topography determined by the Glaucoma-Scope was compared with stereophotogrammetric measurements by

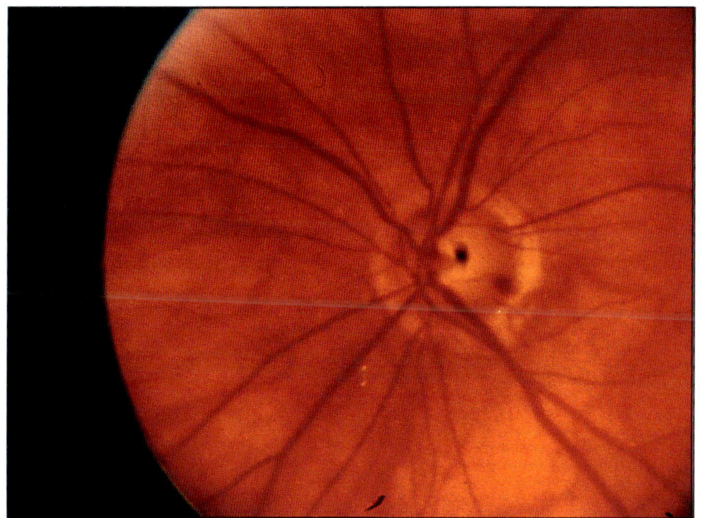

**Figure 2-16a.** A 73-year-old man with low-tension glaucoma developed a disc hemorrhage.

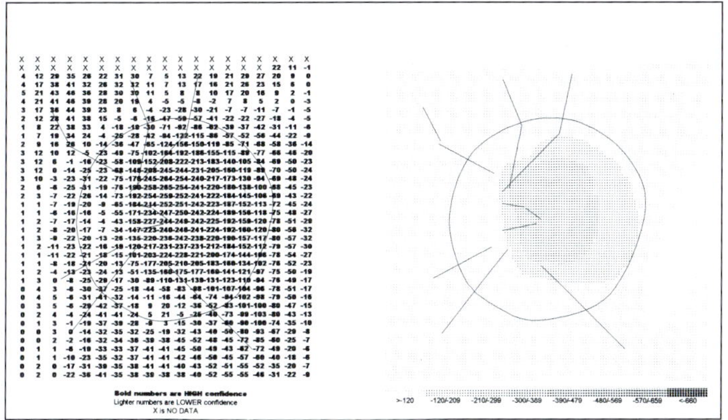


**Figure 2-16b.** The Glaucoma-Scope analysis at the time of the disc hemorrhage showed no apparent change in the contour of the disc in the area corresponding to the hemorrhage. Disc hemorrhages are documented most effectively with clinical observations, drawings, and disc photographs.

Takamoto and associates.[11] Mean±SD for isocontour slopes of Glaucoma-Scope plots was 0.272±0.071 and for photogrammetry was 0.287±0.063 (P=NS). The cup slopes computed by both methods showed a significant correlation ($r_s$=0.908, p<0.01). These findings indicate that both the Glaucoma-Scope and stereophotogrammetry provide similar measurement of cup area versus depth. Shields and coworkers[12] used a model eye to evaluate the accuracy of Glaucoma-Scope depth measurements, with the greatest accuracy of measurements at 22-mm axial length. More recent versions of Glaucoma-Scope software have included a correction factor for magnification error.

The measurement of the relative height of the retinal surface 200 microns outside the disc margin ("nerve fiber analysis" on the Glaucoma-Scope report) was compared to histological estimates of the NFL by Quigley and Pease.[9] In normal monkey eyes, the peripapillary retinal surface was higher superiorly and inferiorly than nasally and temporally. With chronic elevation of intraocular pressure (IOP) in monkey eyes, the retinal height at the upper and lower positions was markedly flattened. In monkey eyes, the nerve fiber area measured by the Glaucoma-Scope correlated well with the number of nerve fibers estimated histologically ($r^2$=0.75, P=0.003, n=9).

## LIMITATIONS

All ONH analyzers may not be capable of measuring ONH topography in certain patients. Dan and coworkers[13] found that Glaucoma-Scope analysis was not achieved in 14% of a total of 336 eyes of 168 patients. The conditions associated with inability to obtain a satisfactory image were hyperpigmented fundi, pseudophakia, aphakia, corneal opacities, cataract, and contact lenses. There may be variability among operators in the rate of unsuccessful analysis of ONH topography using the Glaucoma-Scope.

The minimum pupil size is approximately 4 mm, although image capture may be possible in patients with smaller pupils. Dilation of the pupil is required for most patients. Optic disc hemorrhages may not be detected by the Glaucoma-Scope or other ONH analyzers (Figures 2-16a and 2-16b). Disc hemorrhages are most effectively documented with careful clinical observations or conventional optic nerve photographs. Other ONH analyzers, such as laser scanners, may generate a greater number of data points than the

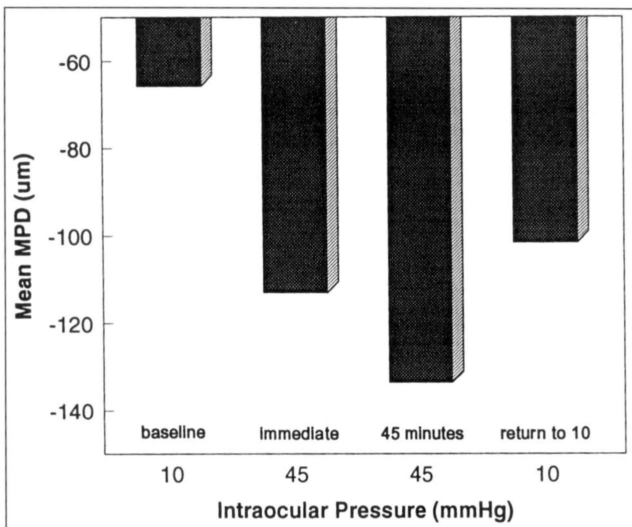

**Figure 2-17.** Glaucoma-Scope measurements of movement of the disc during acute changes of IOP in the monkey eye. The MPD was measured in seven cynomolgus monkey eyes at 10 mmHg, then the IOP was acutely raised to 45 mmHg for 45 minutes. The MPD was significantly different compared to baseline immediately and 45 minutes after raising the IOP to 45 mmHg. The MPD returned to a position that was not significantly different compared with baseline MPD when the IOP was returned to 10 mmHg. These findings indicate that the disc may show acute changes in contour with changes of the IOP, which may be detected with the Glaucoma-Scope. Reprinted with permission from Quigley HA, Pease ME. Change in the optic disc and nerve fiber layer estimated with the Glaucoma-Scope in monkey eyes. *J Glaucoma.* 1996;5:106-116.

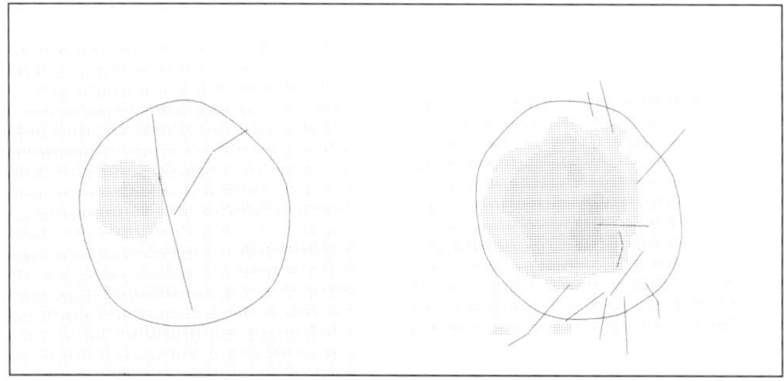

**Figure 2-19.** The Glaucoma-Scope grayscale provides a rapid assessment of the extent of optic nerve cupping. The grayscale analysis of the right eye from a normal subject with a small optic nerve cup (left) is contrasted with the analysis from a patient with pigmentary glaucoma and a large optic nerve cup (right).

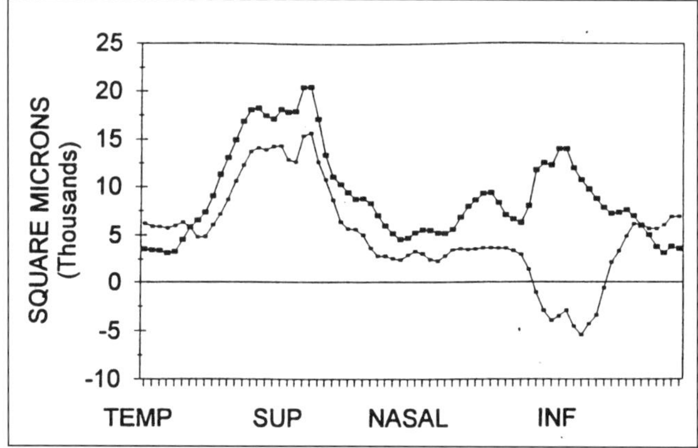

**Figure 2-18.** Glaucoma-Scope measurement of "NFL" area of monkey eyes prior to chronic glaucoma injury (upper darker, larger boxes) and after chronic glaucoma injury with localized inferior NFL atrophy (lower, smaller boxes). The "NFL" area was determined by measuring the retinal height relative to the reference plane at 5° intervals around the disc in four cynomolgus monkey eyes before and after a 4-month period of laser-induced elevation of IOP. Note that the normal values are highest in the superior (Sup) and inferior (Inf) retina in a double-humped pattern. In this model, the Glaucoma-Scope identified changes in the retinal height that occurred after chronic elevation of the IOP. Reprinted with permission from Quigley HA, Pease ME. Change in the optic disc and nerve fiber layer estimated with the Glaucoma-Scope in monkey eyes. *J Glaucoma.* 1996;5:106-116.

Glaucoma-Scope, but many of the data points measured by these other devices are in areas that are not of interest for topographic measurements. Variability observed around blood vessels and in areas of steep slopes is observed in the Glaucoma-Scope, as well as other ONH analyzers.

## CLINICAL APPLICATIONS

The Glaucoma-Scope achieved up to a 91% sensitivity and 90% specificity in identifying patients with glaucoma compared with normals.[14] Due to the relatively low prevalence of glaucoma, this level of specificity is still not satisfactory for glaucoma screening, but suggests possible application for the Glaucoma-Scope as an objective adjunctive method for glaucoma diagnosis.

In an experimental setting, mean backward movements of the disc surface of 50 to 60 microns were observed when IOP was elevated to 45 mmHg for 45 minutes (Figure 2-17).[9] The disc position reverted to its original location on normalization of the IOP. Human observers do not consistently detect the small changes of disc position produced by acute elevation of IOP as effectively as image analysis instruments.[15] Quigley and Pease found that chronic elevation of IOP led to changes

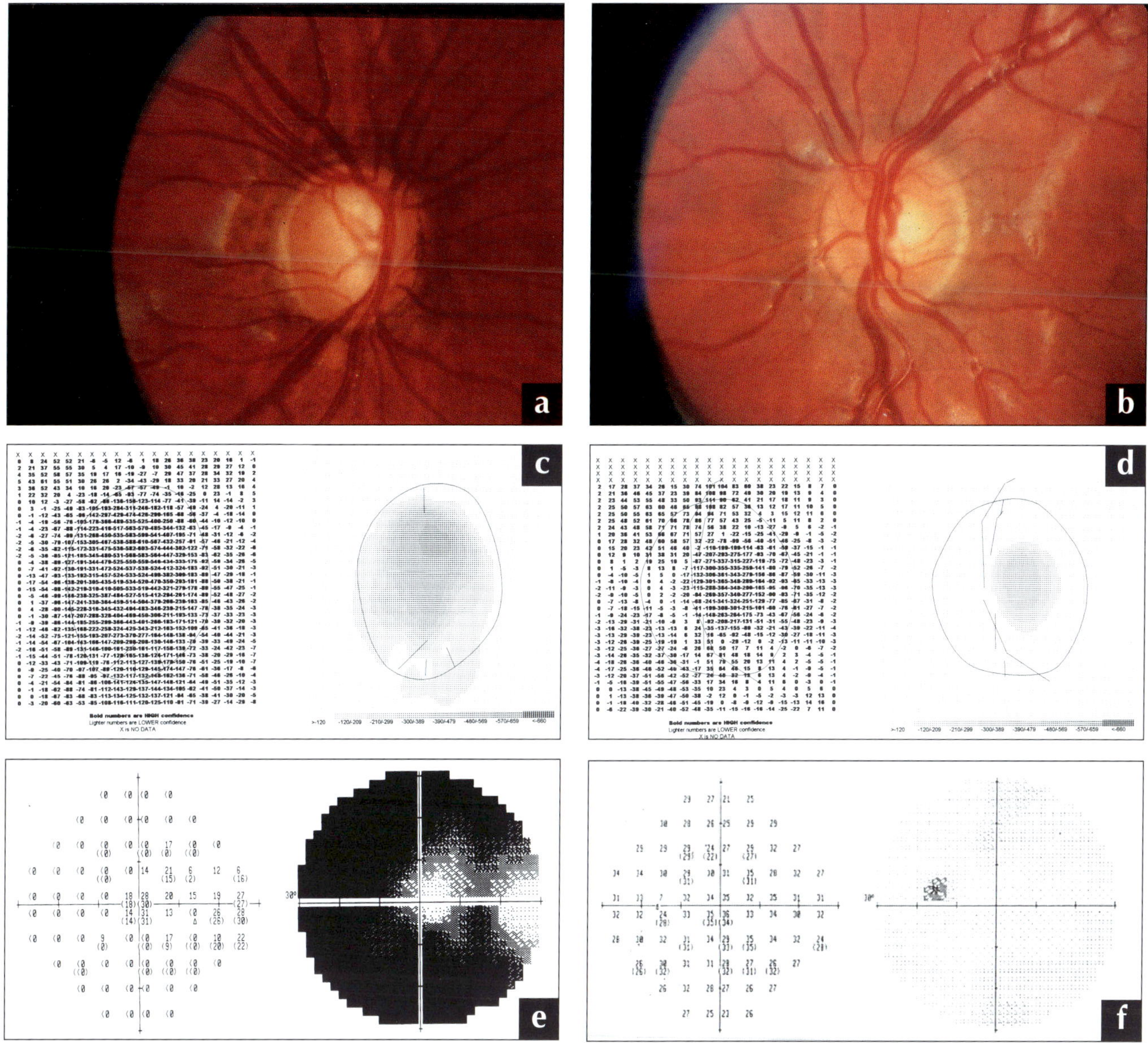

**Figures 2-20a-f.** The Glaucoma-Scope analysis documents differences in the discs in a 9-year-old girl with steroid-induced glaucoma in the right eye and marked cup asymmetry. The optic nerve photographs (a,b), Glaucoma-Scope analysis (c,d), and automated perimetry analysis (e,f) show advanced glaucomatous cupping and visual field loss in the right eye (left) with a relatively normal left eye (right).

in the retinal area as measured by the Glaucoma-Scope (Figure 2-18).[9] Thus, the Glaucoma-Scope may be useful in detecting acute or chronic changes that may represent transient or permanent changes in ONH topography.

The initial exam analysis effectively determines the optic nerve topography. The grayscale report may provide a rapid view of the extent of optic nerve cupping (Figure 2-19). In comparing both eyes, asymmetric optic nerve cupping may be documented (Figures 2-20a through 2-20f). Subtle asymmetry of the optic nerve contour may be detected (Figures 2-21a through 2-21d). Disc elevation may also be demonstrated,

indicated by positive numbers in the Glaucoma-Scope depth analysis (Figures 2-22a and 2-22b). Areas of decreased retinal height in the peripapillary area may be demonstrated, which may correspond with abnormalities of the ONH (Figure 2-23).

Follow-up examinations can determine progressive changes of the optic nerve. In ocular hypertensive patients, disc changes may be documented without visual field changes (Figures 2-24a and 2-24b). Identification of reproducible changes in the ONH contour may be helpful, for example, in the management of low-tension glaucoma patients (Figures 2-25 through 2-26d) and non-compliant

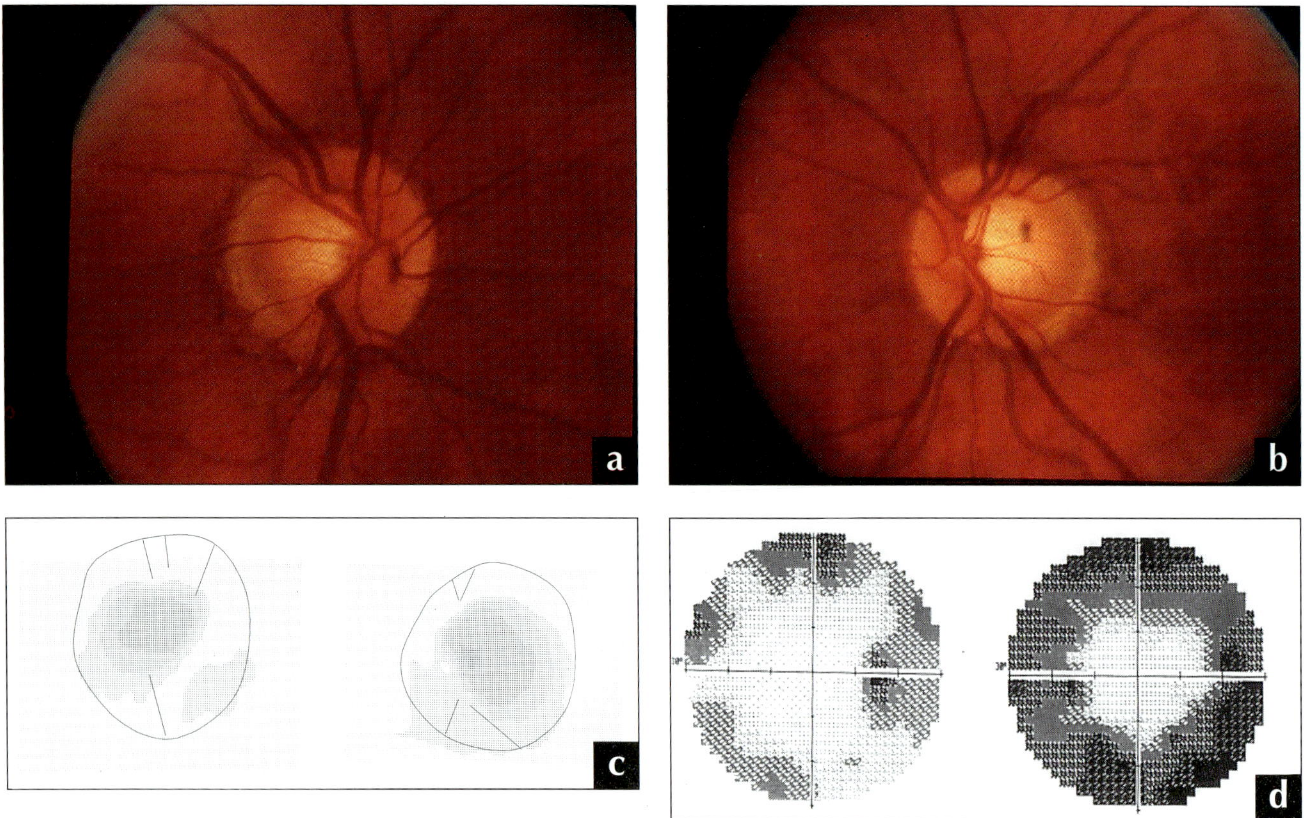

**Figures 2-21a-d.** Optic nerve photographs of the right (a) and left (b) eyes of a 57-year-old man with low-tension glaucoma and mild asymmetry of the IOP, higher in the left eye. The Glaucoma-Scope analysis shows the mild asymmetry of the cupping, worse in the left eye (c,right) compared with the right eye (c,left). Automated perimetry shows greater visual field loss in the left (d,right) compared with the right (d,left) eye.

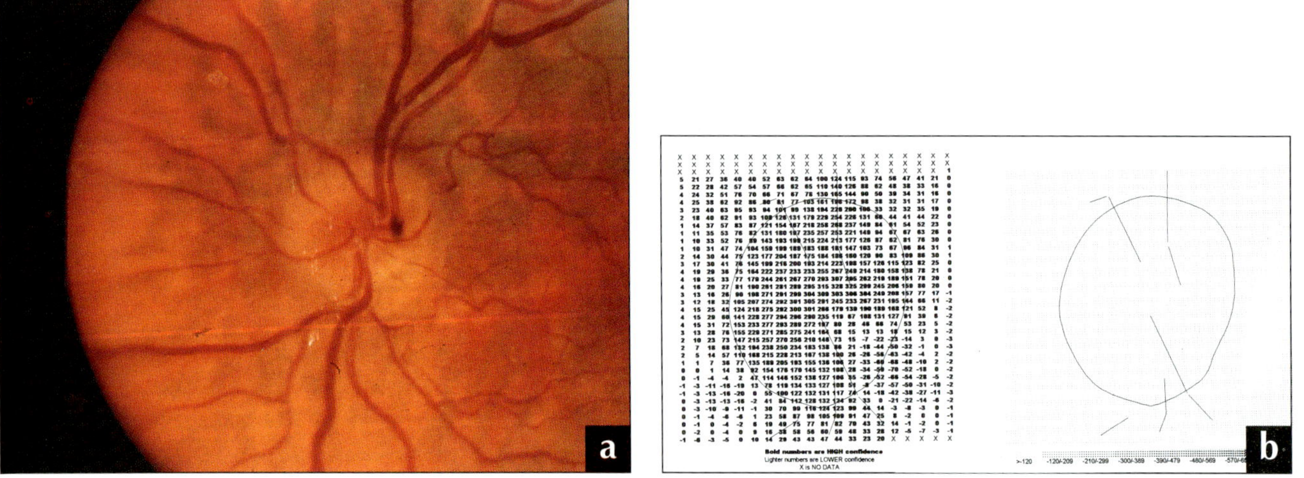

**Figures 2-22a-b.** A 47-year-old woman with pseudotumor cerebri with disc edema (a). The height of the disc is shown on the Glaucoma-Scope analysis (b). Note that positive numbers indicate disc elevation.

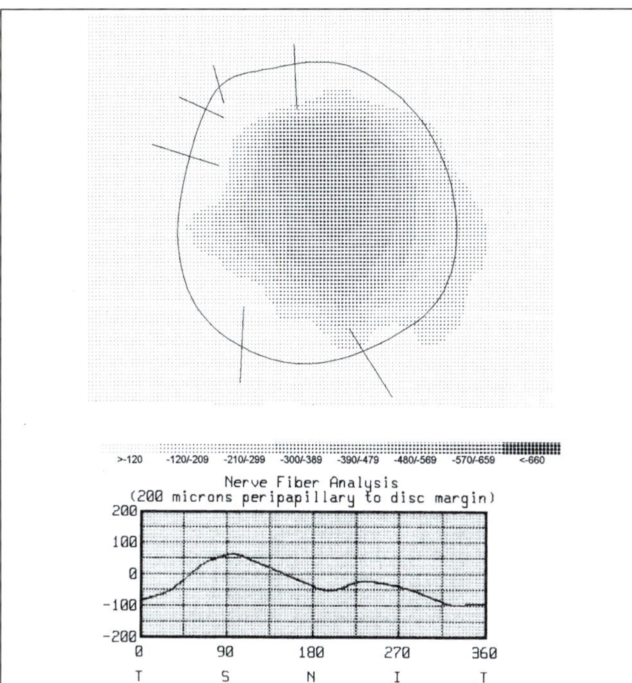

**Figure 2-23.** A 45-year-old woman with open-angle glaucoma with a sloping thin inferotemporal neural rim of the left ONH evident in the Glaucoma-Scope grayscale analysis (top). The retinal height analysis (bottom) showed asymmetry of the double-hump pattern, with a lower retinal height inferior to the disc compared with the height superior to the disc. Courtesy of Dr. D.S. Greenstein, West Roxbury, Mass.

patients (Figures 2-27a and 2-27b). Further investigational work is required to assess the capability of the Glaucoma-Scope and other ONH analyzers to monitor for progressive changes of the optic nerve contour. Areas of variability can occur, usually in areas of steep slopes or areas around blood vessels. Comparison of multiple images during the same sitting will usually distinguish areas of reproducible change from areas of artifactual variability. On follow-up examinations compared with baseline measurements, repeatable changes of depth measurements suggest changes of contour of the ONH. It is also reassuring to both patients and physicians alike when the Glaucoma-Scope documents stable topography of the ONH during follow-up examinations (Figures 2-28a and 2-28b).

## CONCLUSIONS

The Glaucoma-Scope is a computerized ONH analyzer that is based on a technique of computed raster stereography. Line projection analysis provides a quantitative assessment of ONH and peripapillary topography. The measurements appear to be reproducible and accurate, although areas of variability can occur in areas of steep slopes or around blood vessels. The Glaucoma-Scope may be used clinically to quantitatively determine ONH and peripapillary topography and to detect glaucomatous changes of this topography during follow-up examinations.

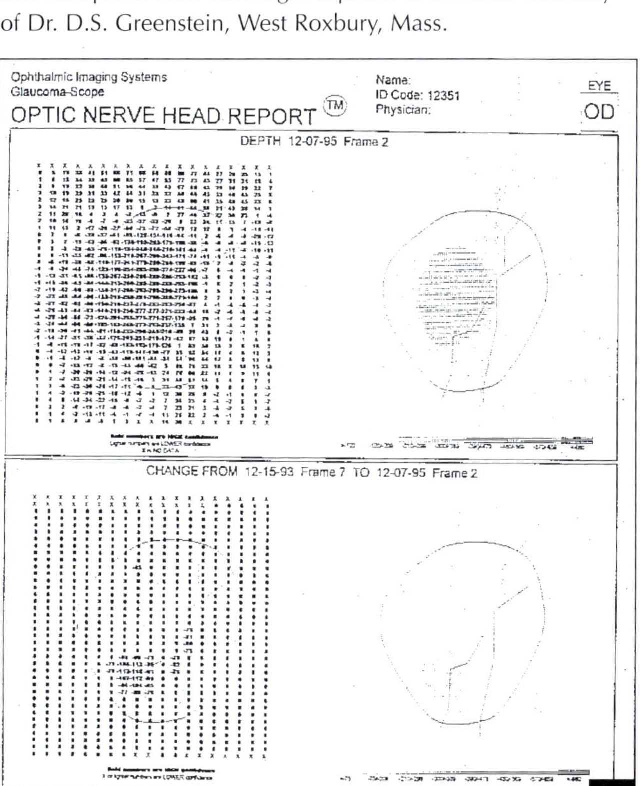

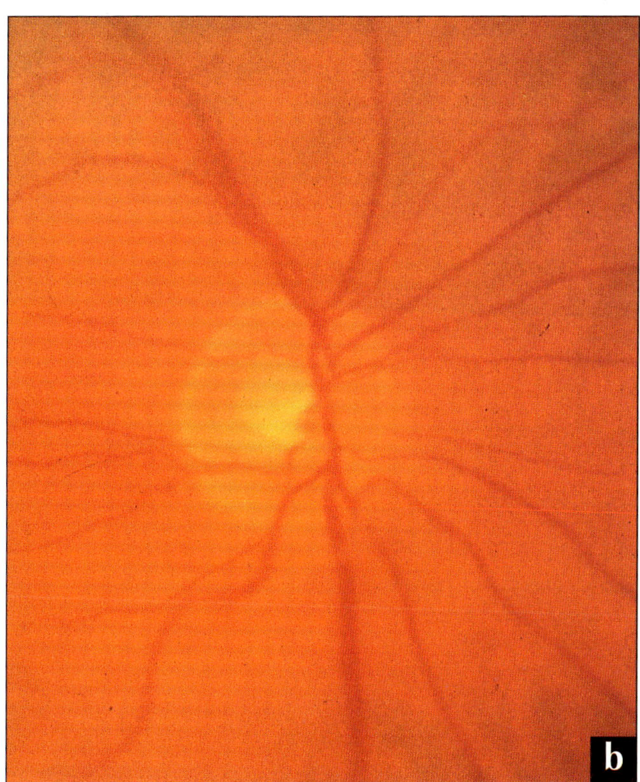

**Figures 2-24a-b.** A 78-year-old man with ocular hypertension developed changes in the contour of the inferotemporal area of the right optic nerve head detected by the Glaucoma-Scope change-from-baseline analysis over a 2-year follow-up period (a). Changes in the optic nerve stereophotographs (b, most recent image shown) corresponded with these changes. Courtesy of Drs. C. Johnson and J.D. Brandt, University of California Davis, Sacramento.

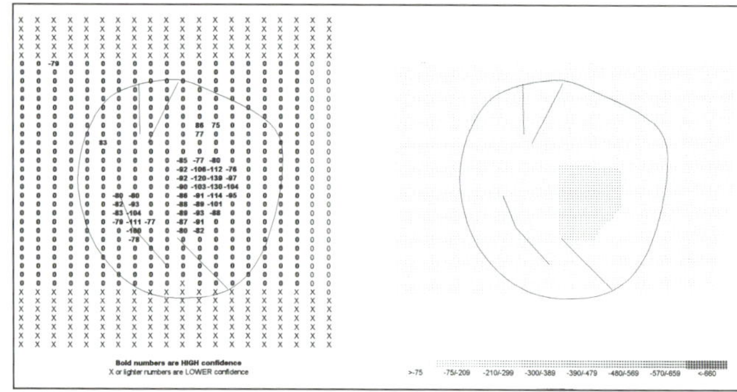

**Figure 2-25.** A 74-year-old man with low-tension glaucoma was noted to have a reproducible change from baseline Glaucoma-Scope analysis over a 6-month period. In response to this change, an additional medication was added to the patient's therapeutic regimen.

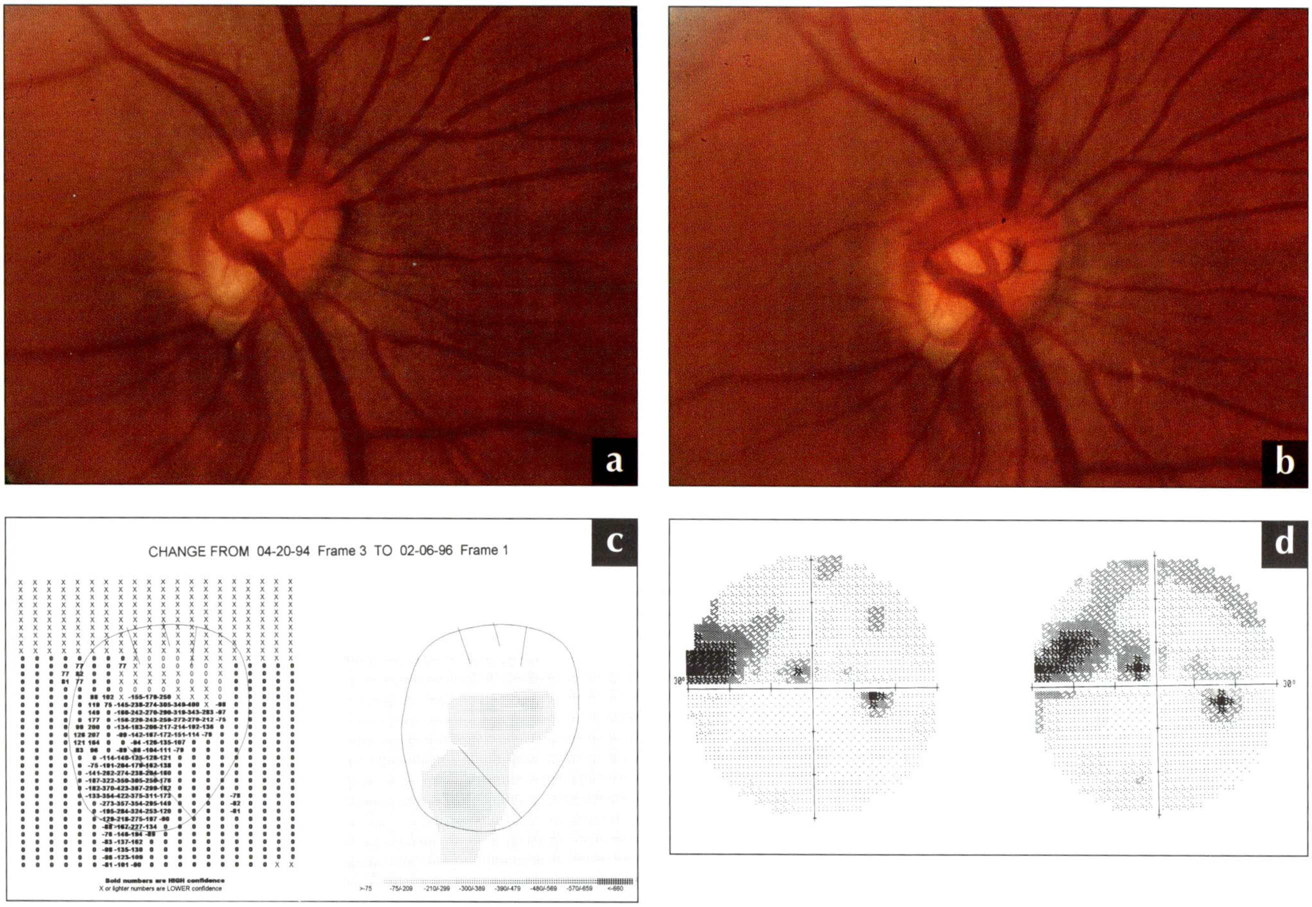

**Figures 2-26a-d.** A 50-year-old woman with low-tension glaucoma and migraine headaches noted a subjective change of her vision over a nearly 2-year follow-up period. The optic nerve photographs showed possible changes in the inferotemporal area of the disc in the right eye during this interval (a,b). The Glaucoma-Scope analysis change-from-baseline showed a reproducible change in the inferotemporal area of the disc (c). Automated perimetry (d) showed progression of visual field loss during this interval. The patient was treated medically in response to these changes.

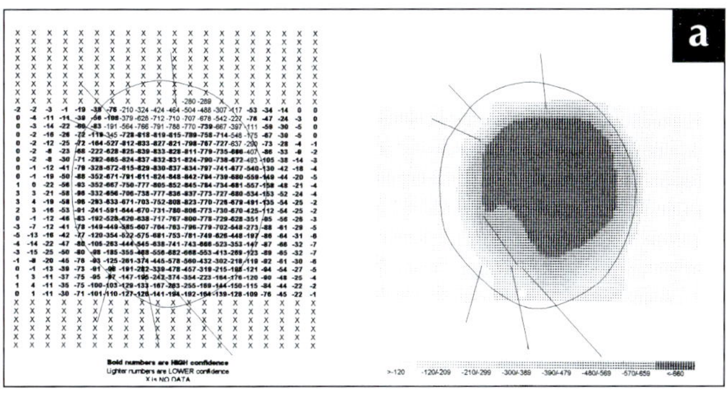
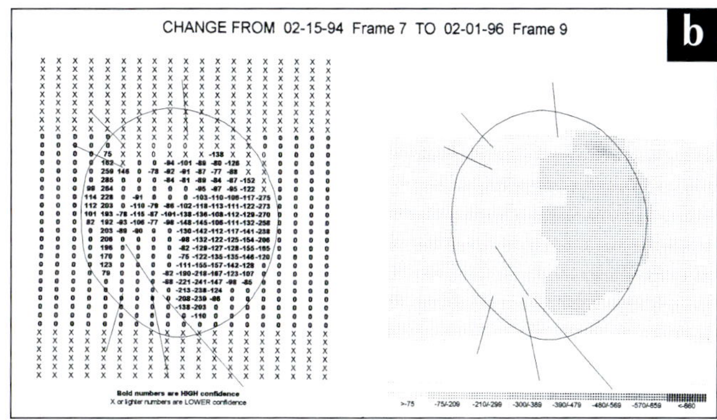

**Figures 2-27a-b.** A 49-year-old woman with open-angle glaucoma was treated with two anti-glaucoma medications. The initial Glaucoma-Scope analysis (a) shows advanced optic nerve glaucomatous atrophy, with a deep cup in the left eye. Although her IOPs were normal during clinic visits, the Glaucoma-Scope change-from-baseline analysis (b) showed reproducible changes in the optic nerve contour over a 2-year follow-up period. Further questioning indicated non-compliance with medical therapy between clinic visits, which was addressed in her subsequent clinical management.

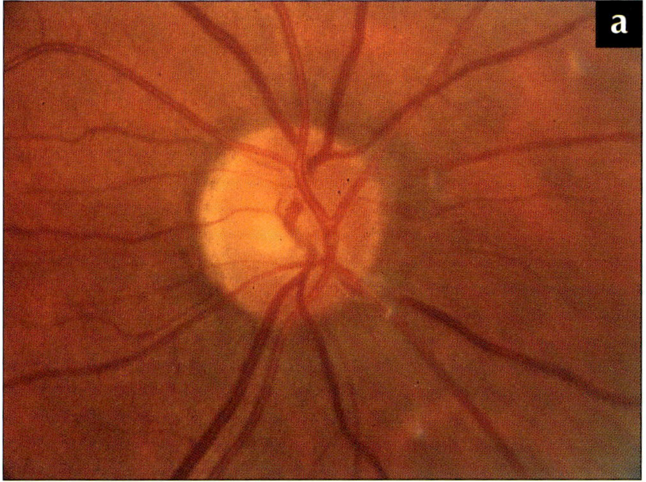
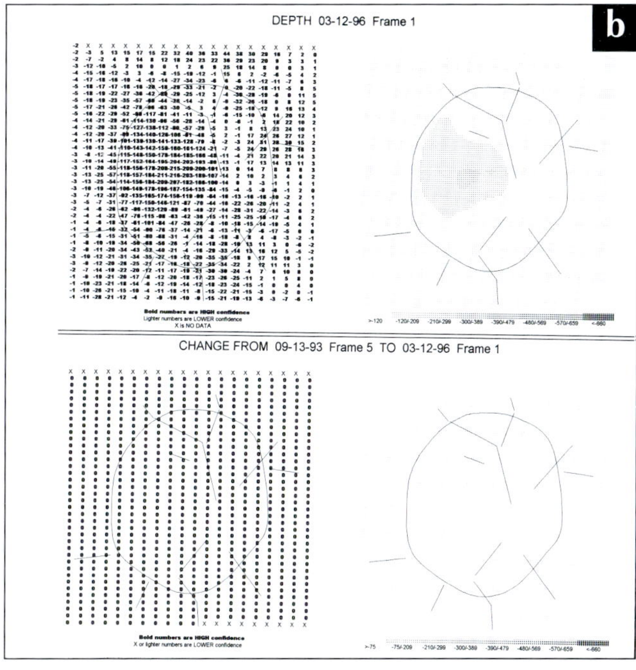

**Figures 2-28a-b.** A 69-year-old man with open-angle glaucoma in both eyes was treated with multiple topical medications. The disc photograph (a) and Glaucoma-Scope analysis (b) of the right eye are shown. During the 2½-year follow-up period, there was no change detected compared with the baseline analysis (b, bottom). The patient was reassured that the glaucoma appeared to be stable at that time with medical therapy.

# REFERENCES

1. Lichter PR. Variability of expert observers in evaluating the optic disc. *Trans Am Ophthalmol Soc.* 1976;74:532-572.

2. Kalina PH, Hutchinson BT, Netland PA. Quantitative assessment of optic nerve head topography. *Int Ophthalmol Clin.* 1994;34:239-253.

3. Holm O, Krakau CET. A photographic method for measuring the volume of papillary excavations. *Ann Ophthalmol.* 1970;1:327-332.

4. Krakau CET, Torlegård K. Comparison between stereo- and slit image photogrammetric measurements of the optic disc. *Acta Ophthalmol.* 1972;50:863-871.

5. Hoskins HD, Hetherington J, Glenday M, Samuels SJ, Verdooner SR. Repeatability of the Glaucoma-Scope measurements of optic nerve head topography. *J Glaucoma.* 1994;3:17-27.

6. Bengtsson B, Krakau CET. Correction of optic disc measurements on fundus photographs. *Graefes Arch Clin Exp Ophthalmol.* 1991;230:24-28.

7. Berríos RR, Chi TSK, Netland PA. Variation of optic nerve head topography measurements during the cardiac cycle. *Invest Ophthalmol Vis Sci.* 1994;35(Suppl):1348.

8. Pendergast SD, Shields MB. Reproducibility of optic nerve head topographic measurements with the Glaucoma-Scope. *J Glaucoma.* 1995;4:170-176.

9. Quigley HA, Pease ME. Change in the optic disc and nerve fiber layer estimated with the Glaucoma-Scope in monkey eyes. *J Glaucoma.* 1996;5:106-116.

10. Hamzavi S, Stewart WC, Jackson GJ, Thompson TL. Reproducibility of the Glaucoma-Scope in cadaver eyes. *Acta Ophthalmol Scand.* 1995;73:264-267.

11. Takamoto T, Netland PA, Schwartz B. Comparison of measurements of optic disc cup by Glaucoma-Scope and stereophotogrammetry. *Invest Ophthalmol Vis Sci.* 1994;35(Suppl):1348.

12. Shields MB, Kim J, White WN II. The accuracy of topographic measurements with the Glaucoma-Scope. *Invest Ophthalmol Vis Sci.* 1995;36:S970.

13. Dan JA, Belyea DA, Lieberman MF, Stamper RL. Evaluation of optic disc measurements with the Glaucoma-Scope. *J Glaucoma.* 1996;5:1-8.

14. Gunderson KG, Heijl A, Bengtsson B. Sensitivity and specificity of structural optic disc parameters in chronic glaucoma. *Acta Ophthalmol Scand.* 1995;73:1-6.

15. Burgoyne CF, Varma R, Quigley HA. Comparison of clinician judgment with digitized image analysis in the detection of induced optic disk change in monkey eyes. *Am J Ophthalmol.* 1995;120:176-183.

# OBJECTIVE ASSESSMENT OF OPTIC DISC FEATURES WITH PERSONAL COMPUTERS

*Philip Lempert, MD*

In the early stages of the computer revolution, the cost and complexity of computer equipment were barriers to the implementation of digital imaging technology. Sophisticated devices employing custom software running on large computers were available only in some medical centers. A watershed was reached in the mid-1980s when personal computers began to have sufficient speed, memory capacity, and graphics resolution to undertake medical tasks.

There has been an almost continuous 25% annual increase in processing speed and memory capacity at constant cost since the mid-1960s. In recent years, graphics equipment for image capture, enhancement, and analysis has become a competitive arena for computer developers. The net effect of the decreasing cost-to-power ratio has been to democratize computerized imaging technology. Cost is no longer a deterrent and computerized optic nerve analysis systems, built around generic modules, may be among the least expensive diagnostic instruments in an ophthalmologist's office.

This chapter illustrates a utilitarian approach to quantitative optic nerve analysis that takes advantage of off-the-shelf hardware and software. The descriptions are limited to IBM-compatible equipment because, at this time, they comprise the overwhelming majority of personal computers. The immediate advantages of participating in this critical mass are low cost and reliability. In the long term, additional benefits accrue. An open architecture system is easy to integrate, modify, or upgrade since all the components are designed around established standards. As needs change, as there is more experience with the system, and as computers evolve, end users can individualize the system in accordance with their particular needs.

## GETTING THE IMAGE INTO THE COMPUTER

Image analysis begins with the acquisition of a digitized image. Slides can be digitized with specialized scanners or captured with a video camera from a slide viewer screen. Real-time direct imaging of the optic disc requires three basic electronic elements:

- A high resolution video camera
- A frame-grabber circuit board
- A computer to carry out commands and store images

Economy and quality are both served by the use of a black and white camera with at least 500 lines of horizontal resolution. Resolution of approximately 800 x 500 lines is required for viewing disc capillaries and other detailed features. The interior of the eye is essentially monochromatic and there are no inherent benefits to color capability for the purpose of making measurements. Modern monochrome cameras require very little light and the fundus camera's viewing light, even with a filter, is sufficient. This sensitivity simplifies the system because the need for flash synchronization is eliminated.

COHU 4800, 4815, and 6500 cameras and their equivalents perform very well and are generally available from specialty scientific suppliers. Consumer-oriented devices do not have sufficient pixel density.

A frame-grabber circuit card is necessary. It must sample the analog video signal from the camera at a minimum of 1/30 second for the entire screen. A slower rate will yield blurred images that are inadequate for medical purposes. There are many vendors of good quality frame-grabbers. These include:

- Data Translation[1]
- Univision[2]

Lower cost options, such as the ComputerEyes/1024[3] and ComputerEyes/PCI, are available. Their major shortcoming is lack of integration with image capture/analysis software packages. Nonetheless, images can still be captured with the software included with the video frame-grabber and then accessed in an intermediate step by the analysis program.

The specific choice of computer is not critical but the processing chip must be at least an 80386. Performance, particularly for filtering or multiple image operations, is significantly enhanced by a faster chip such as the pentium. A VGA color monitor is recommended because the measurement lines are in color, even though the disc image will be black and white. A color monitor also permits pseudo color displays that might be helpful for accentuating certain features.

A retinal camera equipped with a video camera relay attachment permits high quality imaging with minimal patient discomfort. The sensitivity of the monochrome camera allows imaging with the viewing light only. A red-free filter, the type used for nerve fiber layer photographs, makes the light more tolerable for the patient and enhances image quality.

The monitor should be positioned on a shelf or stand behind and above the patient to make it visible to the person operating the camera. Since all of the light is directed to the video camera by the mirror in the relay system, the only way to aim and focus the retinal camera is by watching the monitor. Some additional magnification is induced by the relay system so that locating the disc is easier at the lowest magnification setting. Parallax-related distortions are minimized by positioning the disc in the center of the field. This is particularly important when comparisons or digital subtractions are to be performed because pictures taken at different angles may induce spurious changes in the relative location of blood vessels.

With this optical arrangement, the amount of light entering the camera is adjusted with the intensity control on the fundus camera since there are no aperture controls for the video camera. Begin with the lowest setting that produces a visible image on the screen. Adjust the focus and position and then warn the patient that the light will increase. Increase the light level rapidly until all the disc's features are visible and capture the image.

At this point, by whichever method is most convenient and practical, the disc image has been digitized by the computer. The grist for image processing mill is now ready for the next step.

## IMAGE ENHANCEMENT AND ANALYSIS

Image manipulation is a software function that includes adjustment of brightness and contrast, filtering to remove artifacts, cropping, modification of scale, and measurement of image features. Among the software companies in this arena are Jandel[4] and Media Cybernetics.[5] The cost of their robust and versatile image analysis programs is generally less than $1000. The versions for Microsoft Windows 3.1 and even their DOS predecessors have more modules and features than are actually necessary for ophthalmic applications. Their potential uses are limited only by imagination and patience. Measurement is the immediately relevant task of these systems. The programs provide the means to precisely gauge the length or area of image components in terms of pixels. Conversion to absolute terms, such as millimeters, requires consideration of magnification by the optics of the eye and camera.

The calculations for finding the magnification corrections for the eye/camera optical system assume that the starting image is a 35-mm slide.[6] This requires determining the relationship between image size on the computer monitor and image size on a slide. That value can be established empirically by taking pictures of the same eye, at the same retinal camera magnification, with both the conventional 35-mm camera body and with the computer. When the slides are available, the horizontal and vertical disc diameters can be measured directly with a calibrated loupe or micrometer. A rear projection DOS slide viewer can also be employed and the diameters measured with a ruler on that screen. The magnification of a Kodak rear projection viewer must then be taken into account. For example, if the vertical disc diameter on the projection screen is 47 mm and the magnification of the viewer is 11.5x, then the size on the slide is 4.09 mm. The corresponding vertical and horizontal diameters on the computer image are measured in pixels with the image analysis software. Dividing the values in millimeters on the slide into the equivalent values in pixels will determine the pixel-to-millimeter ratio. In the system I use, this ratio is 31.9 pixels on the computer monitor to 1.0 mm on the slide.

$$\frac{\text{Horizontal diameter in pixels}}{\text{Horizontal diameter in millimeters from slide}} = \text{pixels / mm}$$

There may be differences in the values for the horizontal and vertical measurements. Some computer systems have rectangular rather than square pixels. An imaging system with square pixels will have the same ratio regardless of orientation. Rectangular pixels will produce different pixel counts for the same sized object—diameters of a circle, for example—if the measurement line is placed at different orientations. This requires adjustment of the image before measurement or modification of the formulas to ensure correct size interpretation. A simple way to test the aspect ratio of your system is to take a picture of a circular object and mea-

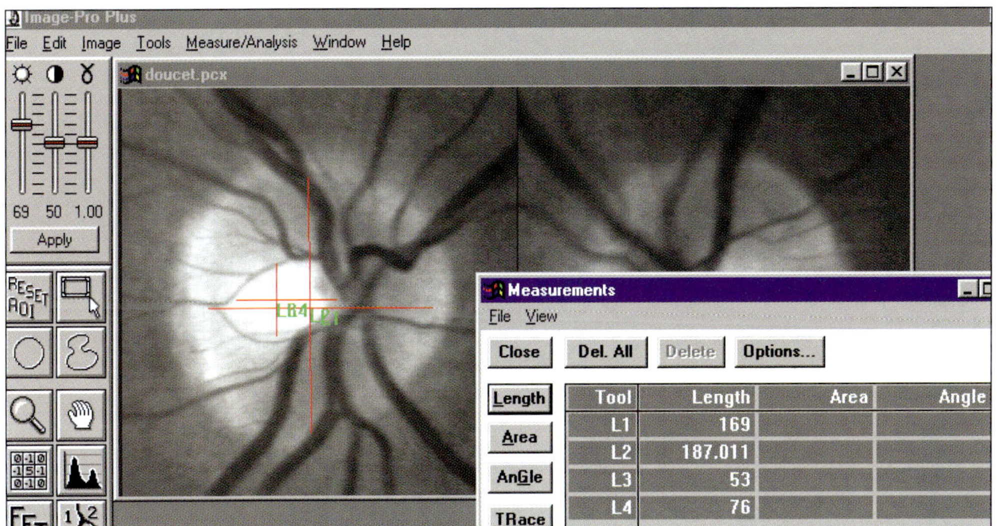


**Figure 3-1.** Linear measurement of the disc diameters with one of the image analysis software programs. The lines are positioned from the inner edge of the scleral ring in the vertical and horizontal positions.

sure the vertical and horizontal diameters. If the horizontal diameter of the circular object is 100 pixels while the vertical is 80 pixels, then an adjustment reducing the initial horizontal value by 20% should be inserted in all the calculations.

Planimetry is a multi-step interactive method for measuring objects within two-dimensional images. The various techniques that have been described combine human judgment with algorithms to correct for magnification.[7,8] In the past, before real-time computer imaging was practical, a photographic print was necessary. Now a digital image can serve as the basis for planimetry and it is measured directly with the computer software.

Figure 3-1 demonstrates linear measurement of the disc diameters with one of the image analysis software programs. The lines are positioned from the inner edge of the scleral ring in the vertical and horizontal positions. Figure 3-2 displays a method for putting the coordinates of the end of each line and the distance between them in a spreadsheet. The data file can be read by conventional spreadsheet programs. Figures 3-3 and 3-4 illustrate another measurement technique. An oval is fit along the scleral rim. This is particularly helpful when the boundaries of the disc are indistinct. The program is then instructed to provide the maximum and minimum diameters, area, shape factor, and a variety of other quantitative expressions which describe the oval.

The criteria for interpreting disc and cup contours from two-dimensional information follow the same concepts for identification of features as were used previously. The inner edge of the scleral canal, visible as a white ring, is recognized to be the boundary of the disc. An equivalent definition of the cup margin is more difficult to achieve. Reliable determinations of the inner margin of the neuroretinal rim may be made by observing the course of disc blood vessels or by pallor changes between the disc and rim.

## Calculating the Magnification Factor

*Nobody would dream of giving a measurement in units of individual body length or fractions thereof. Similarly, the use of the disc diameter as a measurement of fundus structures should be abandoned.[9]*

Performing the calculation of magnification factors is the second area where computers are extremely helpful. Some prior processes, such as templates that are placed over slides, are inherently inaccurate because they assume a fixed disc size—usually 1.5-mm diameter—and magnification factor.[10-12] These presumptions are not supportable in view of the range of disc size in normal eyes[2] and their use is no longer recommended.[13,14] Optic disc diameter, even in normal eyes, is manifestly variable and any method for evaluating the disc or determing the size of intraocular features assuming a constant diameter is inherently inaccurate.[9,15]

The formulas are essentially a collection of straightforward arithmetic steps. However, because there are multiple variables and four-digit optical constants, their manual execution is tedious and prone to error. Either an electronic spreadsheet or database manager program permits accurate calculations and an organized method for collecting data.

Four formulas, all based on the Gullstrand schematic eye, are at hand for calculating the combined magnification effects of the fundus camera and an eye. Their variables are refractive error, axial length, and corneal curvature. The cornea is the least important factor in calculating the magnification factor of the eye/camera combination.[6,16,17] "Both the absolute and the relative magnification depend on 'reduzierte Axenlangenkonvergenz' only."[17] "Measurements of the corneal curvature are therefore hardly rewarding for the present purpose."[13] The optics of the Zeiss and Topcon fundus cameras respectively serve as part of the calculations and the resultant magnification factors apply to the film

**Figure 3-2.** Method for putting the coordinates of the end of each line and the distance between them in a spreadsheet. The data file can be read by conventional spreadsheet programs.

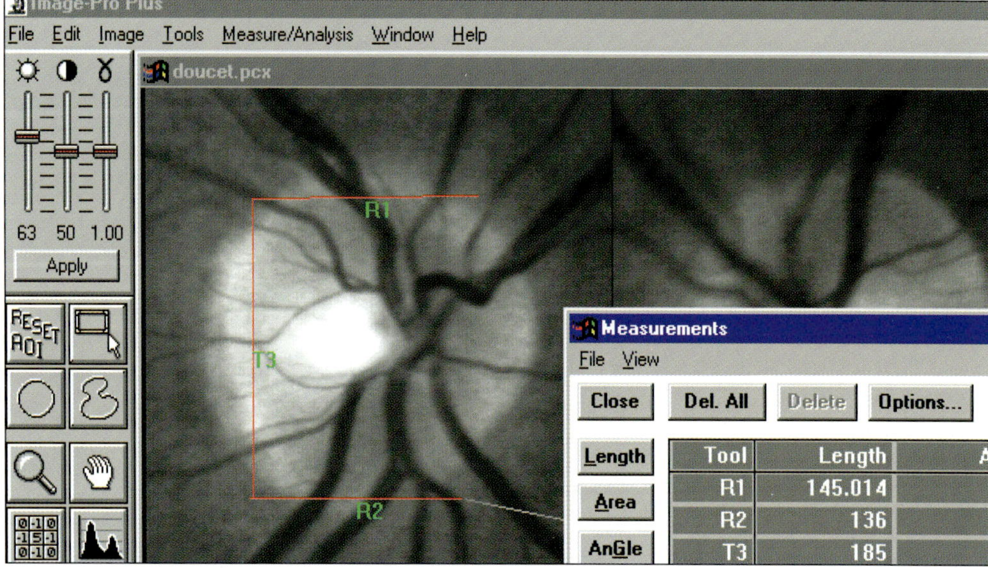

**Figure 3-3.** Another measurement technique. An oval is fit along the scleral rim. This is particularly helpful when the boundaries of the disc are indistinct.

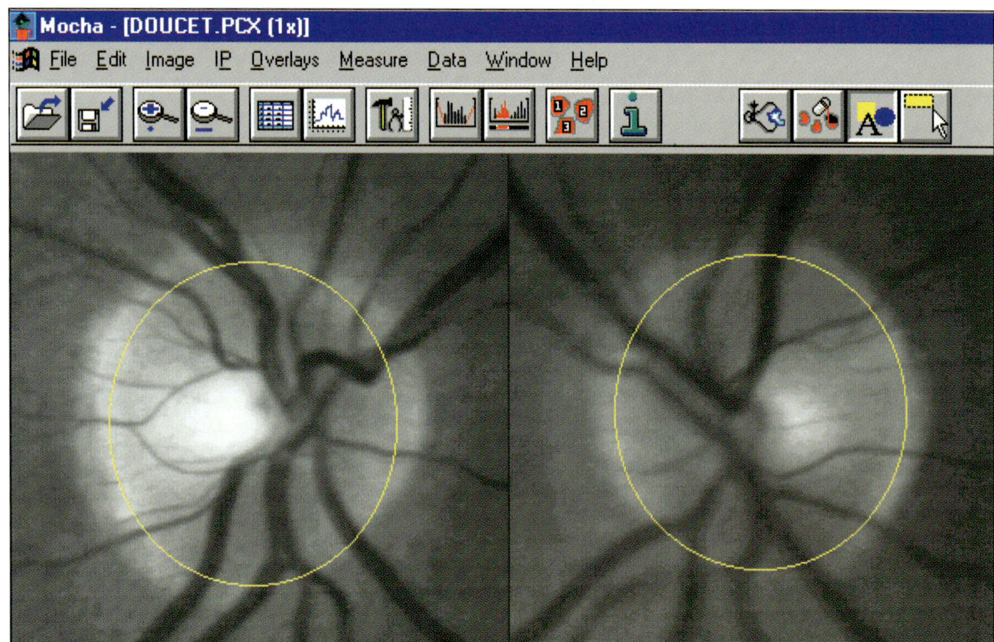

image. The actual size of retinal structures is then determined by dividing the measurements taken from the slide, preferably in millimeters, by the magnification factor. Different imaging accessories require additional compensation. If a Polaroid attachment is used on a Topcon TRC-50VT, it will induce a further 2.72-fold increase in image size. The magnification factor must then be multiplied by 2.72 for Polaroid prints.

Refractive error, axial length, and corneal curvature are the optical variables that determine the contribution of the eye. Though these formulas share a common origin, they utilize alternate optical components to arrive at the magnification factor. The formulas are as follows:

$$M = ((f \times n) / ((axlen - a) \times (1+(L-f) \times (ref\ err))) \times T$$

$$M = 0.056/(axlen - 0.0016)$$

$$M = 2.5 / (1 - 0.017 \times (ref\ err))$$

$$M = 2.5 \times (1 + 0.017 \times B)$$

where:

1. All measurements are in meters and diopters
2. f = focal length of the fundus camera. This is 0.04261 m for a Topcon TRC-50VT and 0.042 m for the Zeiss fundus camera.

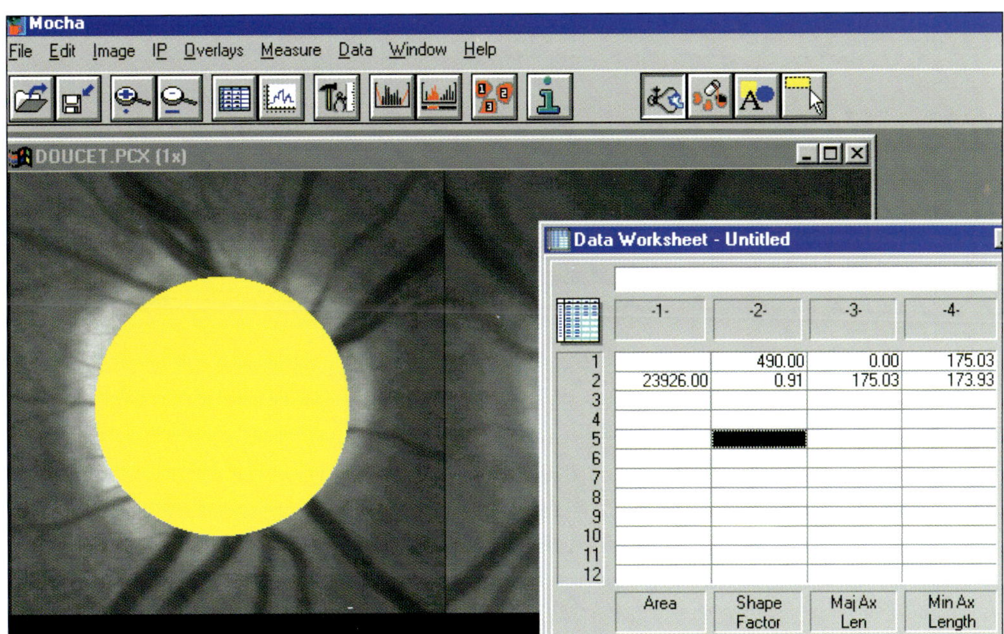

**Figure 3-4.** The program is then instructed to provide the maximum and minimum diameters, area, shape factor, and a variety of other quantitative expressions which describe the oval.

3.  n = index of refraction of the cornea = 1.336
4.  axlen = axial length as measured with ultrasonography
5.  a = distance between the corneal apex and the principal point of the eye = 0.002 m
6.  L = distance between the principal point of the eye and the objective lens of the camera = 0.06344 m
7.  ref err = spherical equivalent of the eye
8.  T = magnification of the Topcon TRC-50VT retinal camera relay optics. They are respectively for each of the field settings:

$$50°=0.74652$$
$$35°=1.02608$$
$$20°=1.48669$$

9.  B = (A + * D)
    where:
    9.1. A = principal point refraction of the eye
         = ref err/(1 - ref err)/("normal" refractive power of the eye)
    9.2. "normal" refractive power of the eye (Gullstrand) = 58.64 D
    9.3. (Stenstrom) = coefficient of regression of (total) refractive power of the eye on refractive power of the cornea
    9.4. D = ($D_1$ - D1) = deviation of refractive power of the cornea from "normal" refractive power of the cornea.

Choosing among the formulas is influenced by clinical realities and the accessibility of other technology. Increasing nuclear sclerosis will change the dioptric power of the lens and introduce error. Incorporation of algorithms based on axial length alone dictates the need for accurate ultrasonography. It may be appropriate, in order to reduce the effect of extreme changes in a single variable, to use an average of the three formulas designed for the Zeiss camera or the initial formula from Topcon that combines axial length and refractive error.

dBASE III or IV or Lotus 1-2-3 are representative electronic tools and each one is abundantly capable of carrying out the necessary calculations. Despite their common logical basis, there are substantial differences between the operations and interfaces of spreadsheets and database managers. Spreadsheets are more flexible and usually have more options for manipulation of data than database managers. Formulas reside in spreadsheet cells and refer to data placed in other cells. In general, mathematical operations are easier to prepare or modify. This capability is particularly helpful when exploring various "what if" scenarios where data and formulas must be changed. Their open construction makes information stored in spreadsheets more vulnerable to contamination or loss. Database managers, more structured and less flexible, keep data in a more organized and secure setting. Once a program with its inclusive formulas is constructed, there is little opportunity to make alterations. Conversely, writing a program in the dBASE language is an exercise in precise syntax and memory use requirements.

dBASE III and Lotus 1-2-3 are applications programs employed for the examples that follow. Most of the office management and billing programs that are encountered in medical offices are aimed at performing a single job. They cannot be employed for anything beyond their immediate context. Applications programs, conversely, are tools that can be applied to almost any aspect of data or numeric manipulation. The key feature is versatility. An applications program can become anything that the user needs. The only limitations are the imagination and linguistic (in the sense of computer languages) skill of the user. These progams have millions of end users and this wide base makes compatibility with other programs likely. Even in those occasions when the program cannot be directly read by a newer program, the principles and concepts remain consistent.

The following example illustrates a method for calculating magnification factors. A second step, finding the actual disc parameters from the measurements, is included that gives the mathematics a clinical context. This model is based on Lotus 1-2-3.

Lotus 1-2-3 is a matrix of cells formed by horizontal rows and vertical columns. The cells can contain labels, numeric data, or formulas. A good first step is to put in a heading identifying the purpose of the spreadsheet template, the programmer, and the date it was prepared. Labels for each item of information should be placed consecutively in the first row or column. The labels should be grouped in the order that you prefer for entering and displaying data. Implicit in this part is some forethought about how to structure the display to fit your preferences. This process should consider the orientation of the data (vertical or horizontal), grouping, and pertinent information to be stored. The format of this sample template is only one of many possible options.

There are conventions for writing in an electronic spreadsheet and understanding them will make the following material more accessible. The cell coordinates are given in the left-hand column and they begin with cell A1 at the uppermost left-hand corner of the sheet. Cell B6 is at the junction of column B—the second along the horizontal axis—and row 6, which is the sixth row on the vertical axis. An apostrophe indicates that the cell entry is text or a label. Entries with an apostrophe cannot be used for calculations. Those entries that begin with a plus sign, parenthesis, or @(function) sign notify the presence of a formula. These contain cell references, in terms of their coordinates, for inclusion into their operations.

The decision-making tree in cell B14 is a nested Boolian logic expression which examines the value in cell B6 (the field of view setting for the Topcon camera) and makes a decision.

B14: @IF(B6=20,1.48669,(@IF(B6=50,0.74652,1.02608)))

The @IF function says that if a certain condition is met, then a specified response will occur, and if the condition is not met, then something else will happen. A shorthand for this is IF, THEN, ELSE. In this instance, the equivalent expression, in English, says that if the value in cell B6 equals 20, then the value appearing in the cell would be 1.48669. If the value does not equal 20, then the computer looks further along to see if it may equal 50, in which case the value in cell

B14 would become 0.74652. If neither of the conditions are met, then the value becomes 1.02608.

Dollar signs in these formulas do not have financial connotations. Rather, they indicate that the cell references will not change if the formula is copied or moved. Ordinarily, in the Lotus 1-2-3 nomenclature, cell references will change automatically to compensate for changes in location.

Parentheses surround mathematical procedures and control the order in which the calculations are carried out. The first step is the one with the most parentheses aound it. For example, in this expression for finding the area of an oval whose maximum and minimum diameters are located in cells B36 and B37, respectively, the first step is the addition of B36 and B37.

$$((((B36+B37)/4)^2)*@PI)$$

The result is the divided by 4, as indicated by the **/,** to find the mean radius. The next step is to find the square, indicated by the caret (^) 2, and surrounded by the third set of parentheses. The last procedure is multiplication by PI. The multiplication operator is an asterisk (*) and is indicated by the function @PI.

The cell location is given on the beginning of each line. The material after the colon is written into the cell exactly as described.

A1: 'Template for calculation of magnification factors
A2: 'March 4, 1996—Philip Lempert, MD
A3: 'Uses Topcon and Zeiss formulas
A4: '
A5: '
A6: 'FIELD OF VIEW
B6: 35
A7: 'SPHERE
B7: 0
A8: 'CYLINDER
B8: 1
A9: 'AXIAL LENGTH
B9: 25
A10: 'K1
B10: 44.7
A11: 'K2
B11: 44.5
A14: 'T=relay optics mag
B14: @IF(B6=20,1.48669,(@IF
    (B6=50,0.74652,1.02608)))
A16: 'MAGNIFICATION
A17: 'TOPCON
B17: ((0.04261*1.336)/(((B9/1000)-0.002)*(1+
    (0.06340.04261)*(B7+B8/2))))*B14
A18: 'ZEISS 1
B18: 0.056/(B9/1000-0.0016)
A19: 'ZEISS 2

B19: 2.5/(1-(0.017*(B7+B8/2)))
A20: 'ZEISS 3
B20: 2.5*(1+0.017*((B7+B8/2)/(1(B7+B8/2))/
(58.64)+(0.84*(58.64((B10+B11)/2)))))
A22: 'SLIDE MEASUREMENT
A24: 'VIEWER MAGNIFICATION
B24: 1
A26: 'VERTICAL DISC DIAM
B26: 5.3
A27: 'HORIZONTAL DISC DIAM
B27: 4.5
A28: 'VERTICAL CUP DIAM
B28: 3.8
A29: 'HORIZONTAL CUP DIAM
B29: 3.6
A32: 'ACTUAL MEASUREMENT—TOPCON
A34: 'VERTICAL DISC DIAM
B34: +B26/$B$24/$B$17
A35: 'HORIZONTAL DISC DIAM
B35: +B27/$B$24/$B$17
A36: 'VERTICAL CUP DIAM
B36: +B28/$B$24/$B$17
A37: 'HORIZONTAL CUP DIAM
B37: +B29/$B$24/$B$17
A38: 'NR RIM AREA
B38: ((((B34+B35)/4)^2*@PI))-((((B36+B37)/4)^2*
@PI)
A40: 'ACTUAL MEASUREMENT—ZEISS 1
A42: 'VERTICAL DISC DIAM
B42: +B26/$B$18/$B$24
A43: 'HORIZONTAL DISC DIAM
B43: +B27/$B$18/$B$24
A44: 'VERTICAL CUP DIAM
B44: +B28/$B$18/$B$24
A45: 'HORIZONTAL CUP DIAM
B45: +B29/$B$18/$B$24
A46: 'NR RIM AREA
B46: ((((B42+B43)/4)^2*@PI))-((((B44+B45)/4)^2*
@PI)
A48: 'ACTUAL MEASUREMENT—ZEISS 2
A50: 'VERTICAL DISC DIAM
B50: +B26/$B$19/$B$24
A51: 'HORIZONTAL DISC DIAM
B51: +B27/$B$19/$B$24
A52: 'VERTICAL CUP DIAM
B52: +B28/$B$19/$B$24
A53: 'HORIZONTAL CUP DIAM
B53: +B29/$B$19/$B$24
A54: 'NR RIM AREA
B54: ((((B50+B51)/4)^2*@PI))-((((B52+B53)/4)^2)
*@PI)

A56: 'ACTUAL MEASUREMENT—ZEISS 3
A58: 'VERTICAL DISC DIAM
B58: +B26/$B$20/$B$24
A59: 'HORIZONTAL DISC DIAM
B59: +B27/$B$20/$B$24
A60: 'VERTICAL CUP DIAM
B60: +B28/$B$20/$B$24
A61: 'HORIZONTAL CUP DIAM
B61: +B29/$B$20/$B$24
A62: 'NR RIM AREA
B62: ((((B58+B59)/4)^2*@PI))-((((B60+B61)/4)^2)
*@PI)

When the template is written it will have the appearance shown in Table 3-1.

The formulas are all in place but are not seen in the cells. Rather, the results of the calculations are displayed. An analogy is a city street in which all of the utility lines are covered and only the end results are visible. In this spreadsheet program, the resulting values for magnification factors and retinal structures will be automatically recalculated.

The appropriate units can be set into the cells in column C. Also, the cell width for column A should be sufficient to display all of the text.

The pertinent features used in this evaluation embrace those recommended by authoritative sources. Another feature, the disc to macula distance to disc diameter ratio (DM:DD), has been included as a means for verification of disc size measurement. The formula for this ratio is:

$$DM:DD = \frac{\text{fovea to disc margin + half of horizontal disc diameter}}{\text{mean disc diameter}}$$

Normal eyes had a DM:DD of $2.67\pm0.29$ while in eyes with hypoplastic nerves the ratio was $3.21\pm0.27$.[18,19] If the absolute optic nerve determination indicates an unusual size, there should be a corresponding finding in this ratio.

A form could be constructed to calculate values for the neuroretinal rim area, disc diameter, cup-to-disc ratio by vertical diameters and area, disparity between the neuroretinal rim areas of the two eyes, and the shape factor. In each, a significant value is selected. For example, a neuroretinal rim area that is smaller than 1.15 mm$^2$ would be considered suspicious. This value is one standard deviation less than the mean area. A meaningful difference between the areas of the two discs is greater than two standard deviations or 0.38 mm$^2$.

Likewise, minimum and maximum disc diameters are defined as 1.28 and 2.28 mm, respectively. A small disc might indicate hypoplasia, possible increased susceptibility to anterior ischemic optic neuropathy, or a warning that there may be damage without apparent cupping. A large disc indicates increased possible vulnerability to pressure effects, or a

Table 3-1

| A | B | A | B |
|---|---|---|---|
| 1. Template for calculation of magnification factors | | 32. ACTUAL MEASUREMENT—TOPCON | |
| 2. March 4, 1996—Philip Lempert, MD | | 33. | |
| 3. Uses Topcon and Zeiss formulas | | 34. VERTICAL DISC DIAM | 2.11 |
| 4. | | 35. HORIZONTAL DISC DIAM | 1.79 |
| 5. | | 36. VERTICAL CUP DIAM | 1.51 |
| 6. FIELD OF VIEW | 35 | 37. HORIZONTAL CUP DIAM | 1.43 |
| 7. SPHERE | 0 | 38. NR RIM AREA | 1.28 |
| 8. CYLINDER | 1 | 39. | |
| 9. AXIAL LENGTH | 25 | 40. ACTUAL MEASUREMENT—ZEISS 1 | |
| 10. K1 | 44.7 | 41. | |
| 11. K2 | 44.5 | 42. VERTICAL DISC DIAM | 2.21 |
| 12. | | 43. HORIZONTAL DISC DIAM | 1.88 |
| 13. | | 44. VERTICAL CUP DIAM | 1.59 |
| 14. T=relay optics mag | 1.03 | 45. HORIZONTAL CUP DIAM | 1.50 |
| 15. | | 46. NR RIM AREA | 1.42 |
| 16. MAGNIFICATION | | 47. | |
| 17. TOPCON | 2.51 | 48. ACTUAL MEASUREMENT—ZEISS 2 | |
| 18. ZEISS 1 | 2.39 | 49. | |
| 19. ZEISS 2 | 2.52 | 50. VERTICAL DISC DIAM | 2.10 |
| 20. ZEISS 3 | 3.00 | 51. HORIZONTAL DISC DIAM | 1.78 |
| 21. | | 52. VERTICAL CUP DIAM | 1.51 |
| 22. SLIDE MEASUREMENT | | 53. HORIZONTAL CUP DIAM | 1.43 |
| 23. | | 54. NR RIM AREA | 1.27 |
| 24. VIEWER MAGNIFICATION | 1 | 55. | |
| 25. | | 56. ACTUAL MEASUREMENT—ZEISS 3 | |
| 26. VERTICAL DISC DIAM | 5.3 | 57. | |
| 27. HORIZONTAL DISC DIAM | 4.5 | 58. VERTICAL DISC DIAM | 1.77 |
| 28. VERTICAL CUP DIAM | 3.8 | 59. HORIZONTAL DISC DIAM | 1.50 |
| 29. HORIZONTAL CUP DIAM | 3.6 | 60. VERTICAL CUP DIAM | 1.27 |
| 30. | | 61. HORIZONTAL CUP DIAM | 1.20 |
| 31. | | 62. NR RIM AREA | 0.90 |

warning that apparent cupping may not be significant.

Another item, the shape factor, is a means of describing the disc's and cup's respective roundness. It is expressed as:

$$(4*PI*area\ of\ the\ oval\ )/circumference^2$$

A perfect circle has a shape factor of 1.000 and a line is 0.00. The disc's vertical and horizontal diameters usually have a ratio of 1.0/0.9 while the cup is usually round. A decreased disc shape factor could indicate dysplasia. A vertical ovalization of the cup could be indicative of glaucoma. The program will automatically report a cup or disc shape factor <0.988 which corresponds to 8/10 oval.

IF, ELSE is the command used to construct these evaluation and warning modules. The condition to be indentified (eg, a vertical diameter cup-to-disc ratio >0.5) is demarcated and the response, if that condition is met, is stated.

An example would consist of setting a phrase such as CUP TO DISC RATIO IS EXCESSIVE into cell F25 so that it is remote from the immediate working area. The formula:

$$@IF(B24/B22>.5,F25,0)$$

The advantage of this module is that questionable or potentially abnormal results are automatically brought to the attention of the technician.

Application programs with mathematical abilities offer many possibilities for clinical practice. Their extreme versatility permits them to perform in every setting. Researchers can employ the statistical functions to process large databases while practicing clinicians can prepare selective recall notices for patients in particular risk groups. Another benefit, from a different perspective, is the power to personally create and modify programs. Communication problems between the user and programmer and the high cost of custom programming are eliminated. Armed with some knowledge of the dBASE or Lotus 1-2-3 languages, highly personal programs designed around specific needs can be created and refined.

## REFERENCES


1. Data Translation, 100 Locke Drive, Marlboro, MA 01752-1192.
2. Univision Technologies, Inc, Three Burlington Woods, Burlington, MA 01803.
3. Digital Vision Inc, 270 Bridge Street, Dedham, MA 02026.
4. Jandel Scientific, 2591 Kerner Blvd, San Rafael, CA 94901.
5. Media Cybernetics, 8484 Georgia Avenue, Silver Springs, MD 20910.
6. Bengtsson B, Krakau CET. Correction of optic disc measurements on fundus photographs. *Graefe Arch Clin Exp Ophthalmol.* 1992;230:24-28.
7. Jonas JB, Fernandez MC, Naumann GOH. Correlation of the optic disc size to glaucoma susceptibility. *Ophthalmology.* 1991;98:675-680.
8. Tuulonen A, Airaksinen J, Schwartz B, Alanko HI, Juvala. Neuroretinal rim area measurements by configuration and by pallor in ocular hypertension and glaucoma. *Ophthalmology.* 1992;99:1111-1116.
9. Bengtsson B. The variation and covariation of cup and disc diameters. *Acta Ophthalmol.* 1976;54:804-817.
10. Bloom SM. Subfoveal neovascular lesions in age-related macular degeneration. *Arch Ophthalmol.*1993;111:900-901.
11. Bressler NM, Alexander J, Hawkins BS, Maguire MG, Fine SL. In reply. *Arch Ophthalmol.*1993;111:901.
12. Macular Photocoagulation Study Group. Laser photocoagulation of subforveal neovascular lesions in age-related macular degeneration. *Arch Ophthalmol.* 1991;109:1220-1231.
13. Lempert P. The natural history of idiopathic subfoveal choroidal neovascularization. *Ophthalmology.* 1995;102:1411. Letter.
14. Lempert P. Optic disc size. *Ophthalmology.* 1996;103:248-249. Letter.
15. Airaksinen PJ, Drance SM, Mikelberg FS. Nerve fibre layer and neuroretinal rim area in glaucoma. Course 306, American Academy of Ophthalmology meeting, 1988
16. Mansour AM. Measuring fundus landmarks. *Invest Ophthalmol Vis Sci.* 1990;31:41-42.
17. Bengtsson B, Krakau CET. Some essential optical features of the Zeiss fundus camera. *Acta Ophthlmol.* 1977;55:123-131.
18. Zeki SM, Dudgeon J, Dutton GN. Reappraisal of the ratio of disc to macula/disc diameter in optic nerve hypoplasia. *Br J Ophthalmol.* 1991;75:538-544.
19. Wakakura M, Alvarez E. A simple clinical method of assessing patients with optic nerve hypoplasia. The disc-macula distance to disc diameter ratio. *Acta Ophthalmol.* 1967;65;612-617.

# Confocal Scanning Laser Ophthalmoscopy to Detect Glaucomatous Optic Neuropathy

*Linda Zangwill, PhD, Marcia de Souza Lima, MD,*
*Robert N. Weinreb, MD*

Assessment of changes in the optic nerve head (ONH) is essential for diagnosing glaucoma and monitoring its progression. Photography can be used to obtain a permanent record for assessment of the optic nerve. As photographs are obtained using cameras with conventional optical systems, pupil dilatation and clear media are required for acquisition of good quality images. These conditions cannot always be met, particularly in an aging population. Results from the Baltimore Eye Study illustrate the potential magnitude of this problem: good quality stereoscopic photographs could not be obtained in 47% of the glaucoma patients and 22% of normal subjects.[1] In addition, photographs require laborious development and their evaluation must take place at a later time, clinical decisions often waiting until a subsequent patient visit.

In contrast, instruments using confocal scanning systems, the confocal scanning laser ophthalmoscope (CSLO), provide real-time images of the human fundus that can be evaluated at the time of the patient visit. Confocal laser scanning devices, with their minimal depth of focus, improve the ability to obtain good quality images with reduced need for pupil dilation and clear media. Confocal scanning systems obtain higher contrast than nonconfocal systems because only light reflected from the area of the retina or ONH to be scanned is detected. In addition, tomographic or layer by layer imaging within the ONH is possible.

Recent research using confocal scanning laser ophthalmoscopy measurements highlights its potential for clinical use. Studies have shown:

- Good agreement between cup-to-disc ratio measurements by glaucoma expert evaluation of stereoscopic photographs and CSLO measurements.[2]
- Mean topographic optic nerve parameter measurements of ocular hypertensive eyes are intermediate between those of both normal and glaucomatous eyes.[3]
- Differences in topographic optic nerve parameters by ethnic group in young healthy eyes.[4]
- Correlation between CSLO measurements and global and regional indices of visual field loss.[5-7]

## INSTRUMENTATION

Confocal laser scanning ophthalmoscopy has been shown to be an objective and reproducible method for acquiring and analyzing real-time three-dimensional images of the optic disc.[8-10] Details of one CSLO, the Heidelberg Retina Tomograph (HRT, Heidelberg Engineering, Heidelberg, Germany), have been described previously.[8,9] In brief, this instrument employs a diode laser (670-nm wavelength) to scan a surface in x, y, and z directions. A three-dimensional image is acquired as a series of optical section images at 32 consecutive focal planes. The topography image determined from the acquired three-dimensional image consists of 256 by 256 pixel elements, each of which is a measurement of height at its corresponding location. Image acquisition and processing takes approximately 1.6 seconds. In clinical practice, we obtain three images of each eye and create a mean topography image for analysis. Acquired images are stored and analyzed using a standard personal computer. Another confocal scanning laser ophthalmoscope, the Topographic Scanning System (TopSS, Laser Diagnostic Technologies, San Diego, Calif), employs a laser with a different wavelength (780 nm). Differences between the HRT and TopSS systems have not been studied.

## DATA ANALYSIS

Confocal scanning laser ophthalmoscopy instruments include comprehensive software packages that facilitate image acquisition, storage, retrieval, and quantitative analysis. Topographic optic nerve parameters measured include area cup disc ratio, cup volume, rim volume, disc area, cup area, rim area, cup depth, peripapillary retinal height, and indirect estimates of retinal nerve fiber layer (RNFL) thickness and area. To obtain topographic optic nerve parameter measurements, an operator outlines the optic disc margin of the mean topographic images. The resulting outline around the disc margin is called the contour line. The contour line is corrected by the software for local elevations caused by peripapillary blood vessels.

Several topographic optic nerve parameters, including cup area, cup-disc area ratio, cup volume, rim area, rim volume, RNFL thickness, and RNFL cross-section area are calculated relative to a reference plane. With the HRT, the standard reference (HRT operating software version 1.11) is defined as a plane 50 microns posterior to the mean height of the peripapillary retinal height along the contour line at a temporal segment between 350° and 356° below the horizontal line. Other topographic optic disc parameters (cup volume below the surface, mean cup depth, maximum cup depth, and cup shape) are measured relative to the curved surface calculated by the HRT operating software. The curved surface is not a plane. It has the height along the corrected contour line as its boundary. The center of the curved surface is the mean height of the peripapillary retinal surface along the corrected contour line. Each section of the curved surface from its center to its boundary point is a straight line.

Included in the standard HRT software package are two quantitative methods that facilitate longitudinal analysis of the topographic information:
1.   Evaluation of topographic difference images
2.   Evaluation of changes of stereometric parameters

Topographic difference images are determined from the mean topography images of two examinations after automatic correction for shift, rotation, and tilt between the images. Based on multiple image acquisition during each visit, the software also determines the reproducibility for each individual examination. This allows the significance of a detected local height change to be determined and displayed in false color codes. Areas in red are significantly deeper in the follow-up examination than in the baseline examination. Areas where the surface is significantly higher (toward the vitreous) are displayed as green. The sensitivity for detecting changes is influenced by the reproducibility of the height measurements. The mean reproducibility (mean standard deviation of each pixel) for the 256 by 256 height measurements with the latest HRT software has been reduced by approximately 30% and is often less than 25 microns (unpublished data) in glaucoma patients.

Despite the existence of these and other quantitative analysis tools, the development of clinical methods for distinguishing between normal and glaucomatous eyes using these measurements has been difficult for two major reasons.[11] First, there is considerable variability in the appearance of normal ONHs. Second, there is considerable overlap in the appearance of normal and glaucomatous ONHs.

Techniques are under development, however, that assist the clinician in interpreting information obtained from CSLO images to differentiate between a normal and glaucomatous eye. One of these techniques, the ranked-segment distribution (RSD) curve technique,[12] is an adaptation of the cumulative defect curve of Bebie used in automated visual field analysis.[13] It is based on the assumption that the pattern of measurements, rather than their specific location, is similar among normal individuals. Given the variability of the optic nerve among normal individuals, a mean measure of a neuroretinal rim area, for example, may be within normal limits even though there is localized thinning of the rim (ie, small local reductions in area may not be apparent from the overall mean value). With visual inspection of an RSD curve, one can determine whether a topographic parameter is within normal limits. In addition, an RSD curve may differentiate between diffuse or localized abnormality, as well as indicate its location.

Details of the RSD method have been described previously.[12] This technique can be used to evaluate topographic optic nerve parameters. (Examples of this technique for analyzing rim area and RNFL cross-section area are included in Cases 2 and 3.) In brief, optic nerve parameters are measured in 10° segments from 1° to 360° around the disc margin to obtain 36 segment values. The 36 10° segments are ranked in descending order. To calculate normal limits, the 5th percentile of each ranked segment for rim area and RNFL cross-section area are from measurements of 39 age-matched healthy eyes. The 5th percentile value is used as baseline normal limits for comparison with age-matched glaucoma patients. The normal RSD curves of each parameter for each age group are constructed by plotting the 5th percentile data along the y axis and the rank number of the segment along the x axis. To evaluate a glaucomatous eye, the RSD curve is plotted for the topographic optic nerve of interest and compared to a normal RSD curve from the same age group to identify segment values that are outside normal limits. RSD curves are identified as "abnormal RSD curves" if there are three or more consecutive ranked segments outside normal limits.

Evaluation of RSD curves of glaucoma patients is done automatically using a computer algorithm and also can be visualized from the plotted curves. Any segments that have values below the 5th percentile baseline value of the normal

RSD curve are classified as "outside normal limits" by the computer. RSD curves that have three or more consecutive ranked segments outside normal limits are defined as "abnormal RSD curves."

The location of the segment that is outside normal limits is identified by reading the angle value directly from the angle-bar. The angle of the midpoint of the segment is used to identify the location of the 10° segment. For example, segment 1 from 1° to 10° is assigned as 5°, segment 2 from 11° to 20° was assigned as 15° and so forth. With 0° as temporal, angles of the superior segments are assigned as positive values from 5°, 15°, 25°, through 175°; angles of the inferior segments are assigned as negative values from -5°, -15°, -25°, through -175°. A downward angle-bar (negative angle value) indicates a location that is below the horizontal plane in the inferior region. The value of the angle also is shown above each bar identifying the segment location. The position of the bar (upward or downward) helps to quickly identify whether a segment is in the superior or inferior region.

## CASE STUDIES

The following case studies describe the clinical application of qualitative and quantitative evaluation of glaucomatous optic neuropathy using confocal scanning laser ophthalmoscopy, using standard analysis and the RSD curve technique They highlight both benefits and limitations of the instrument, and areas for future development and research. Normal values used for comparison are based on evaluation of 39 normal subjects between the ages of 50 and 79 years. Outside normal limits describes a global (360°) measurement that is either less than (for rim and RNFL parameters) or greater than (for cup area, cup volume, cup disc ratio, and cup depth parameters) the 95th percentile of normal values.

Each case is illustrated using measurements obtained from the mean topography created from three original image series. Corneal curvature measurements were utilized to correct for magnification error. Computerized visual fields are displayed with Peridata version 6.3b (Interzeag Inc., Schlieren, Switzerland).

### Case 1

A 70-year-old white female primary open-angle glaucoma patient was evaluated in 1993. Superior notching of the neuroretinal rim OS was observed with both photography (Figure 4-1a) and CSLO image (Figure 4-1b). In 1993, CSLO topography indices, including cup area (1.88 mm$^2$), cup disc area ratio (0.677), mean cup depth (0.354 mm), cup volume (0.622 mm$^3$), rim area (0.900 mm$^2$), and rim volume (0.185 mm$^3$) were outside of normal values. Visual fields indicated an inferior arcuate defect (Figure 4-1c).

Comment: Characteristic appearance of glaucomatous optic nerve is outside normal limits for CSLO disc parameters and consistent with stereophotograph assessment of the optic disc.

### Case 2[12]

A 55-year-old female primary open-angle glaucoma patient demonstrated a wedge-shaped NFL defect in the inferotemporal quadrant OS with both disc photograph (Figure 4-2a) and CSLO image (Figure 4-2b). The height variation diagram of the CSLO image showed a depressed double-hump pattern in the inferotemporal quadrant (see Figure 4-2b). Computerized visual field confirmed a nasal step (Figure 4-2c).

Global (360°) measurement of RNFL cross-sectional area (0.989 mm$^2$) was within 95th percentile values for normal eyes, and rim area was just outside normal limits of the global value (1.14 mm$^2$).

The RSD curves of rim area and RNFL cross-section area were outside normal limits using the previous criteria. This also can be seen from the plotted curves for both rim area (Figure 4-2d) and RNFL cross-section area (Figure 4-2e) which were lower than the normal RSD curve (the 5th percentile curve) of this age group. For rim area, the deviated segments, reading from the angle-bar, were from segment 13 to 36 with marked drop of values from segment 26 to 36. The angles associated with the deviated segments from 13 to 24 were scattered in both superior and inferior regions (the bar graphs had both positive and negative values) indicating that the defects were partially diffuse. Segments 26 to 36 (-5° to -85°) were markedly deviated; their location in the inferotemporal quadrant corresponded to the location of the NFL defect. The RSD curve of RNFL cross-section area showed the same values and trend that were outside normal limits; there were scattered defects from segment 17 to 23 and localized defects from segment 29 to 36 (-5° to -75°, inferotemporal quadrant).

Comment: Wedge-shaped RNFL defects can be identified by visual inspection of the CSLO image and height variation diagram and quantitatively using the RSD curve technique.

### Case 3[12]

A 57-year-old female primary open-angle glaucoma patient demonstrated a wedge-shaped NFL defect in the inferotemporal quadrant OS with both NFL photograph (Figure 4-3a) and CSLO image (Figure 4-3b). The height variation diagram of the CSLO image showed a depressed normal double-hump pattern in both the superior and inferior region with marked depression in the inferior region (Figure 4-3c, arrows). Visual field demonstrated a superior arcuate defect (Figure 4-3d).

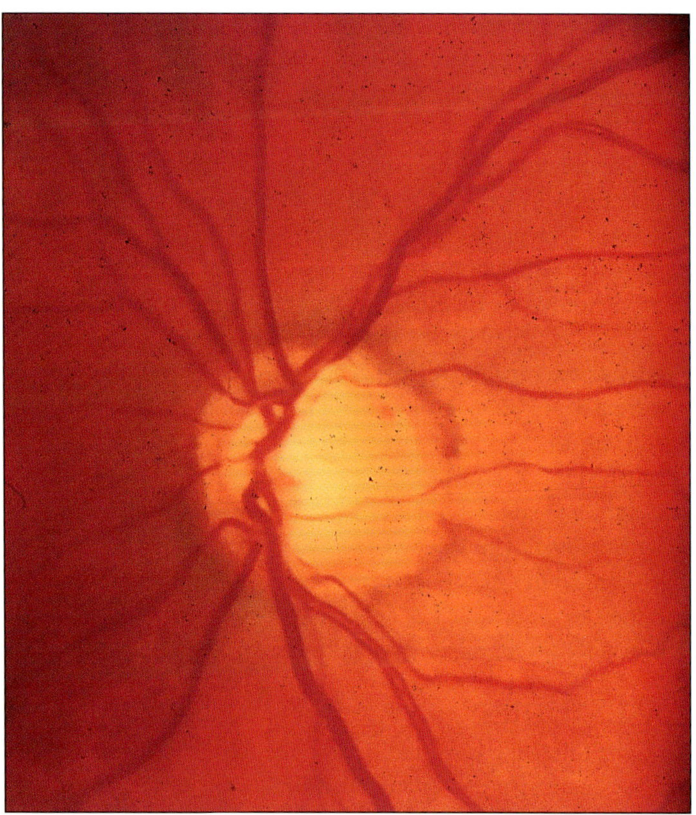

**Figure 4-1a.** Case 1 (left eye). Disc photograph shows notching in the superior region (1993).

The RSD curves of rim area (Figure 4-3e) and RNFL cross-section area (Figure 4-3f) were outside normal limits. These were obvious from visual inspection of the plotted RSD curves, both of which were below the normal 5th percentile curve limit for all segments suggesting the diffuse nature of the defects. However, the marked abnormal segments from segment 34 to 36 (-85° to -105°) for rim area and segment 31 to 36 (-65° to -115°) for RNFL cross-section area indicated the localized nature of the defect in the inferotemporal region corresponding to the NFL photographic defect. Measurement of rim area and RNFL cross-section area as global 360° parameters were both outside the 95th percentile of normal eyes.

Comment: Diffuse optic nerve damage of the RNFL and neuroretinal rim can be detected by analysis of CSLO topography.

## Case 4

A 66-year-old male with ocular hypertension was evaluated in 1991 with persistent elevated intraocular pressure (IOP) OD 30 mmHg and OS 32 mmHg with pilocarpine. In 1993, standard visual fields remained normal (Figure 4-4a) and optic discs also were not considered glaucomatous with horizontal and vertical cup disc ratios of 0.5 and 0.6, respectively (Figure 4-4b). Analysis of CSLO topography of the right eye (Figure 4-4c) indicated that most topographic optic

disc parameters were within the 95th percentile of age-specific normal eyes. Mean height contour appeared to have a normal double-hump pattern. Rim volume (0.198 mm³) and RNFL cross-section area (0.766 mm²) measurements were lower than normal values. Visual field testing of the right eye in 1993 using short wavelength automated perimetry[14] showed a local defect in the superior and inferior nasal regions (Figure 4-4d). Between 1993 and 1995, treated IOP fluctuated between 24 mmHg and 34 mmHg. Clinical evaluation of the optic disc (and assessment of stereoscopic photographs) was unchanged. In 1995, standard visual fields of the right eye showed progressive loss in the inferior nasal region (Figure 4-4e). Changes in some topographic optic nerve parameters were found, including RNFL cross-section area (from 0.766 to 0.622 mm²) and cup volume (below reference) (from 0.065 to 0.106 mm³). CSLO difference image showed deepening in retinal topography, particularly in the superior temporal region (Figure 4-4f).

Comment: It is difficult to determine whether the topographic optic nerve parameters which were outside normal limits in 1993 were measuring structural damage that contributed to the SWAP defect in that same year. Changes in optic nerve topography identified by evaluation of the CSLO difference image corresponded to the development of a glaucomatous visual field defect detected using standard perimetry.

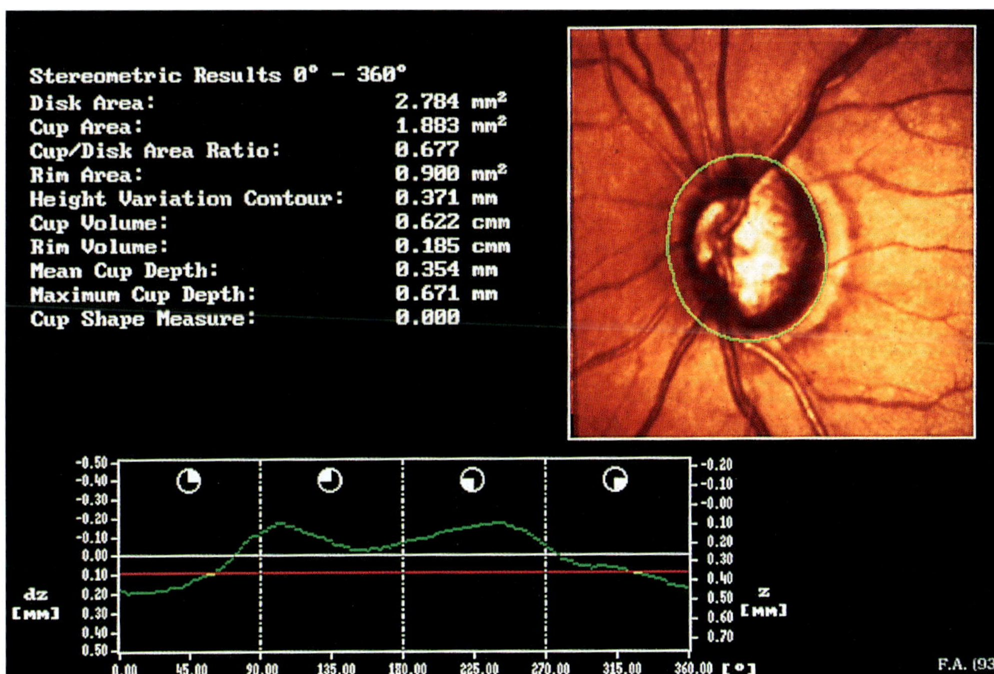



**Figure 4-1b.** CSLO image shows notching and thinning of the neuroretinal rim as indicated by low rim area and low rim volume. Mean height contour around disc margin (below) was non-diagnostic (1993).

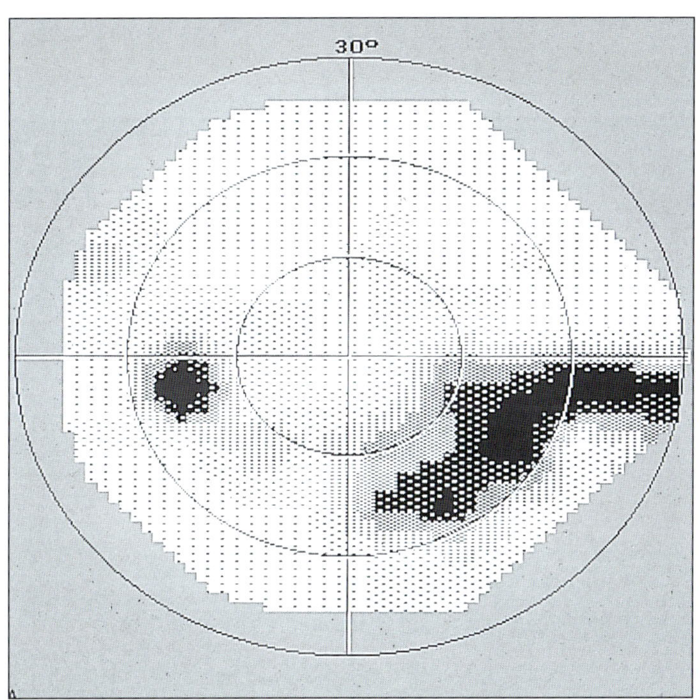



**Figure 4-1c.** Visual field inferior arcuate defect (1993).

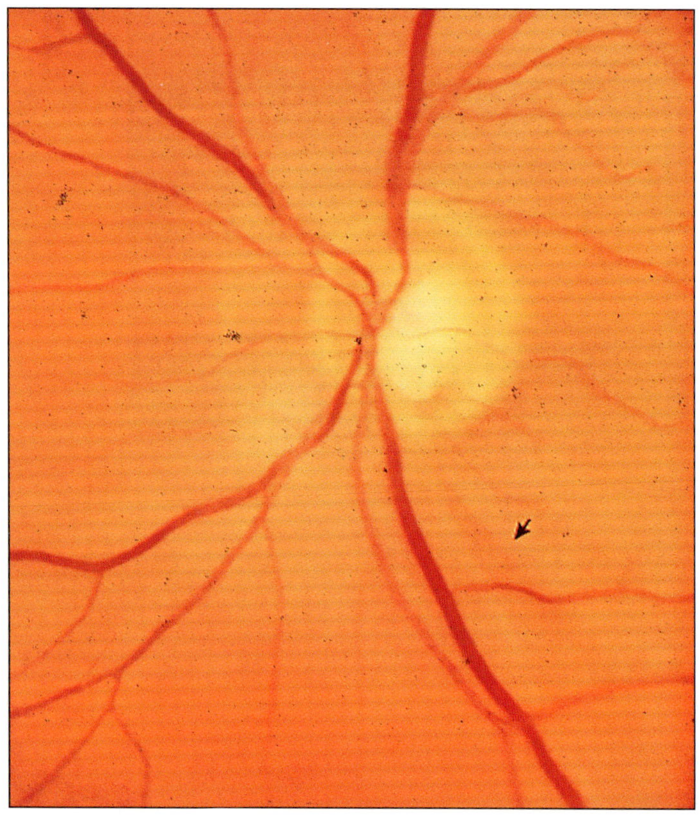

**Figure 4-2a.** Case 2 (left eye). Disc photograph shows wedge-shape NFL defect (arrow). Reprinted with permission from Asawaphureekorn S, Zangwill L, Weinreb RN. Ranked-segment distribution curve for interpretation of optic nerve topography. *J Glaucoma.* 1996;5:79-90.

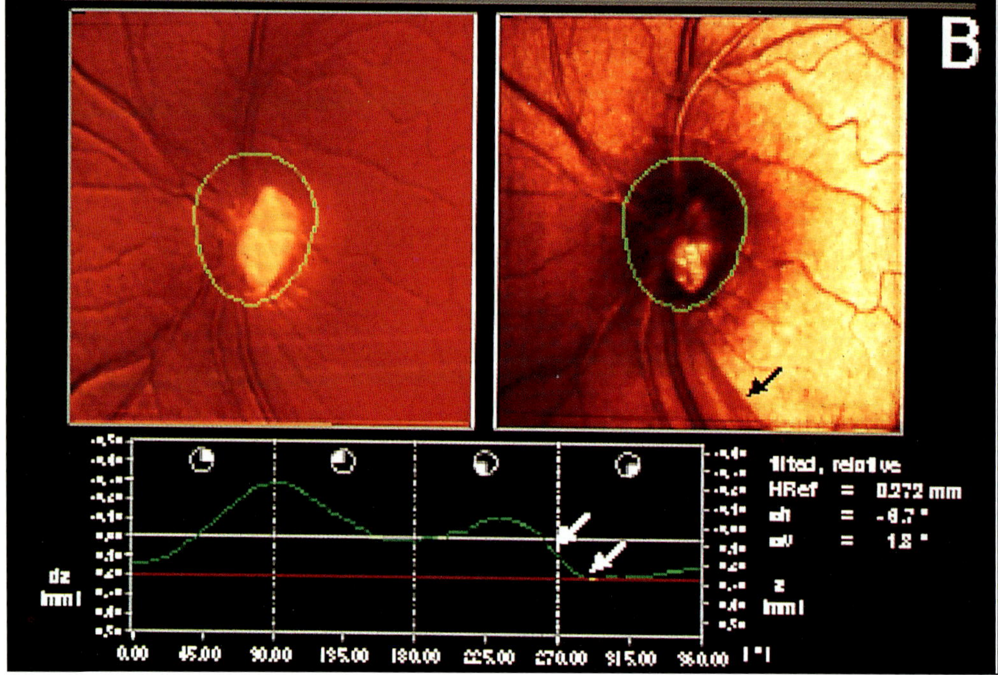

**Figure 4-2b.** CSLO image shows NFL defect in reflectivity image (arrow) and depressed double-hump pattern in the height variation diagram (arrow). Reprinted with permission from Asawaphureekorn S, Zangwill L, Weinreb RN. Ranked-segment distribution curve for interpretation of optic nerve topography. *J Glaucoma.* 1996;5:79-90.

## Case 5

A 39-year-old white female with a prominent family history of glaucoma was diagnosed with primary open-angle glaucoma approximately 19 years prior to her evaluation in August 1993. Visual acuity was OD 20/20 (-5.50 sph) and OS 20/20 (-6.50 +1.25 x 180). Gonioscopy showed wide open angles and IOPs were OD 26 mmHg and OS 31 mmHg on maximum tolerated medication. Slit lamp examination was within normal limits for both eyes. Discs appeared excavated with superior thinning of rim and no notching or hemorrhage (Figure 4-5a).

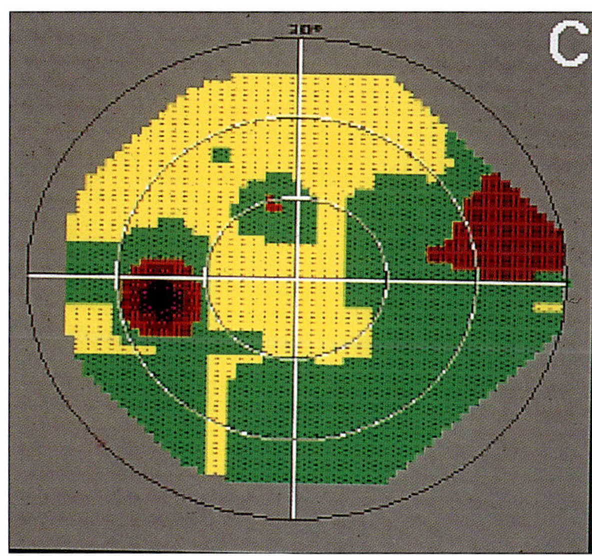

**Figure 4-2c.** Computerized visual field shows nasal step (brown indicates 5 to 10 dB sensitivity loss compared to age-matched normal subjects; yellow and green are within ±5 dB of normal sensitivity values). Reprinted with permission from Asawaphureekorn S, Zangwill L, Weinreb RN. Ranked-segment distribution curve for interpretation of optic nerve topography. *J Glaucoma.* 1996;5:79-90.

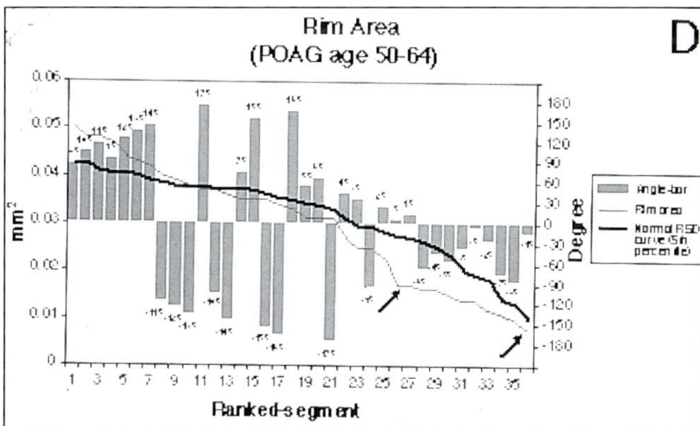

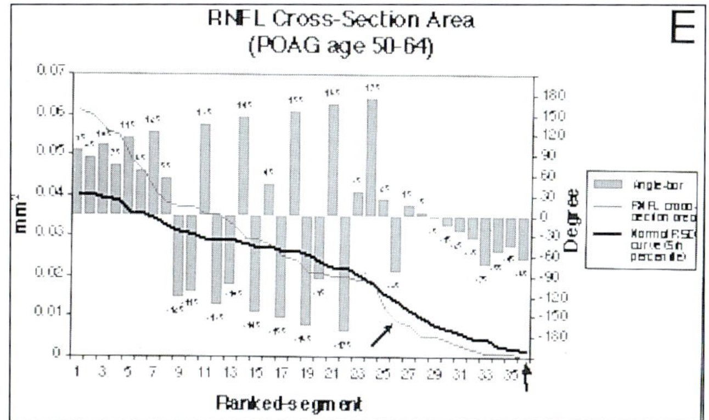

**Figure 4-2d.** RSD curve of rim area has abnormal segments from segment 13 to 36 with marked abnormal values (sharp drop of the curve) from segment 26 to 36 (arrow). The location of this localized defect is inferotemporal from -5° to -85° (reading from the bar graphs). Reprinted with permission from Asawaphureekorn S, Zangwill L, Weinreb RN. Ranked-segment distribution curve for interpretation of optic nerve topography. *J Glaucoma.* 1996;5:79-90.

**Figure 4-2e.** RSD curve of RNFL cross-section area has abnormal segments from segment 17 to 23 with marked abnormal values (sharp drop of the curve) from segment 26 to 36 (arrow). The location of this localized defect is inferotemporal from -5° to -85° (reading from the bar graphs). Reprinted with permission from Asawaphureekorn S, Zangwill L, Weinreb RN. Ranked-segment distribution curve for interpretation of optic nerve topography. *J Glaucoma.* 1996;5:79-90.

Compared with age-matched normals, visual field (December 1993) showed OD: inferior arcuate defect (Figure 4-5b). CSLO (Figure 4-5c) measurements of cup volume and mean cup depth were outside the 95th percentile of normal values. Mean height contour around the disc margin was reduced superiorly. On January 1995, IOPs were OD 42 mmHg and OS 24 mmHg. Progression of characteristic glaucomatous optic nerve damage was apparent from 1995 disc photograph (Figure 4-5d) with additional thinning of the neuroretinal rim and excavation superiorly. A general reduction in visual field sensitivity in the right eye also was detected (Figure 4-5e). Progression of glaucomatous optic neuropathy was suggested by the difference image within the optic disc and inferior peripapillary region (Figure 4-5f) and change in cup volume (below the surface) and mean cup depth (from 0.493 to 0.691 mm$^3$ and from 0.306 to 0.414 mm,

respectively). Other topographic optic nerve parameters, including rim area and area cup disc ratio showed little change, from 1.40 to 1.42 mm$^3$ and 0.37 to 0.40, respectively.

Comment: Changes in the optic nerve with corresponding progression in the visual fields can be detected by evaluation of the difference image and evaluation of some, but not necessarily all, topographic optic nerve parameter measurements obtained with the CSLO.

## DISCUSSION

The CSLO shows potential as a clinical tool for examining and monitoring the health of the optic nerve in glaucoma and other optic neuropathies. These cases provide examples of how information obtained with confocal scanning laser ophthalmoscopy can be used in a clinical setting. Glaucoma

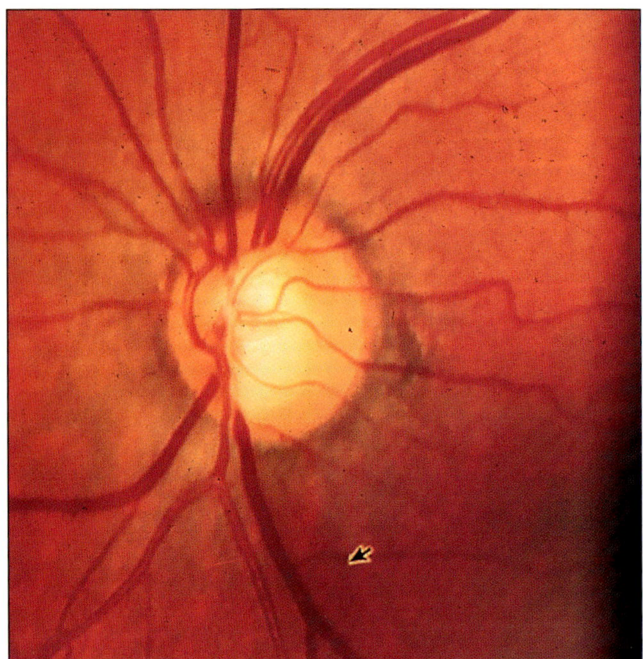

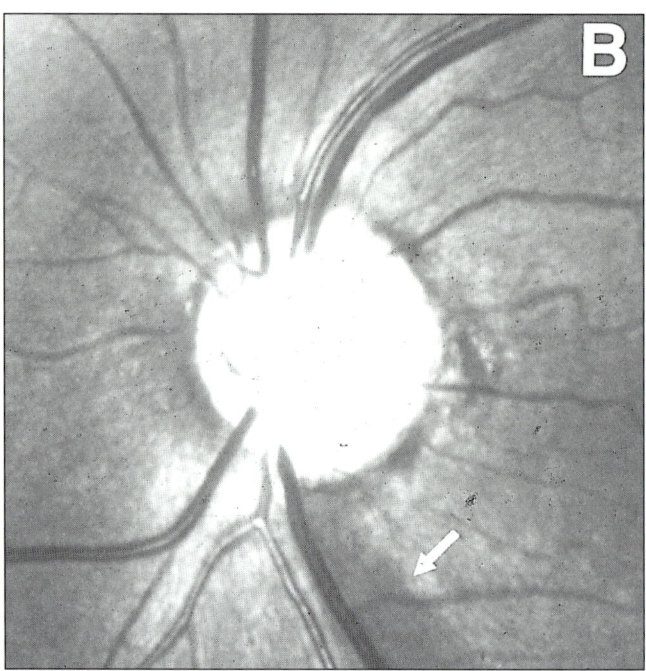

**Figure 4-3a.** Case 3 (left eye). Disc photograph shows wedge-shaped NFL defect. Reprinted with permission from Asawaphureekorn S, Zangwill L, Weinreb RN. Ranked-segment distribution curve for interpretation of optic nerve topography. *J Glaucoma.* 1996;5:79-90.

**Figure 4-3b.** NFL photograph shows wedge-shaped NFL defect (arrows). Reprinted with permission from Asawaphureekorn S, Zangwill L, Weinreb RN. Ranked-segment distribution curve for interpretation of optic nerve topography. *J Glaucoma.* 1996;5:79-90.

**Figure 4-3c.** CSLO image shows NFL defect in reflectivity image (arrow) and depressed normal double-hump pattern in both superior and inferior region with marked depression in the inferior region (arrow). Reprinted with permission from Asawaphureekorn S, Zangwill L, Weinreb RN. Ranked-segment distribution curve for interpretation of optic nerve topography. *J Glaucoma.* 1996;5:79-90.

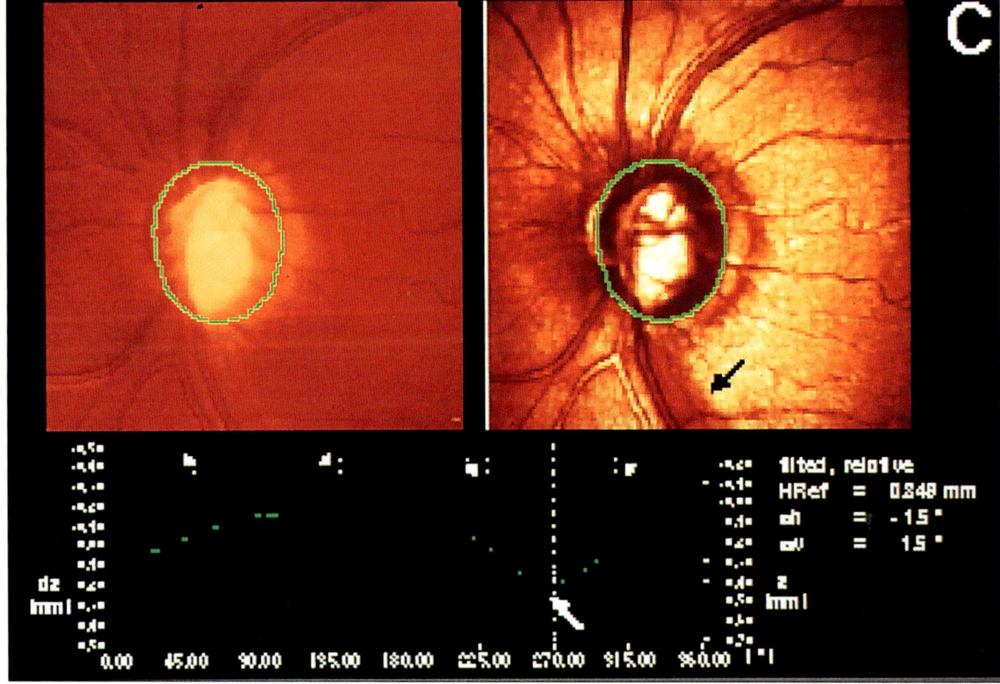

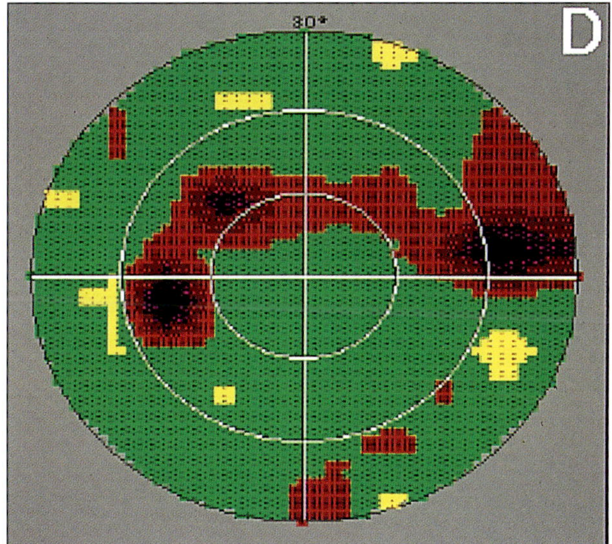

**Figure 4-3d.** Computerized visual field shows superior arcuate defect (sensitivity loss compared with age-matched normal subjects: brown [5 to 10 dB] to black [20 to 25 dB]; yellow and green are within ±5 dB of normal sensitivity values). Reprinted with permission from Asawaphureekorn S, Zangwill L, Weinreb RN. Ranked-segment distribution curve for interpretation of optic nerve topography. *J Glaucoma.* 1996;5:79-90.

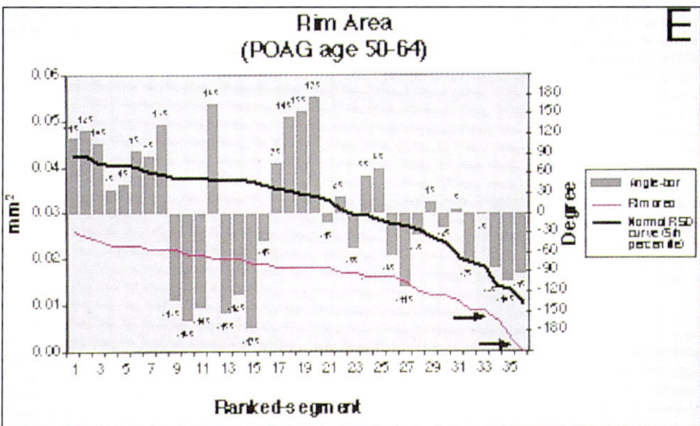

**Figure 4-3e.** All segments of the RSD curve of rim area are outside normal limits with marked abnormal values (sharp drop of the curve) from segment 34 to 36. The location of this localized defect is from -85° to -105° (arrow). Reprinted with permission from Asawaphureekorn S, Zangwill L, Weinreb RN. Ranked-segment distribution curve for interpretation of optic nerve topography. *J Glaucoma.* 1996;5:79-90.

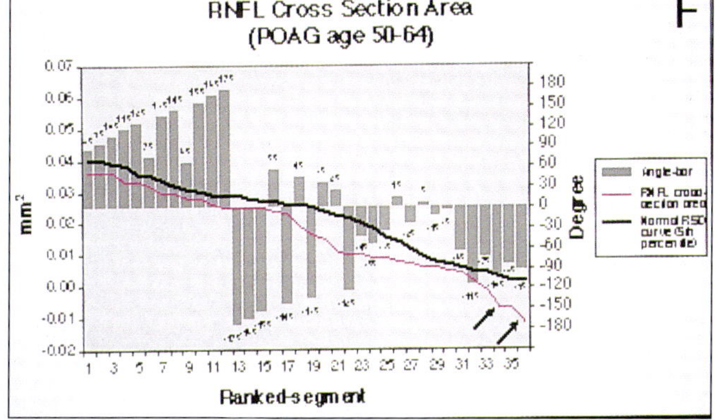

**Figure 4-3f.** All segments of the RSD curve of RNFL cross-section area are outside normal limits with marked abnormal values (sharp drop of the curve) from segment 34 to 36. The location of this localized defect was from -85° to -115° (arrow). Reprinted with permission from Asawaphureekorn S, Zangwill L, Weinreb RN. Ranked-segment distribution curve for interpretation of optic nerve topography. *J Glaucoma.* 1996;5:79-90.

Case 1 highlights how CSLO topographic measurements characterize glaucomatous optic nerve damage. In Cases 2 and 3, the RSD curves of rim area and RNFL cross-section area demonstrated glaucomatous defects more consistently than analysis of the global optic nerve parameters and computerized visual fields. In both Case 2 and Case 3, the extent of RNFL defects demonstrated by the RSD curves was wider than demonstrated by qualitative evaluation of optic disc photographs or RNFL photographs. These cases also illustrate that RNFL defects can be detected in some eyes by qualitative evaluation of CSLO images.

Cases 4 and 5 demonstrate that detection of progression of glaucomatous optic neuropathy can be detected by CSLO topo-graphic measurements and difference images. In Case 4, changes in some topographic optic nerve measurements were identified, despite apparent stability of optic nerve photography. Case 5 illustrates progression in both the optic nerve (CSLO topography and photographic assessment) and visual field.

In order for a new instrument to be accepted and implemented into clinical practice, it must be superior to existing instruments in clinically relevant ways. One advantage of confocal scanning laser ophthalmoscopy is that it provides real-time quantitative measurements of optic nerve topography with reduced need for pupil dilation and clear media. Unlike photography, which requires an ophthalmic photographer, film, and processing time, confocal scanning laser ophthalmoscopy

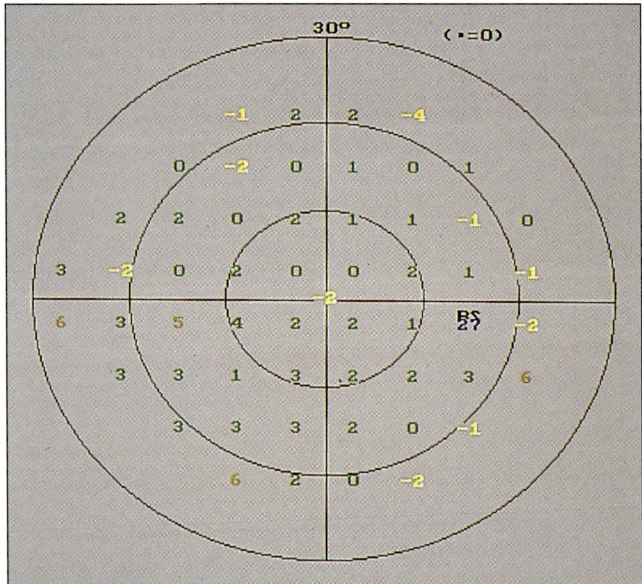

**Figure 4-4a.** Case 4 (right eye). Visual field was within normal limits (1993) (values represent sensitivity loss compared to age-matched normal subjects).

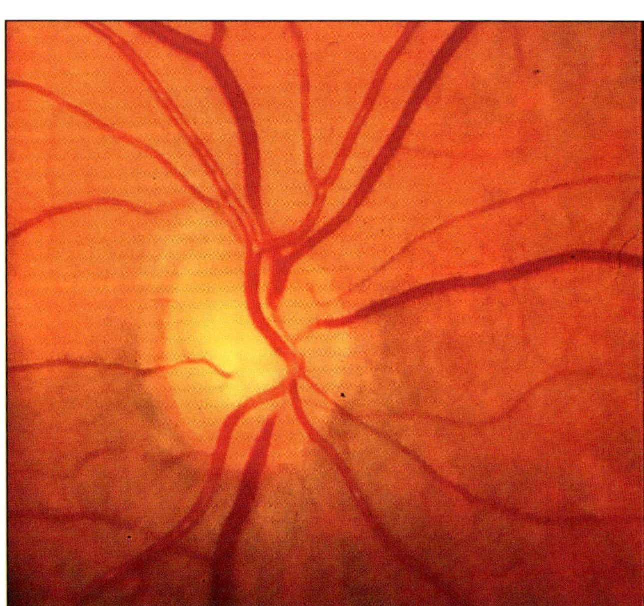

**Figure 4-4b.** Normal-appearing optic disc photograph (1993).

**Figure 4-4c.** CSLO topography indicated that except for rim volume and RNFL cross-section area, optic disc parameters were within normal limits (1993).

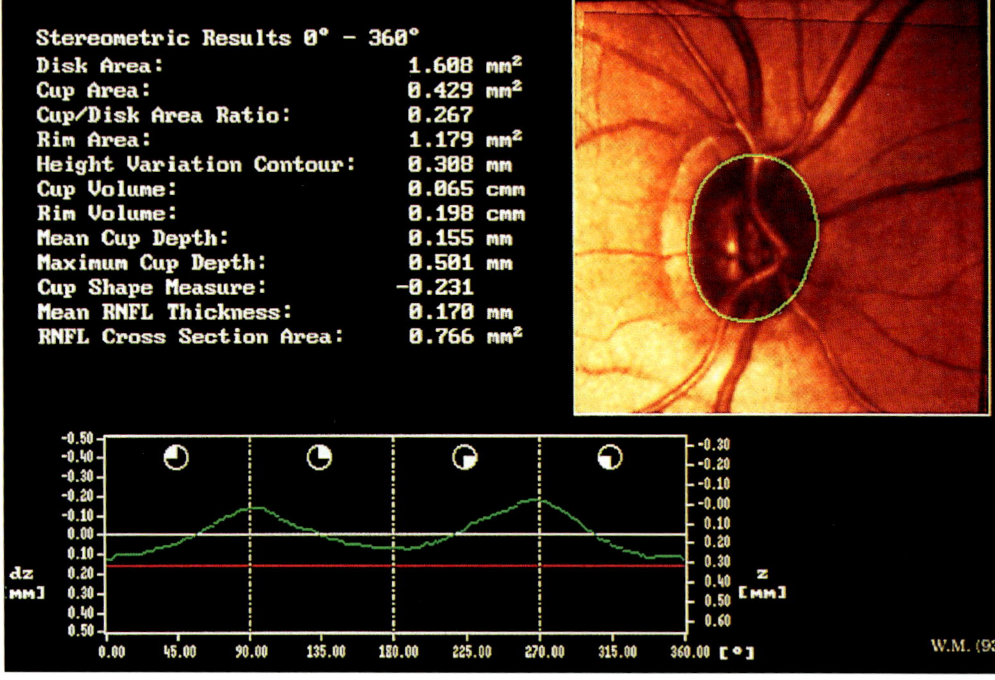



allows assessment of the optic nerve during the clinic visit. As these cases illustrate, CSLO topographies can assist the clinician in identifying glaucomatous optic neuropathy. Because of wide variability of optic nerve topography among normal eyes, this instrument, or any other instrument that measures ONH topography, may have limited usefulness as a single and definitive diagnostic test. In contrast, CSLO, with its objective and reproducible measurements, is well suited for detecting topographic change in the ONH and peripapillary retina.

Further development of analysis methods to better assist the clinician in interpretation of relatively small but perhaps clinically significant change in topography optic nerve parameters is needed. Several analytic methods, including condensed pixel analysis[15] and the RSD curve,[12] show promise for identifying glaucoma change over time. Techniques that identify the location and provide information on the proba-

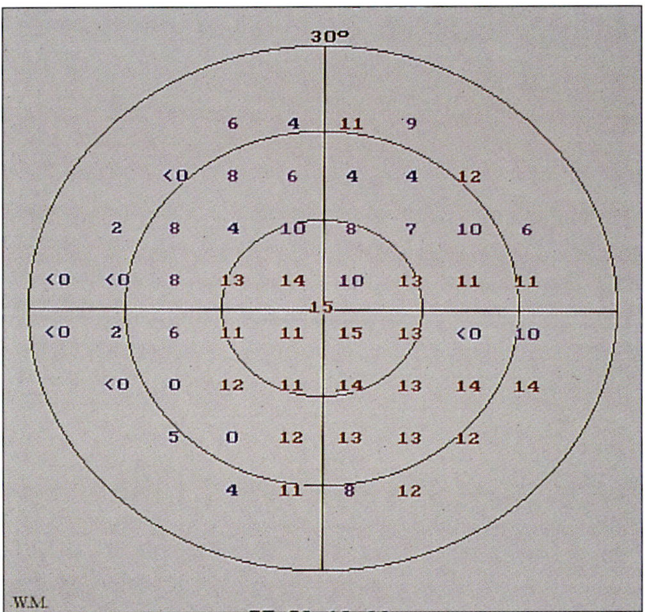

**Figure 4-4d.** Short wavelength automated perimetry shows inferior arcuate defect (values represent absolute sensitivity [dB]; blue indicates absolute defect).

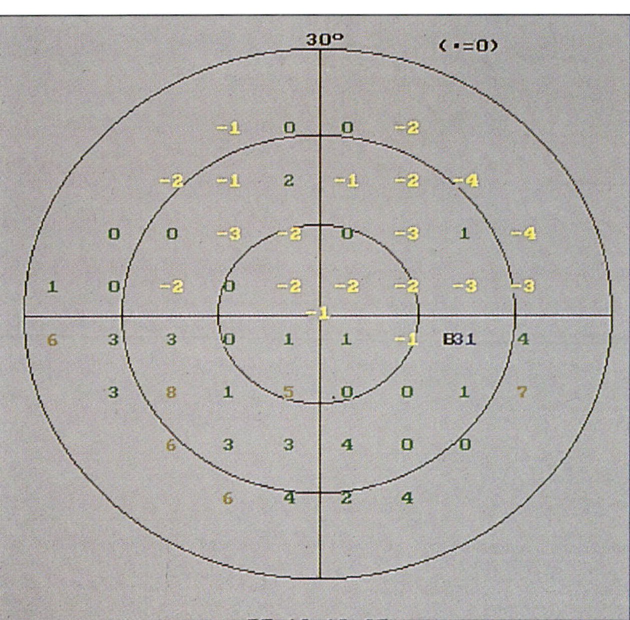

**Figure 4-4e.** Visual field shows progressive loss in the inferior region (1995) (values represent sensitivity loss [dB] compared to age-matched normal subjects).

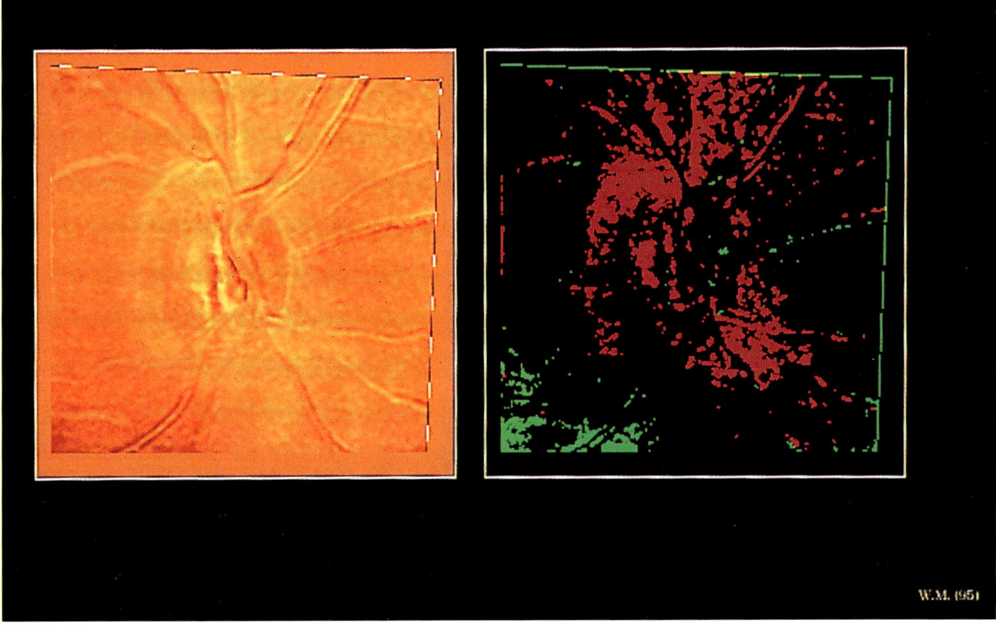

**Figure 4-4f.** CSLO difference image indicates deepening of surface (red) corresponding to increasing cup volume and reduced peripapillary RNFL height (1993-1995).

bility of change are of particular interest. Whether ONH topography can improve the precision with which we can detect glaucomatous progression over time needs to be determined with well-designed longitudinal studies and comparison with established diagnostic techniques for evaluating glaucomatous optic neuropathy.

It should be noted that although there is a reduced need for pupil dilation and clear media for obtaining CSLO images, pupil dilation may be necessary to obtain good quality images in some eyes with small (≤3 mm) pupil diameters, and/or lens opacities.[16] As glaucoma is a disease that affects the elderly, who often have some lens opacity, and since miotic treatment may be used to control IOP, the quality of CSLO images obtained should be evaluated systematically. Given that good quality photographs are often unavailable in these patients, CSLO images may play an important role in providing clini-

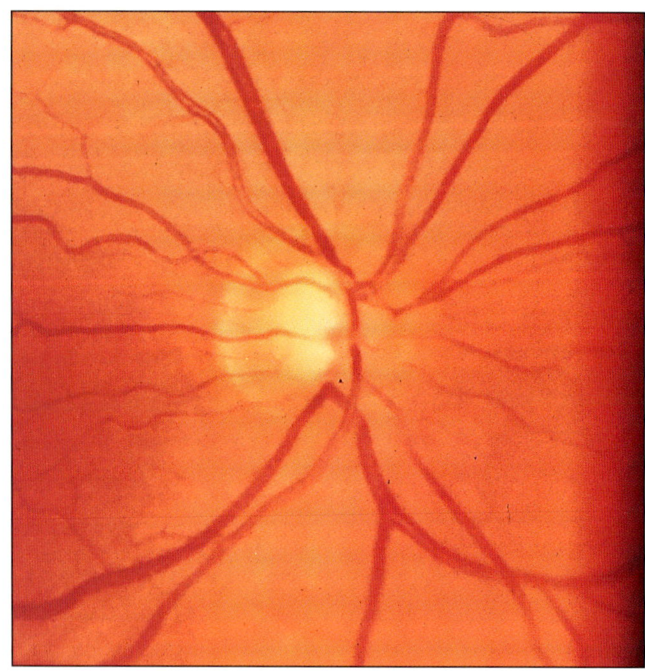

**Figure 4-5a.** Case 5 (right eye). Optic disc photograph shows glaucomatous damage (1993).

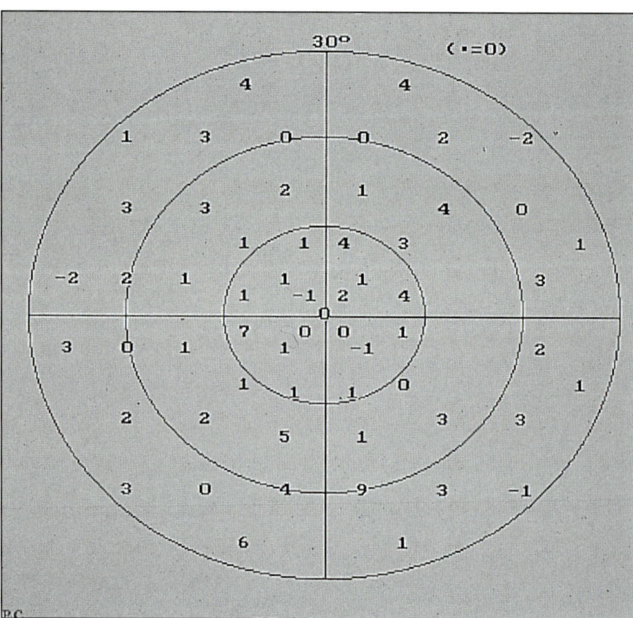

**Figure 4-5b.** Visual field defect in the inferior region (1993) (values represent deviation in threshold sensitivity compared with age-matched normals).

**Figure 4-5c.** CSLO topography cup and volume measurements were outside normal limits (1993).

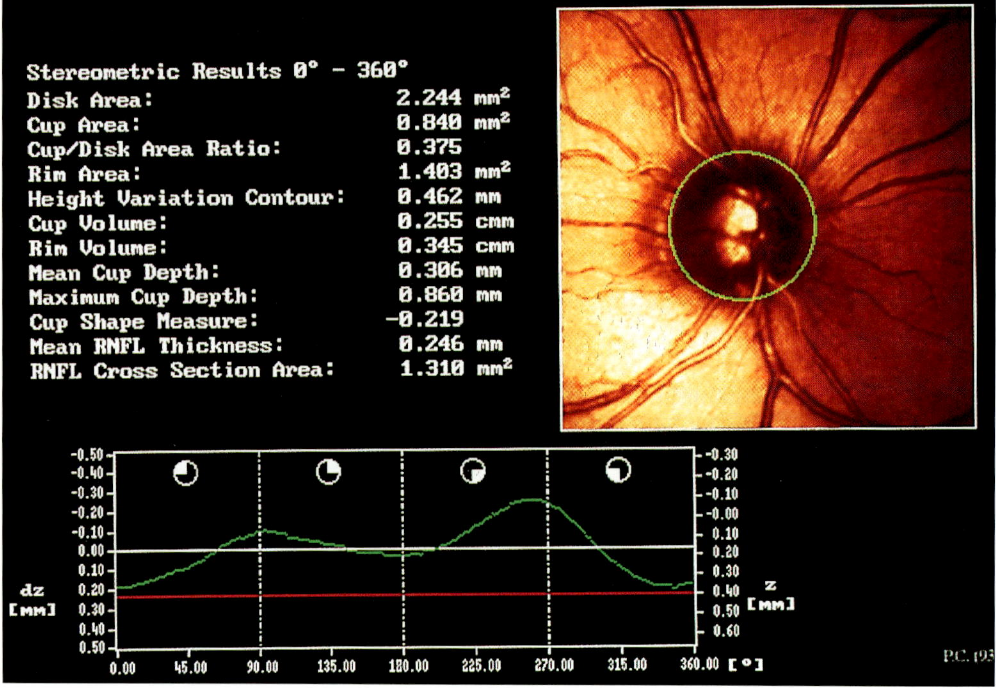



cians with information otherwise impossible to obtain. However, just as limited information can be obtained from a poor quality photograph of the optic disc, caution should be exercised when interpreting information and measurements from poor quality CSLO images. This is particularly important when comparing measurements over time obtained from images of different quality. Since after pupil dilation, good quality images can be obtained in most subjects, even ones with small pupils and/or lens opacities,[16] clinical decisions should be based on the best available information, which may require image acquisition after dilation for some patients.

There are several other issues that must be addressed to improve the clinical utility of CSLO topographic information. First, the establishment of a relatively stable reference plane

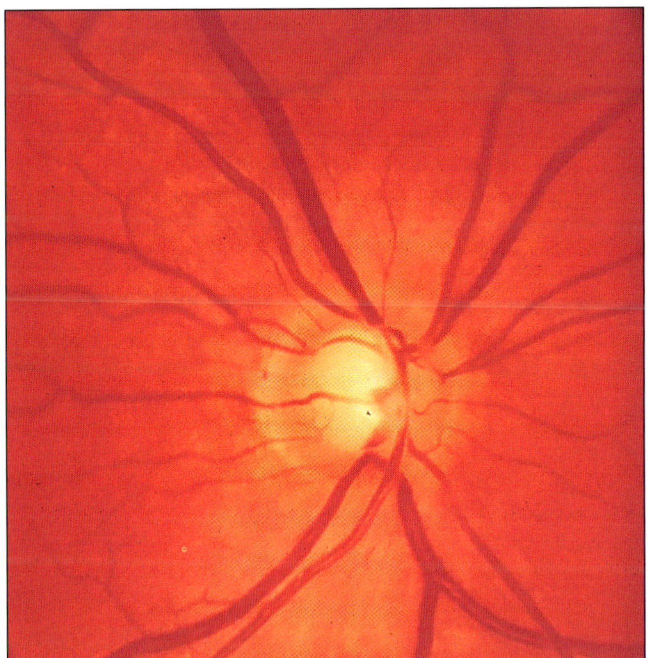

**Figure 4-5d.** Optic disc photograph demonstrates progression of optic disc damage (1995).

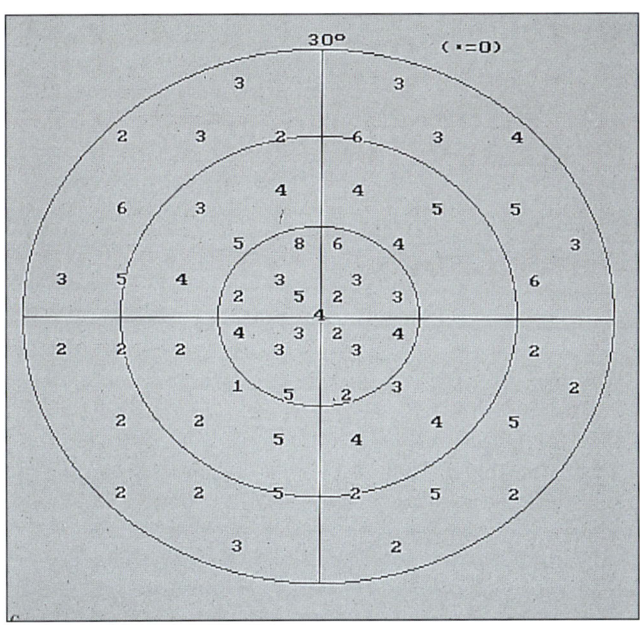

**Figure 4-5e.** Visual field shows general reduction in sensitivity (1995) (values represent sensitivity loss [dB] compared to age-matched normal subjects).

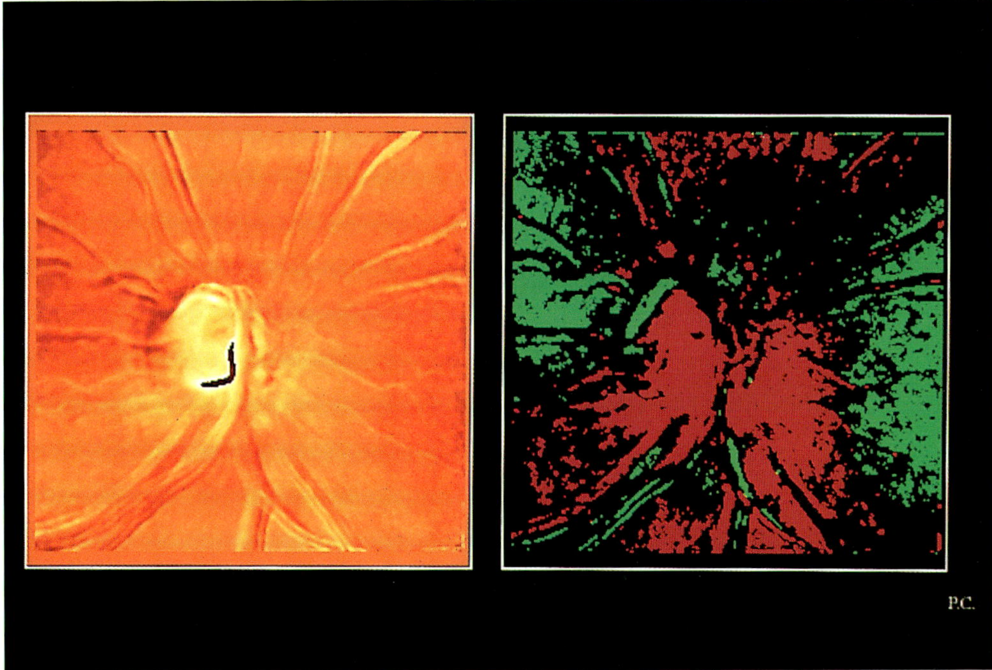

**Figure 4-5f.** CSLO difference image indicates change in optic nerve topography (1993-1995).

for determining topographic ONH parameters which, ideally, would be independent of retinal or ONH topography that changes with the course of glaucoma. In the cases presented, for comparison of topographic optic nerve parameter measurements over time, the reference plane for follow-up images was set to the standard reference plane of the first image. Second, for comparison of information obtained with different CSLOs, standardized outlining of the disc margin used to define many topographic optic nerve parameters is needed. Third, automated methods for evaluation of image quality currently under development should improve our ability to accurately interpret change in CSLO topography over time.

Confocal scanning laser ophthalmoscopy shows promise for improving our ability to detect glaucomatous optic nerve damage and change. Continued study is needed to understand its role in clinical decision making.

## REFERENCES

1. Tielsch JM, Katz J, Singh K, et al. A population-based evaluation of glaucoma screening: the Baltimore Eye Survey. *Am J Epidemiol.* 1991;134:1102-1110.

2. Zangwill L, Shakiba S, Caprioli J, Weinreb RN. Agreement between clinicians and a confocal scanning laser ophthalmoscope in estimating cup/disk ratios. *Am J Ophthalmol.* 1995;119:415-421.

3. Zangwill L, Van Horn S, de Souza Lima M, Sample PA, Weinreb RN. Optic nerve head topography in ocular hypertensive eyes using confocal scanning laser ophthalmoscopy. *Am J Ophthalmol.* In press.

4. Tsai C, Zangwill L, Gonzalez C, et al. Ethnic differences in optic nerve head topography. *J Glaucoma.* 1995;4:248-257.

5. Weinreb RN, Shakiba S, Sample PA, et al. Association between quantitative nerve fiber layer measurement and visual field loss in glaucoma. *Am J Ophthalmol.* 1995;120:732-738.

6. Mikelberg FS, Parfitt CM, Swindale NV, Graham SL, Drance SM, Gosine R. Ability of the Heidelberg Retina Tomograph to detect early glaucomatous visual field loss. *J Glaucoma.* 1995;4:242-247.

7. Tsai CS, Zangwill L, Sample PA, Garden V, Bartsch D, Weinreb RN. Correlation of peripapillary retinal height and visual field in glaucoma and normal subjects. *J Glaucoma.* 1995;4:110-116.

8. Weinreb RN, Lusky M, Bartsch D, Morsman D. Effect of repetitive imaging on topographic measurements of the optic nerve head. *Arch Ophthalmol.* 1993;111:636-638.

9. Mikelberg FS, Wijsman K, Schulzer M. Reproducibility of topographic parameters obtained with the Heidelberg Retina Tomograph. *J Glaucoma.* 1993;2:101-103.

10. Rohrschneider K, Burk ROW, Kruse FE, Volcker HE. Reproducibility of the optic nerve head topography with a new laser tomographic screening device. *Ophthalmology.* 1994;101:1044-1049.

11. Weinreb RN. Diagnosing and monitoring glaucoma with confocal scanning laser ophthalmoscopy. *J Glaucoma.* 1995;4:225-227.

12. Asawaphureekorn S, Zangwill L, Weinreb RN. The ranked-segment distribution curve for interpretation of optic nerve topography. *J Glaucoma.* 1996;5:79-90.

13. Bebie H, Flammer J, Bebie T. The cumulative defect curve: separation of local and diffuse components of visual field damage. *Graefes Arch Clin Exp Ophthalmol.* 1989;227:9-12.

14. Sample PA, Taylor JD, Martinez GA, Lusky M, Weinreb RN. Short-wavelength color visual fields in glaucoma suspects at risk. *Am J Ophthalmol.* 1993;115:225-233.

15. Chauhan BC, LeBlanc RP, McCormick TA, Rogers JB. Test-retest variability of topographic measurements with confocal scanning laser tomography in patients with glaucoma and control subjects. *Am J Ophthalmol.* 1994;118:9-15.

16. Irak I, Zangwill L, de Souza Lima M, Garden V, Weinreb RN. Effect of pupil dilation on optic disc topography in cataract patients. *Invest Ophthalmol Vis Sci.* 1996;37(Suppl):S1089.

# Evaluating the Nerve Fiber Layer

# CLINICAL EXAMINATION OF THE NERVE FIBER LAYER

*Cynthia Mattox, MD*

The clinical examination of the nerve fiber layer (NFL) can be an important way of detecting glaucoma damage. Hoyt and Newman[1] first noted that characteristic changes of the NFL accompanied glaucoma damage. Further investigations have helped to delineate important features of glaucomatous damage to the NFL. Evaluating the NFL during examination of the patient will enable the clinician to make correlations with the optic disc and visual field and will aid in diagnosis. Leisurely examination of the NFL can be accomplished with NFL photography. This valuable technique of nerve fiber evaluation can be performed with the equipment most ophthalmologists already have in their offices.

## ANATOMY

The NFL is composed of the axons from the ganglion cells, neuroglia, and astrocytes. There are an estimated 700,000 to 2 million ganglion cells in the human retina and a similar number of nerve fibers found in the optic nerve.[2-4] The ganglion cells are arranged in layers of four to six cells in the macula, and are only two cells thick in the retinal periphery. At the present time, three cell types are identified. P cells are small and compose 90% of all ganglion cells. They are sensitive to low contrast testing methods and have a fast axonal conduction rate. M cells are large, comprise only 10% of ganglion cells, have a slower conduction rate, and are sensitive to low contrast testing methods. W cells are rare, are sensitive to on-off centers, and have slow conduction rates. There has been some work in trying to distinguish if certain types of ganglion cells are preferentially damaged in glaucoma.[5]

The axons of the ganglion cells travel towards the optic nerve in an organized fashion[6-9] (Figure 5-1). Superior ganglion cell axons travel to the superior and superotemporal disc, while inferior ganglion cell axons project to the inferior and inferotemporal disc. The temporal retinal raphe is an imaginary horizontal line that bisects the disc and fovea and separates the superior NFL from the inferior. Axons traveling from the temporal side of the fovea arc around the fovea to enter the disc at its superior pole. Axons from ganglion cells between the fovea and disc course directly to the disc and are termed the papillomacular bundle.

The axons are also organized in a layered fashion.[6-9] Axons of ganglion cells from the peripheral retina lie deep in the NFL, or closer to the choroid. Axons from ganglion cells closer to the disc cross over these and come to lie more superficially in the NFL, or closer to the vitreous. Concomitantly, the axons from the peripheral retina end up closer to the disc rim as they turn to make up the optic nerve. The peripapillary axons lie more centrally in the optic disc head.

Obviously, as the NFL builds up with more and more axons, it becomes thicker closer to the disc. The superior and inferior poles contain the most nerve fibers. In non-human primates, it has been measured histologically and found to be 228 to 320 microns thick at the superior peripapillary region and 194 to 320 microns at the inferior peripapillary region.[9] The nasal and papillomacular bundles are much thinner, measuring only 60 microns. This arrangement results in a characteristic double-hump pattern if the NFL is viewed histologically or measured in a circumferential section, with the thickest humps at the superior and inferior regions. The NFL also thins dramatically as it is measured farther away from the disc, down to 40 microns only two disc diameters away from the disc rim.

The axons are gathered in bundles and are surrounded by neuroglia. The axon bundles reflect light and therefore become visible as silvery striations with the proper viewing technique.[1,10] Green and blue light reflects from the NFL bet-

**Figure 5-1.** Representation of the typical arrangement of the human RNFL. Lower drawing represents the topography of the NFL where the more distal ganglion cell axons project to the more peripheral area of the optic disc rim.

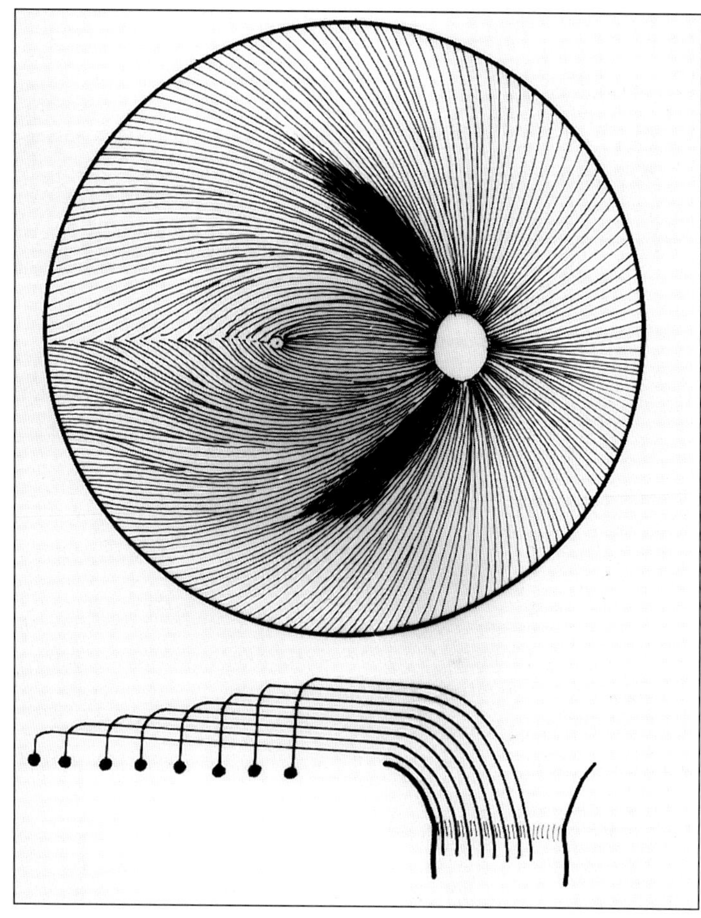

ter than other color light. The green or blue wavelengths are more highly absorbed by the retinal pigment epithelium and choroid, and, therefore, the reflected light allows more contrast and easier viewing of the NFL. In patients with more pigmented retinal pigment epithelium and choroid, the NFL is more easily viewed due to this contrast effect.

## PATHOLOGIC CHANGES IN THE NERVE FIBER LAYER

Loss of NFL visibility has been investigated experimentally. Radius and Anderson, Minckler, and Quigley et al have all induced experimental optic nerve or retinal damage in nonhuman primates and found histologic correlation with the clinical or photographic evidence of loss of NFL.[6-9] In humans, Hoyt and Newman first reported the NFL abnormalities in patients with glaucoma, and other reports followed.[1,11-14] The NFL atrophy has also been found to correlate with the decrease of the neuroretinal rim area of the optic disc.[15-17] NFL defects have been found to correlate with statistical indices on automated perimetry.[18-20] Focal NFL defects have correlated with focal visual field defects as well. NFL atrophy has been shown to progress after optic disc hemorrhage.[21] So, evaluating the NFL is a valid way of determining if glaucoma damage is present.

## TECHNIQUES FOR VIEWING THE NERVE FIBER LAYER CLINICALLY

The NFL is best visualized using a red-free or green light as described earlier. A good stereoscopic image of the NFL is preferred, and can be achieved with many types of lenses at the slit lamp biomicroscope.[22] The optimal lens is probably a Goldmann or other contact fundus lens. This allows for easier and more controlled viewing. However, the drawback is the requirement of methylcellulose or other viscous contact solutions and this may interfere with subsequent fundus photography. The 78 D indirect non-contact fundus lens used with the slit lamp also allows an excellent magnification and stereoscopic view of the NFL. Others may use a 90 D lens, which allows a larger field of view with less magnification, or a Hruby lens. Some prefer a direct ophthalmoscope with the red-free light for high power examination of the NFL, however, this does not provide a stereoscopic image. In some patients with miotic pupils, the direct ophthalmoscope may be the only way to view the NFL. Using any of the lenses, the red-free light should be oriented as a wide, short slit beam, and a systematic examination of the NFL can then be performed.

The advantages of the clinical exam are that it is quick and inexpensive and can be performed even in the presence

Table 5-1
## Photography Techniques

| | Airaksinen | Quigley | NEEC* | NEEC* |
|---|---|---|---|---|
| | | | | **Topcon 501A** |
| **Camera** | **Canon** | **Zeiss** | **Canon 6F60Z** | **Digital System** |
| Field | 60° | 1.6x magnifier | 60° | 55° |
| Filter | Blue filter | Filter transmits <1% of light, >580 nm, and 70% of light between 400 and 555 nm | Barrier filter out, exciter filter in | 495 nm exciter filter only |
| Film | Kodak Pantomic-X | Kodak Technical Pan | T-Max 400 | Digital |
| Settings | | 480 to 720 watt-seconds | Flash on 3 or 4 | Gain 6 dB, flash 25 |
| Processing | 7 minutes in Kodak HCl 10 mix 1:3 | 12 minutes at 70°F in D-11, 1:1 mix | 8.5 minutes in D-19 process | Digital to prints or slides |

*NEEC=New England Eye Center, Boston, Mass*

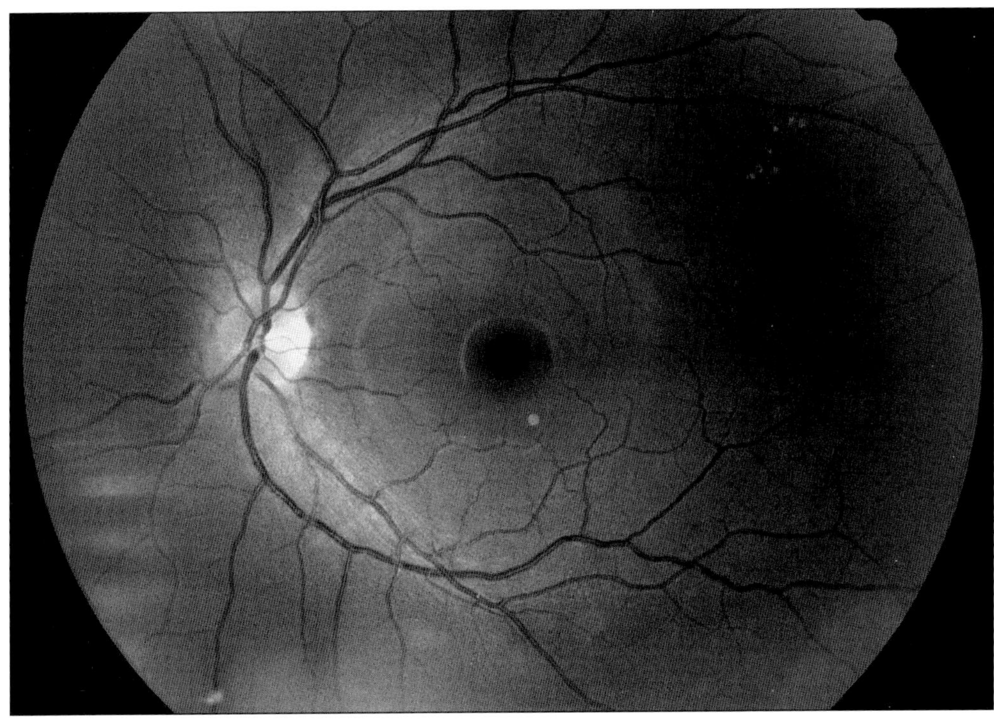

**Figure 5-2.** Normal NFL appearance with red-free light. Note the bright striations at the superior and inferior arcuate areas which transition to less bright striations toward the papillomacular bundle.

of miotic pupils in most cases. However, it does require some practice and patience to become adept with the technique.

## NERVE FIBER LAYER PHOTOGRAPHY

Various methods of NFL photography have been described (Table 5-1).[10,23] Photography allows for a more leisurely evaluation of the NFL than during a live patient examination. It also allows for better comparisons of fellow eyes. Some experience on the part of the photographer is required before reliable photographs can be obtained.

## EVALUATING THE NFL CLINICALLY AND IN PHOTOGRAPHS[1,10,22]

Examination should begin with the striations. The brightest striations should be most prominent in the superior and inferior poles, and should transition to less bright stria-

**Figure 5-3.** Normal NFL appearance using higher magnification and red-free light. Notice the characteristic grainy texture to the striations.

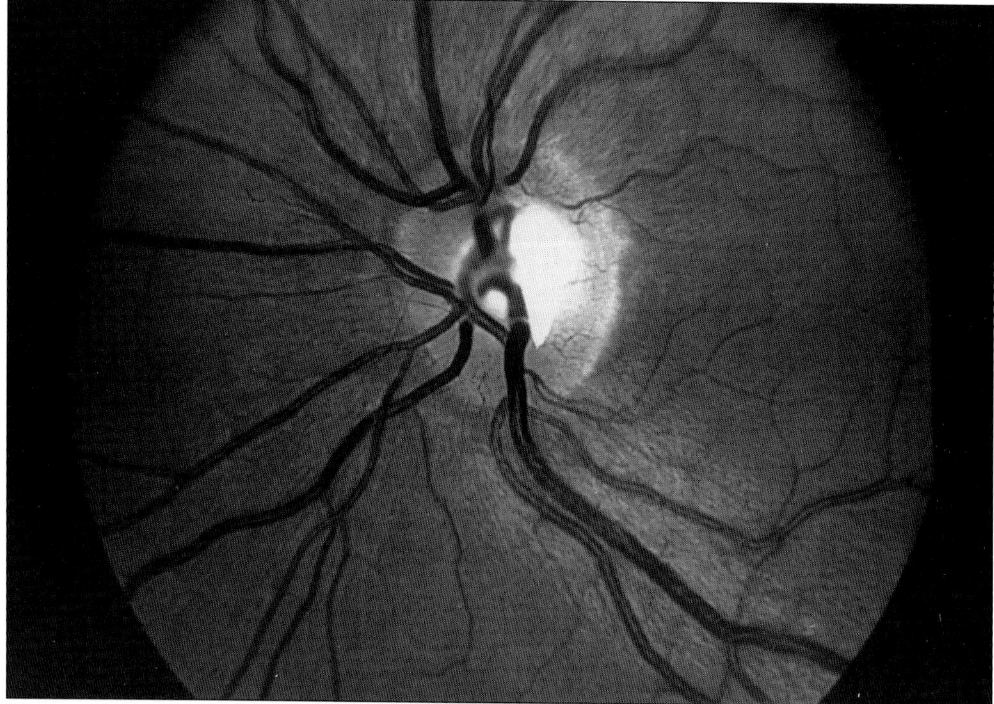

**Figure 5-4.** This demonstrates a poorly focused NFL photograph. However, notice that the lightly pigmented fundus can also make viewing the NFL difficult.

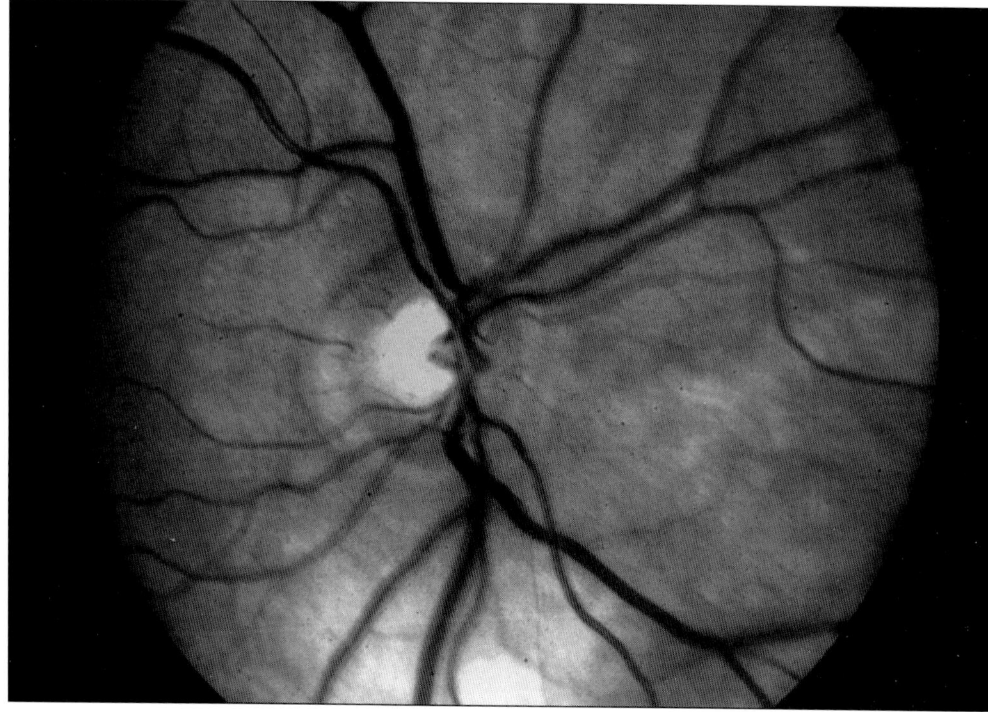

tions as the viewer examines the papillomacular bundle[24] (Figure 5-2). The examiner should compare the superior to the inferior striations and fellow eyes, watching for any abrupt gaps or any diffuse differences.

The striations should have a characteristic texture, described as rice grains laid end to end (Figure 5-3). This texture should be most visible at the superior and inferior poles, and will be noticeable as the striations cross over the retinal blood vessels. A decrease in the visibility of the texture may indicate thinning of the NFL.

The medium-sized retinal blood vessels are normally covered by a thin layer of nerve fibers as they course to the disc. This causes the blood vessels to appear slightly blurred at the margins (see Figure 5-3). As the NFL thins, these medium-sized blood vessels will appear sharper and more distinct.

The NFL may be difficult to see for several reasons

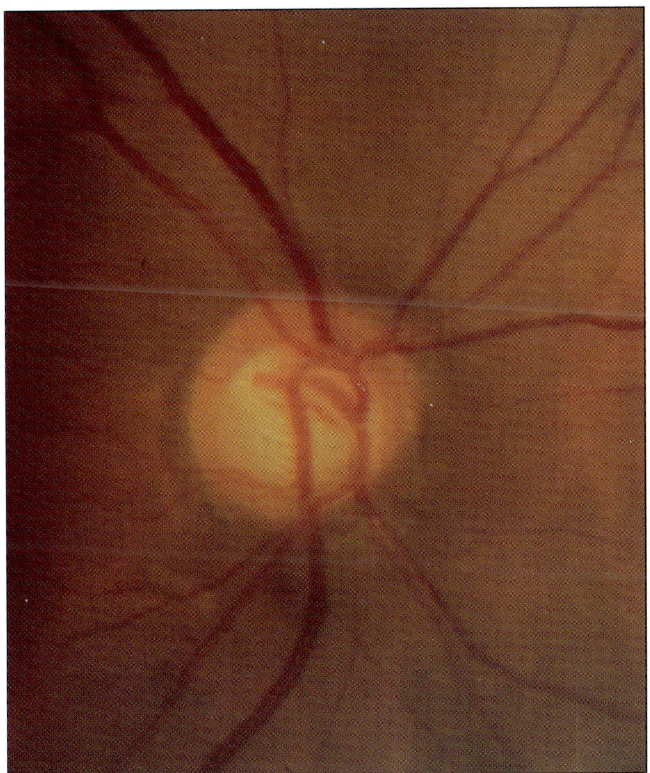

**Figure 5-5a.** Color photograph of right optic disc.

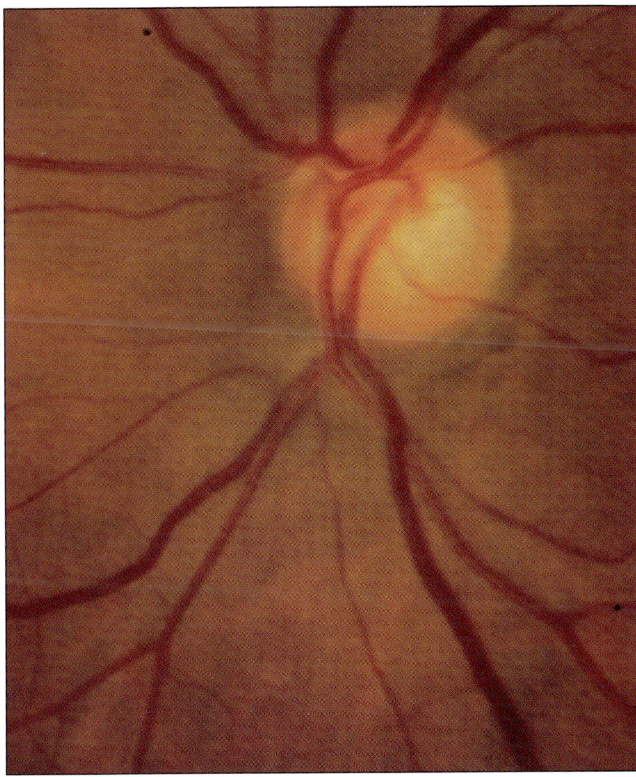

**Figure 5-5b.** Color photograph of left optic disc.

(Figure 5-4). The image may be blurred by media opacity such as cataract. Poorly focused photographs are detected by the blurring of the large retinal vessels. Poor contrast may also occur due to a lightly pigmented fundus. Glare from a cataract or a slit lamp beam that is too bright or wide will also impair the view. Of course, photographs need to be centered on the peripapillary area, since the thinner peripheral NFL is difficult to see. In advanced cases of glaucoma, the NFL may be so thin as to be undetectable.

## PATTERNS OF NERVE FIBER LAYER LOSS IN GLAUCOMA

The NFL loss may be detected as diffuse or localized NFL defects. Localized loss, although easier to detect, is actually less common than diffuse loss in glaucoma.[1,9,12,13,16,25,26] Diffuse loss can be detected by comparing the superior and inferior regions in one eye and also to the fellow eye (Figures 5-5a through 5-6b). The examiner will notice loss of striations, less texture, and more prominent appearing medium-sized vessels in an entire region. The striations in the superior and/or inferior pole may have the same brightness as the papillomacular bundle when there is diffuse loss.

Localized, or wedge, defects are more striking and more easily recognized (Figures 5-7a through 5-10c). The defect will have an arcuate course, with a wedge shape, thinner in the peripapillary region and fanning out to the periphery. It will be more easily detected when the surrounding NFL is thicker, however, careful observation will note wedge-shaped defects sometimes overlying areas of diffuse loss.

Slit-like defects are relatively common and do not represent pathological NFL loss (Figure 5-11). Slit defects are found in up to 10% of normal eyes.[10] They can be distinguished from wedge defects by their smaller size, usually no larger than a large retinal vein, and by noticing that they do not extend up to the disc rim.

In advanced disease, the superior and inferior NFL striations are lost, while the papillomacular bundle is preserved (Figures 5-12a through 5-12c). This creates an image of darkness at the superior and inferior poles, while the papillomacular area appears brighter. In end-stage disease, even most of these fibers are lost, and the fundus has a uniform dark appearance. Occasionally, a few remaining nerve fibers will be seen and can be monitored for change.

Early in learning the technique of NFL examination, observers may tend to overcall the NFL defects, particularly slit defects, and also may have difficulty detecting mild diffuse loss. Practice will improve the accuracy of the observations.

Both Quigley and Airaksinen have proposed grading scales to quantify the degree of NFL loss (Table 5-2).[12,26] These scales are most helpful as research tools to provide a

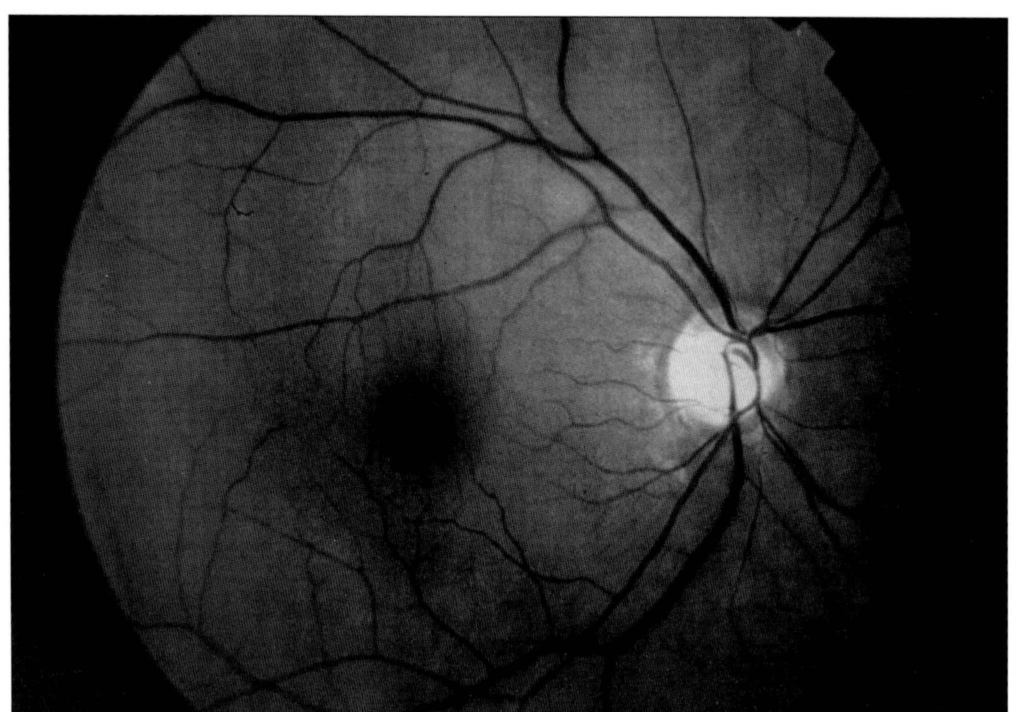

**Figure 5-5c.** Red-free photo of NFL right eye.

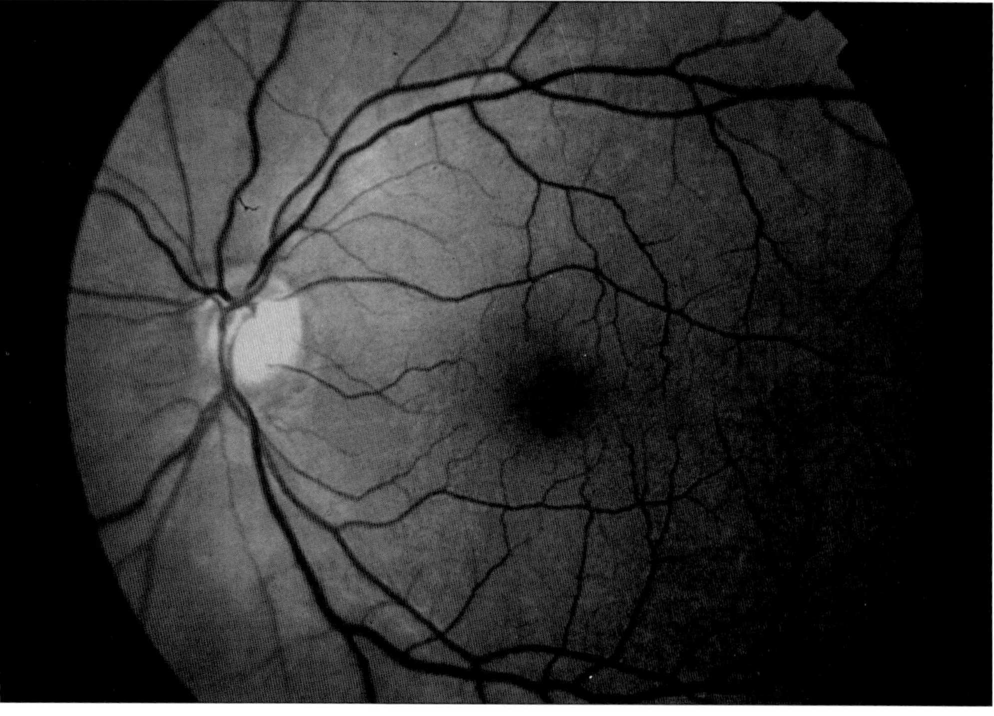

**Figure 5-5d.** Red-free photo of NFL left eye. Notice diffuse loss of NFL striations, prominence of retinal vessels.

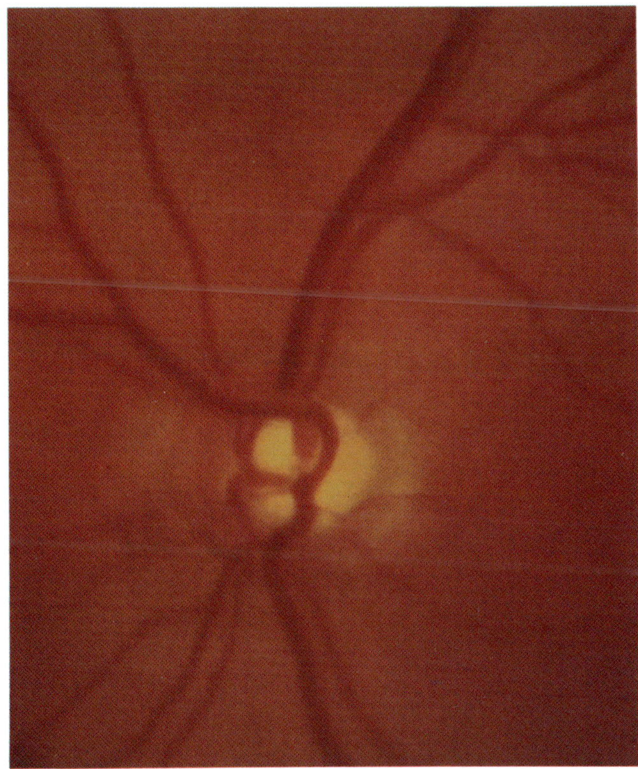

**Figure 5-6a.** Color photograph of patient's left optic disc.

**Figure 5-6b.** Red-free photograph of NFL. Notice mild diffuse loss of NFL.

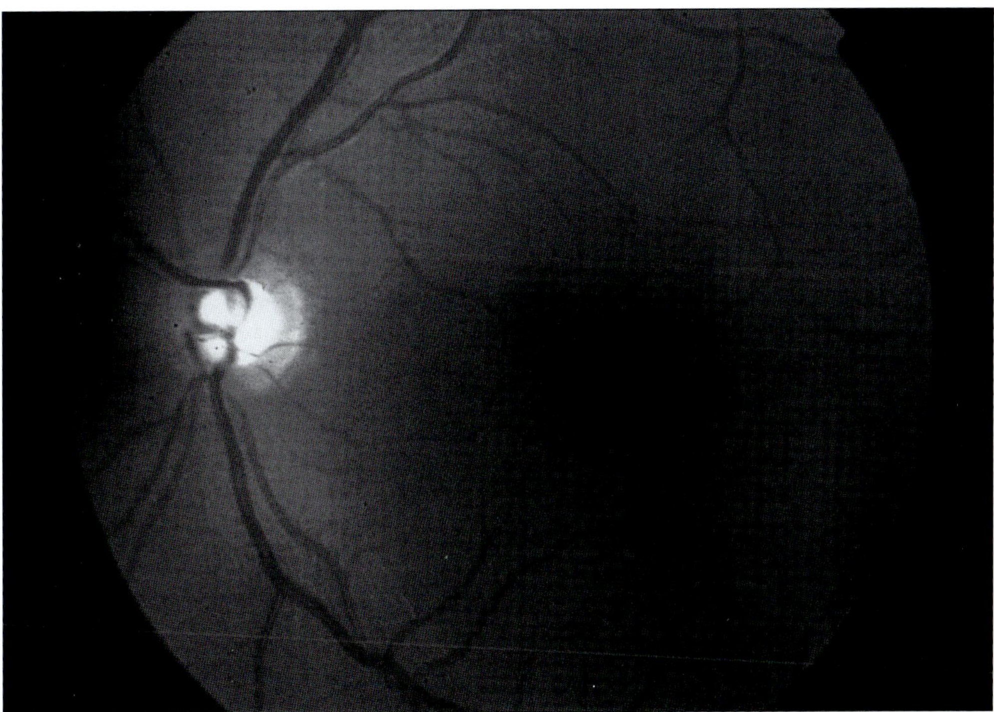

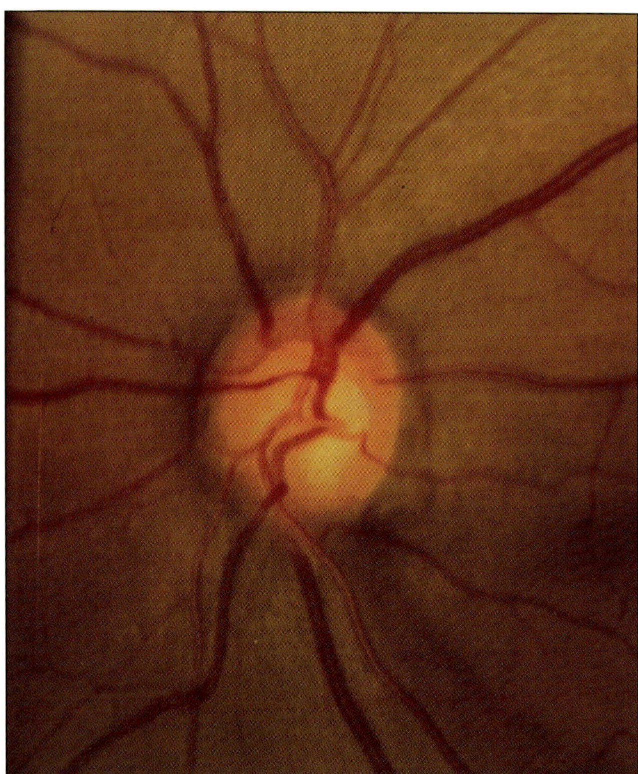

**Figure 5-7a.** Inferior wedge NFL defect, corresponding to notch in the optic disc rim, is visible on color optic disc photo.

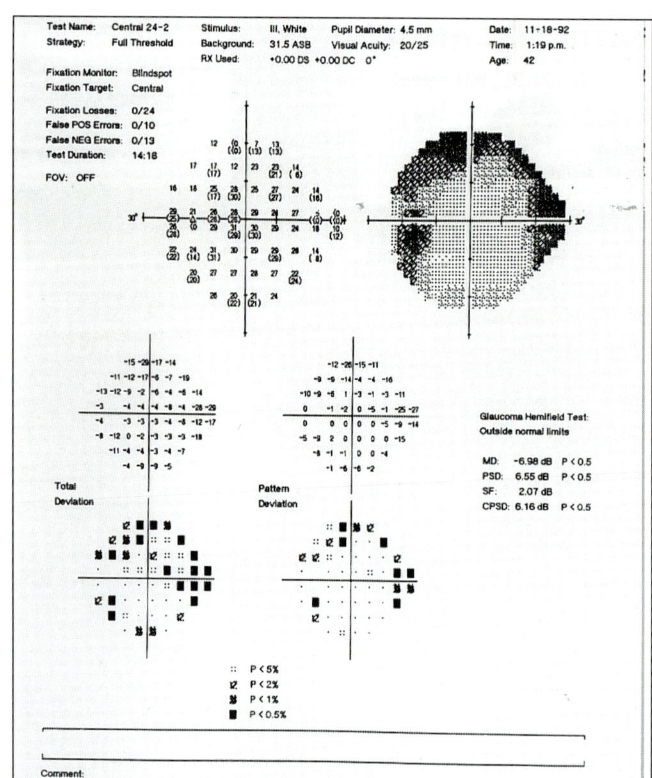

**Figure 5-7b.** Corresponding superior arcuate scotoma on visual field testing.

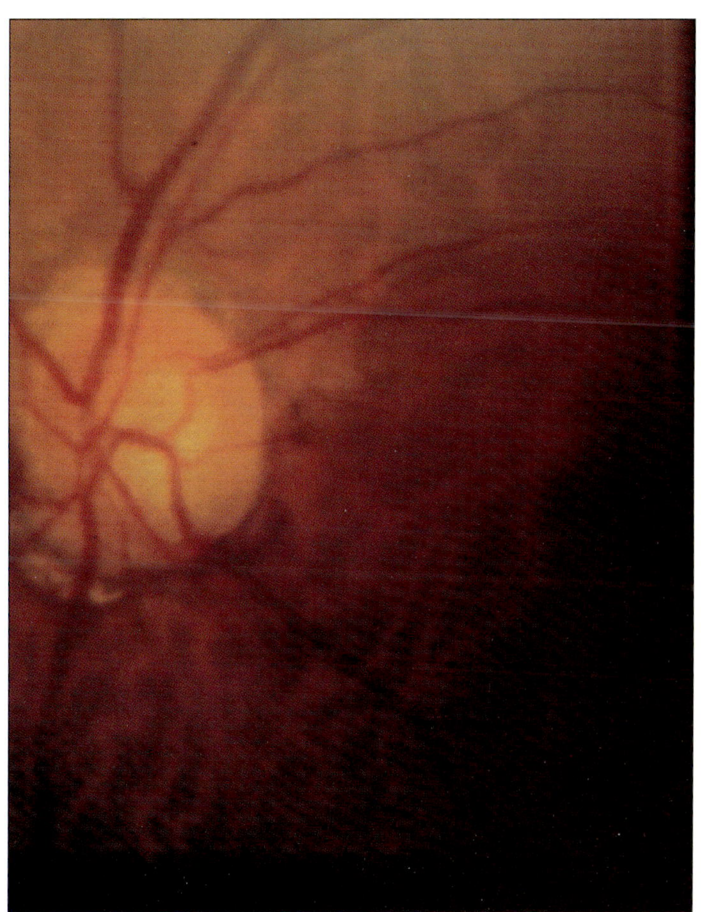

**Figure 5-8a.** Notch in inferior optic disc rim seen in color photo.

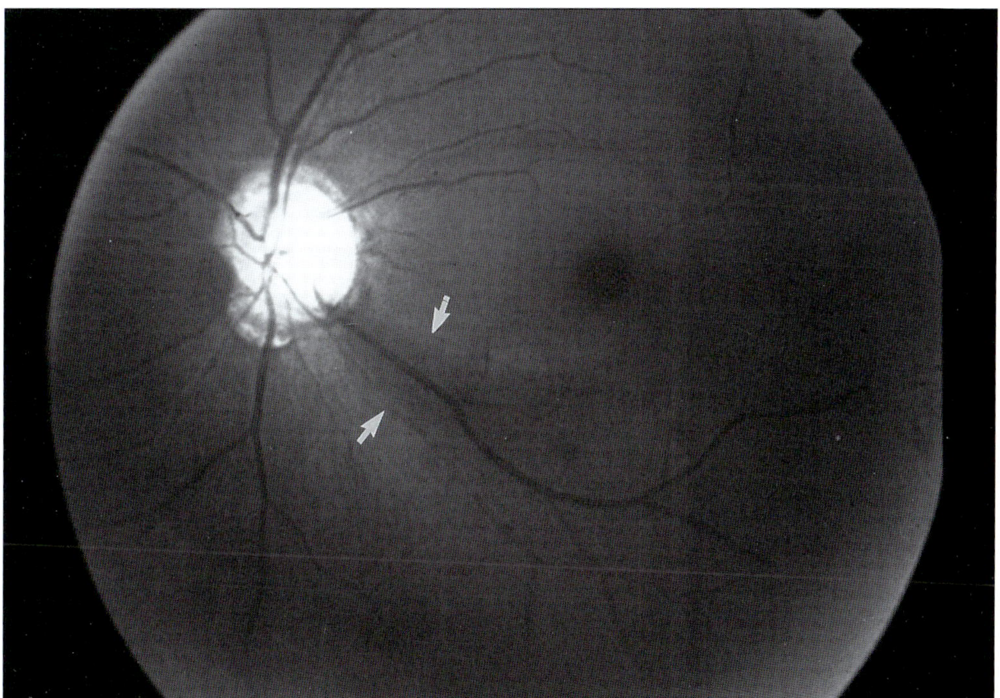

**Figure 5-8b.** Inferior wedge NFL defect seen on red-free photo.

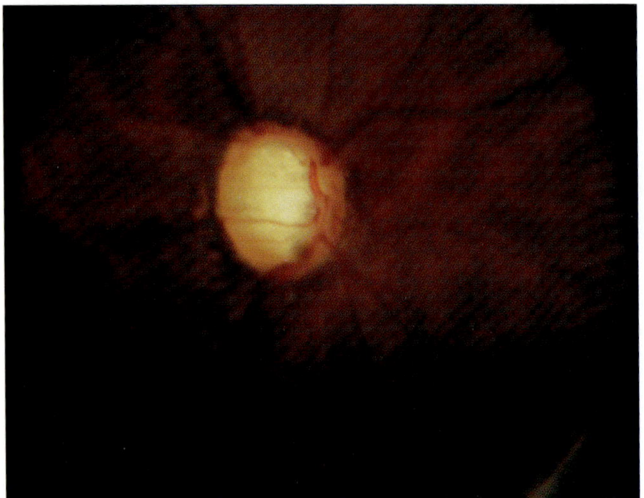

**Figure 5-9a.** Optic disc right eye.

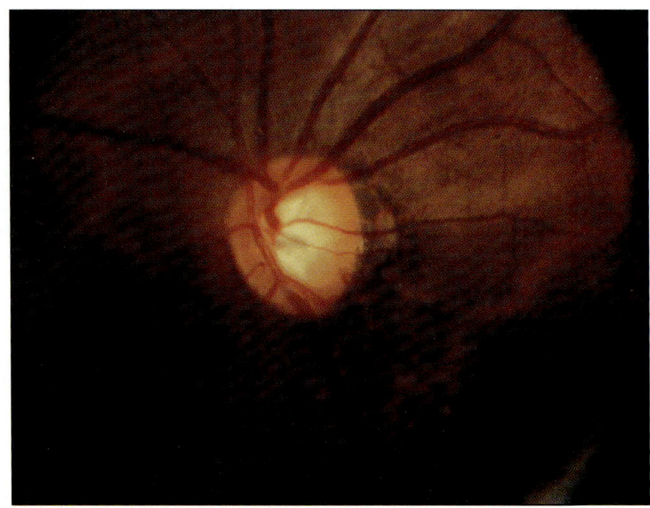

**Figure 5-9b.** Optic disc left eye.

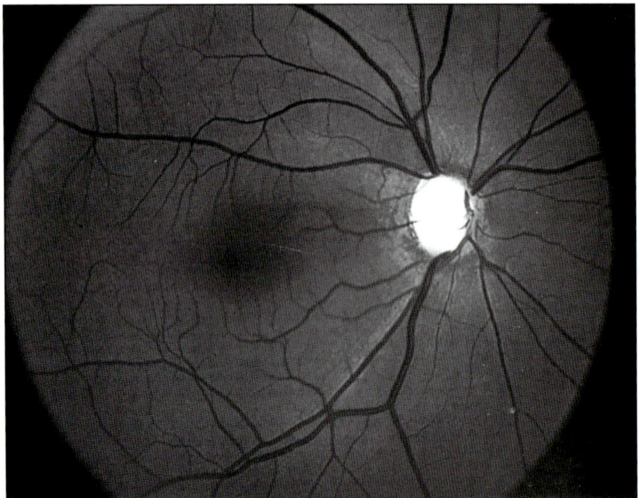

**Figure 5-9c.** Right eye, superior wedge NFL defect.

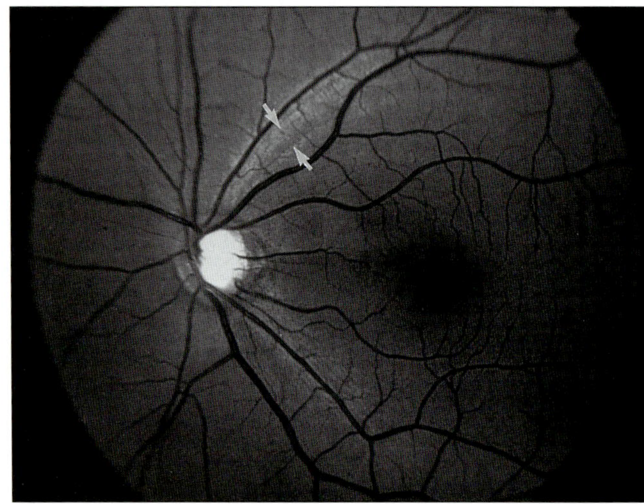

**Figure 5-9d.** Left eye, smaller superior wedge NFL defect.

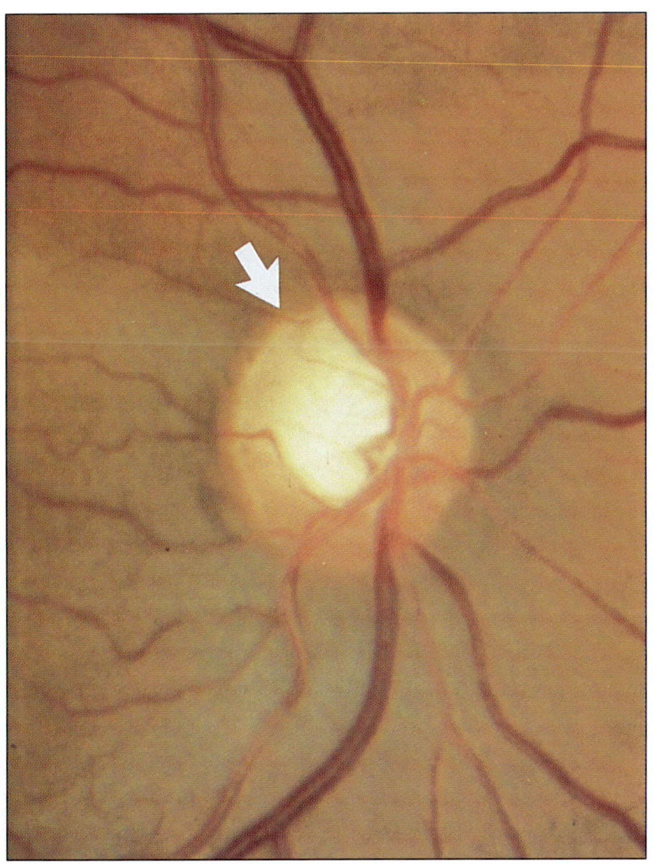

**Figure 5-10a.** Optic disc right eye, with superior rim notching.

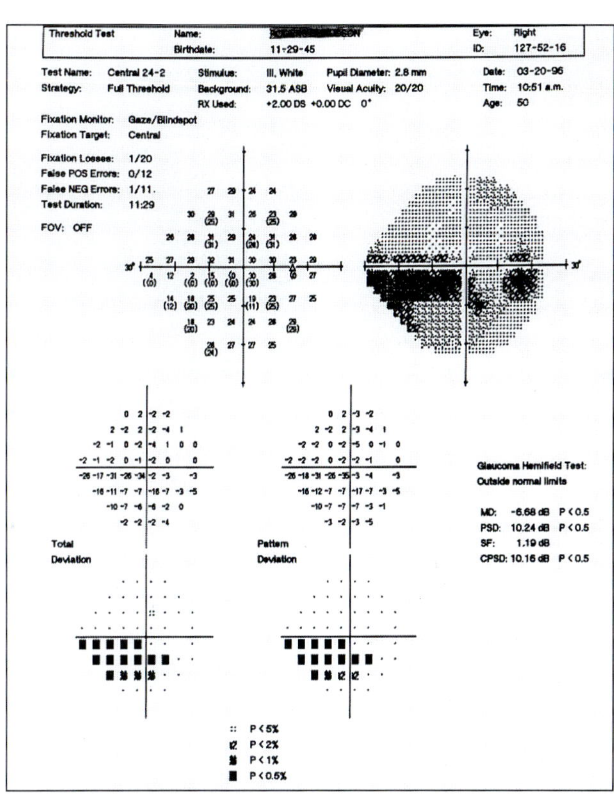

**Figure 5-10c.** Corresponding visual field defect.

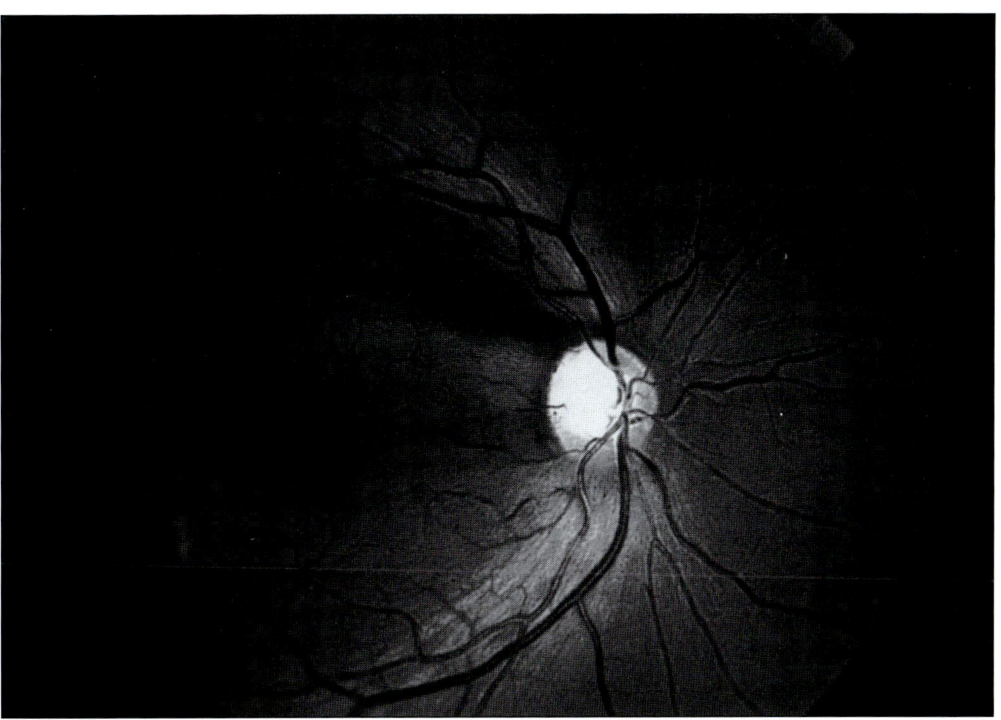

**Figure 5-10b.** Superior wedge defect in NFL.

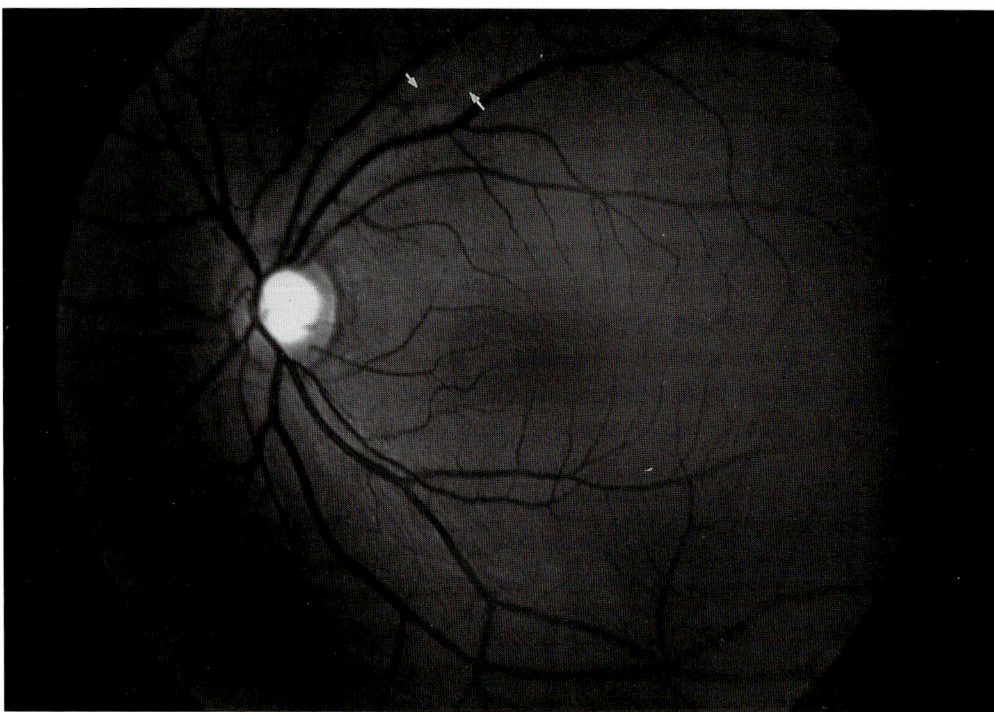

**Figure 5-11.** Two small pseudoslits indicated by arrows. Note small size, less than the width of a retinal vein.

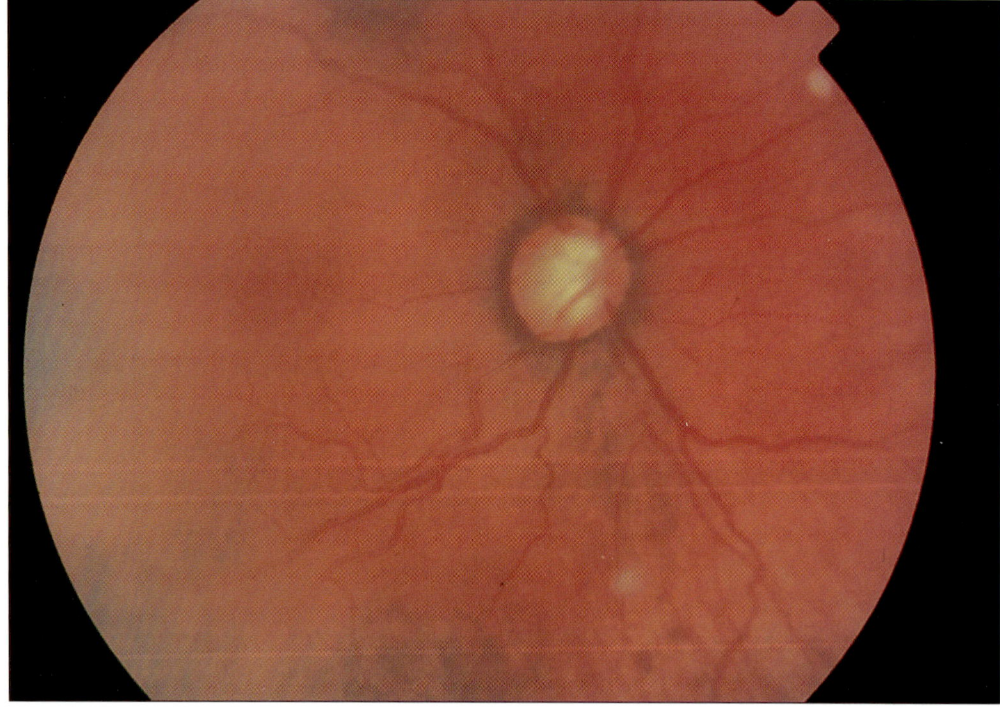

**Figure 5-12a.** Optic disc with severe cupping right eye.

meaningful, standardized system for intra- and interobserver comparisons. Validity and good reliability has been shown for both systems.

## WHY EXAMINE THE NERVE FIBER LAYER?

Examining the NFL is particularly useful in trying to distinguish between glaucoma suspects and true glaucoma damage. Fortunately, this clinical situation is most often encoun-

tered in relatively younger groups of patients, and hopefully, in those who have less cataract change and more easily visualized NFL. Several studies have shown that detecting NFL defects in glaucoma suspects with high intraocular pressure (IOP) but normal visual fields predicts which patients will have or go on to visual field loss.[16,18-20] Sommer et al evaluated 1344 eyes with IOP over 21 mmHg and no visual field loss with serial NFL photography and visual field testing.[19] Eighty-three eyes

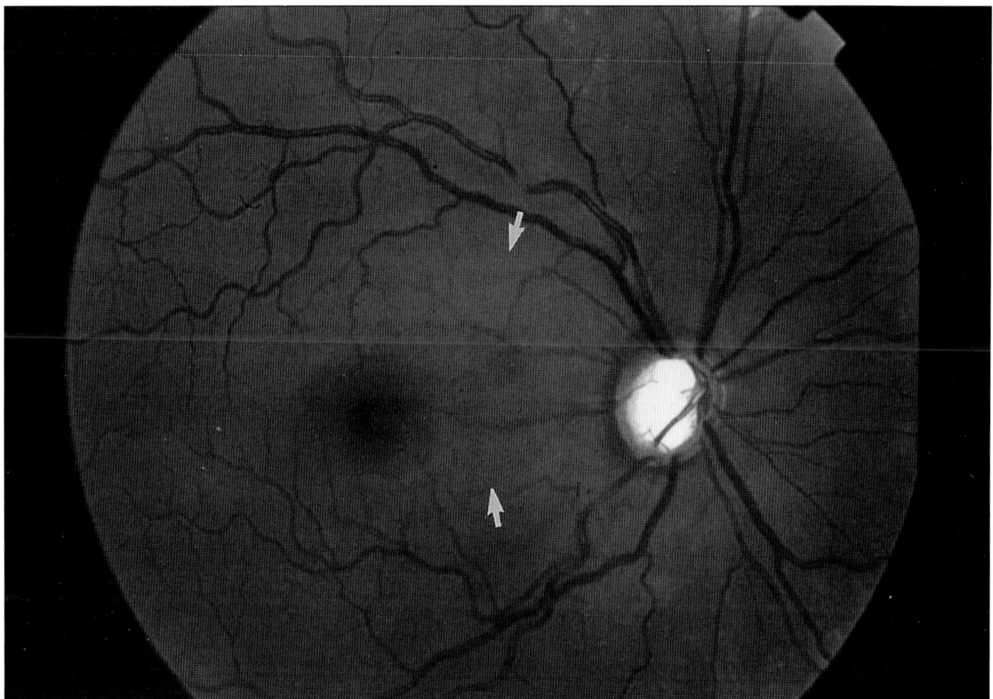

**Figure 5-12b.**
Papillomacular bundle striations (between arrows) are brighter than the superior and inferior arcuate regions.

developed visual field loss during the study period. Of these eyes, 88% had nerve fiber loss preceding or at the time of visual field loss. Six out of 10 eyes followed for 6 years had nerve fiber loss 6 years prior to visual field loss. In addition, Quigley et al investigated whether change in optic disc cupping evaluated by serial stereophotography or nerve fiber loss evaluated by photography was more successful in identifying those ocular hypertensives who went on to visual field loss.[20] An initial abnormality or change to an abnormal NFL was found in 73% of eyes that developed visual field loss compared to only 19% of eyes that had a qualitative change in optic disc cupping.

In clinical practice, once a diagnosis of glaucoma is made, correlation of visual field defects with NFL defects is helpful. NFL inspection is a satisfying, objective way of confirming a subjective finding such as a visual field defect.

Another use of NFL evaluation is in distinguishing between large physiologic cupping in congenitally large discs and actual glaucomatous optic disc cupping (Figures 5-13a through 5-14d). Normal-appearing NFL is a characteristic of these large cups in congenitally large discs, and the patient can be reassured and followed. Conversely, small optic discs often appear "crowded" with nerve fibers and have small cups. In these cases, early damage in the NFL may be detected before the cup enlarges to a suspicious degree.[27]

## SUMMARY

The clinical examination of the NFL is easily learned and can aid in the early diagnosis of glaucoma. The technique requires only the usual tools present in the ophthalmologist's office.

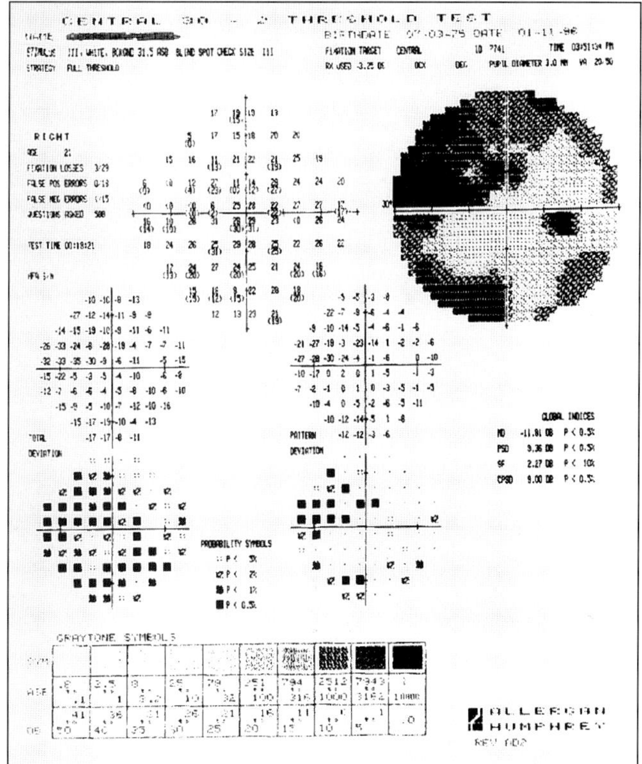

**Figure 5-12c.** Corresponding visual field defect.

<table>
<tr><td colspan="2" align="center">Table 5-2<br>Grading Scales</td></tr>
<tr><td>Airaksinen et al</td><td>Quigley et al</td></tr>
<tr><td>10 sections</td><td>Diffuse NFL atrophy</td></tr>
<tr><td>Diffuse defects</td><td>D0 (normal)</td></tr>
<tr><td>  Score 0 (no damage)</td><td>D1</td></tr>
<tr><td>  Up to Score 4 (total loss)</td><td>D2</td></tr>
<tr><td>Localized defects</td><td>D3 (advanced)</td></tr>
<tr><td>  Score 0 (no damage)</td><td>Wedge NFL atrophy</td></tr>
<tr><td>  Up to Score 4 (total loss)</td><td>W1 (moderate)</td></tr>
<tr><td>Total score of 0 to 40</td><td>W2 (severe)</td></tr>
</table>

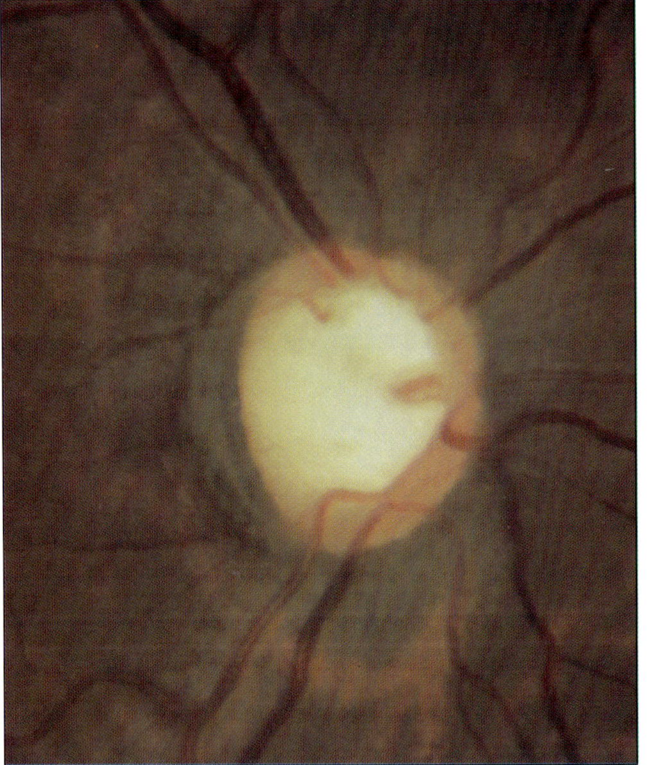

**Figure 5-13a.** Congenitally large optic disc right eye.

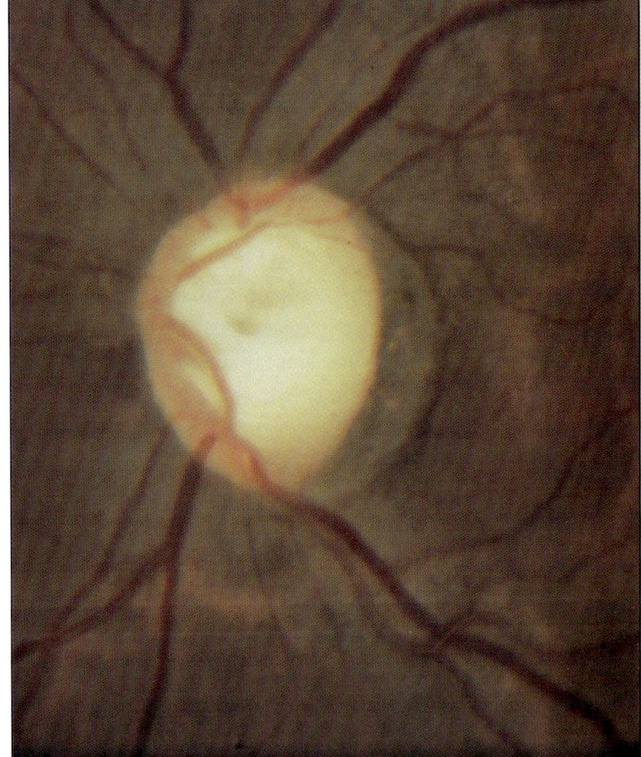

**Figure 5-13b.** Congenitally large optic disc left eye. Note size of disc compared to the size of the retinal veins.

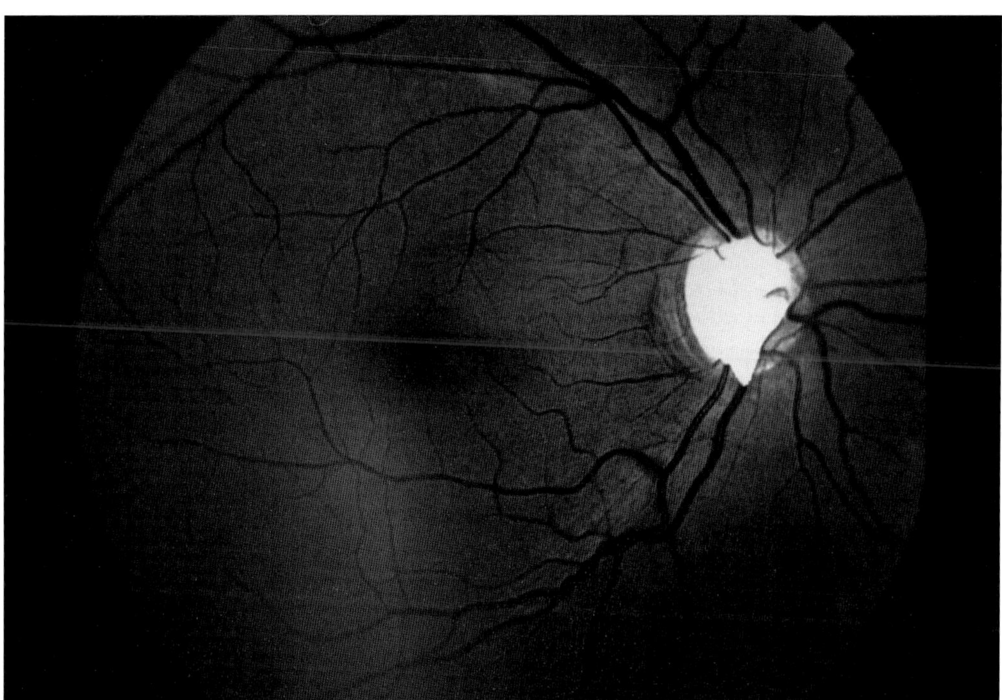

**Figure 5-13c.** Normal NFL right eye.

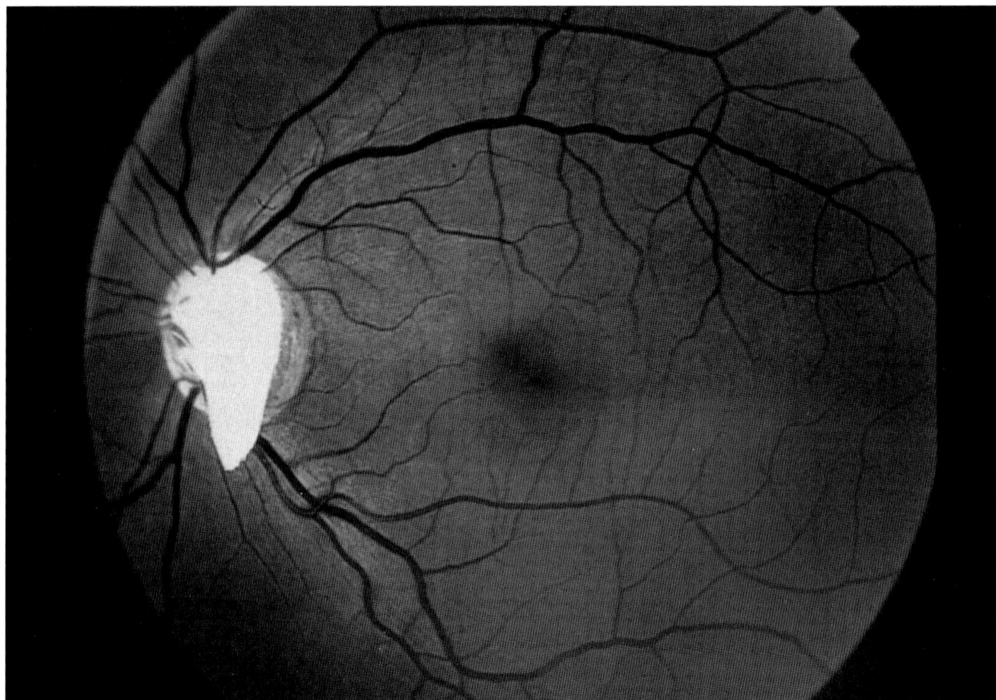

**Figure 5-13d.** Normal NFL left eye.

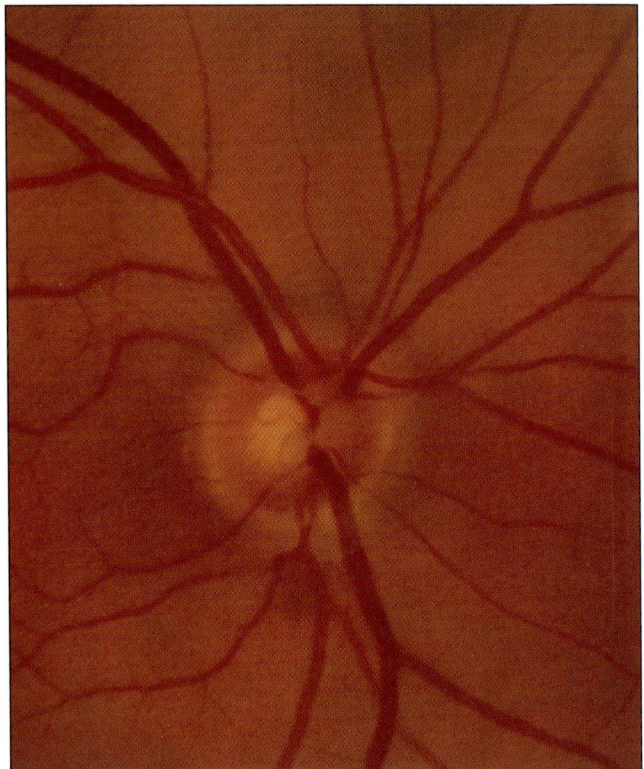

**Figure 5-14a.** Relatively small optic discs with corresponding-ly small cups, right eye.

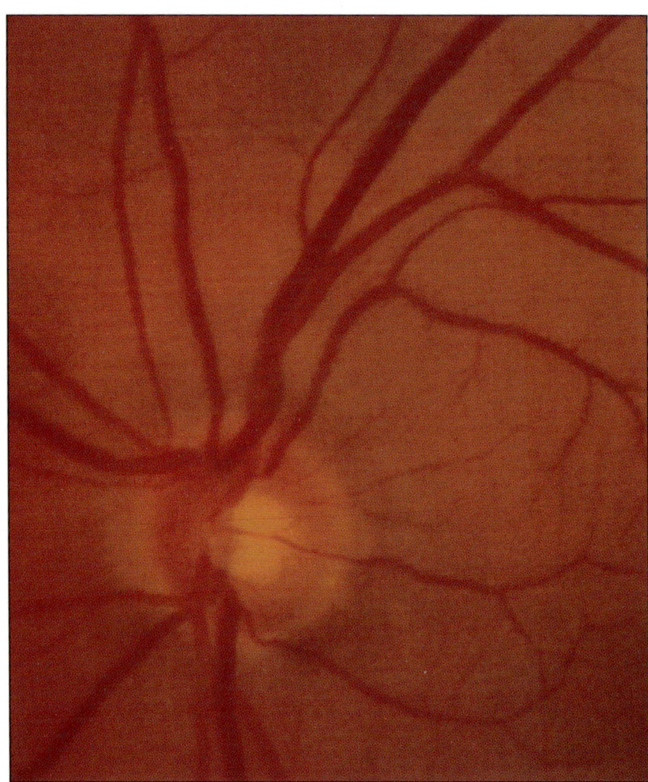

**Figure 5-14b.** Relatively small optic discs with corresponding-ly small cups, left eye.

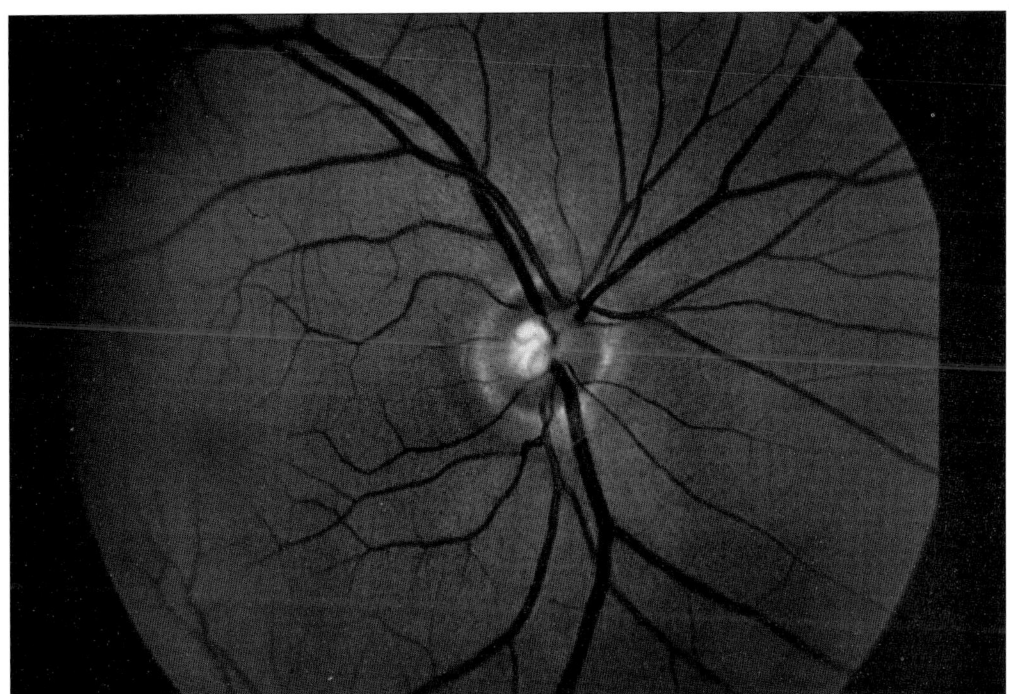

**Figure 5-14c.** Mild generalized decrease in NFL.

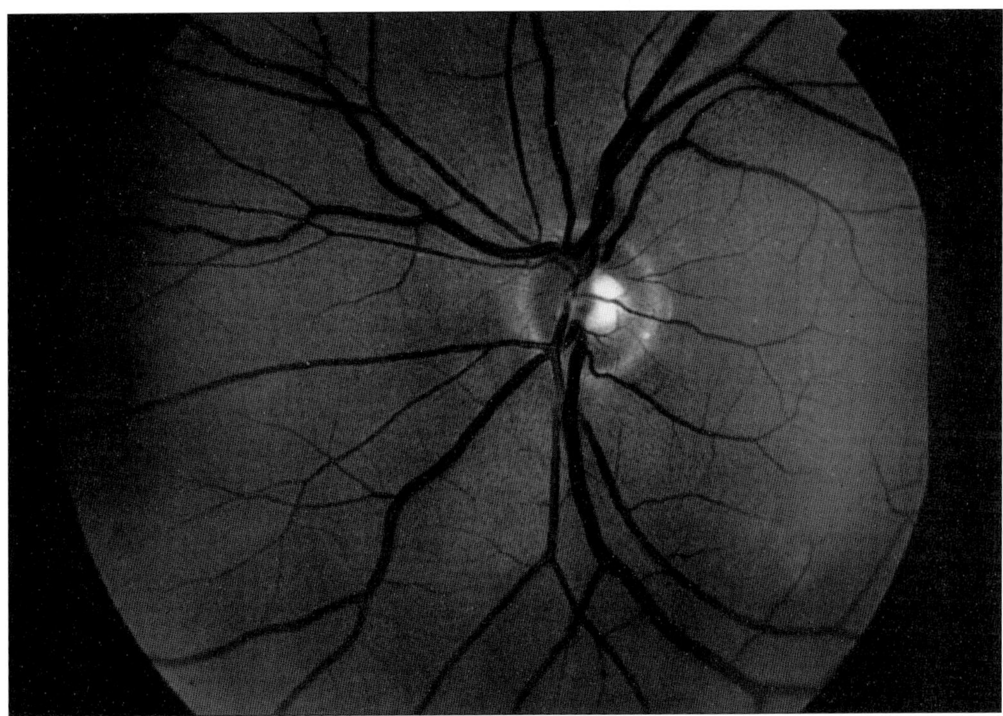

**Figure 5-14d.** Mild generalized decrease in NFL with inferior wedge defect.

## REFERENCES

1. Hoyt W, Frisen L, Newman N. Funduscopy of nerve fiber layer defects in glaucoma. *Invest Ophthalmol Vis Sci.* 1973;12:814-829.

2. Mikelberg F, Drance S, Schulzer M, Yidegiligne H, Wesi H. The normal human optic nerve-axon diameter distribution. *Ophthalmology.* 1989;96:1325-1328.

3. Jonas J, Muller-Bergh J, Schlotzer-Schrehardt U, Naumann G. Histomorphometry of the human optic nerve. *Invest Ophthalmol Vis Sci.* 1990;31:736-744.

4. Repka M, Quigley H. The effect of age on normal human optic nerve fiber number and diameter. *Ophthalmology.* 1989;96:26-31.

5. Quigley H, Sanchez R, Dunkelberger G, L'Hernault N, Baginski T. Chronic glaucoma selectively damages larger optic nerve fibers. *Invest Ophthalmol Vis Sci.* 1987;28:913-920.

6. Radius R, Anderson D. The course of axons through the retina and optic nerve head. *Arch Ophthalmol.* 1979;97:1154-1158.

7. Radius R, Anderson D. The histology of retinal nerve fiber layer bundles and bundle defects. *Arch Ophthalmol.* 1979;97:948-950.

8. Minckler D. The organization of nerve fiber bundles in the primate optic nerve head. *Arch Ophthalmol.* 1980;98:1630-1636.

9. Quigley H, Addicks E. Quantitative studies of retinal nerve fiber layer defects. *Arch Ophthalmol.* 1982;100:808-814.

10. Quigley H. *Diagnosing Early Glaucoma with Nerve Fiber Layer Examination.* New York: Igaku-Shoin; 1996.

11. Hitchings R, Poinoosawmy D, Poplar N, Sheth G. Retinal nerve fiber layer photography in glaucomatous patients. *Eye.* 1987;1:621-625.

12. Airaksinen P, Drance S, Douglas G, Mawson D, Nieminen H. Diffuse and localized nerve fiber loss in glaucoma. *Am J Ophthalmol.* 1984;98:566-571.

13. Quigley H, Miller N, George T. Clinical evaluation of nerve fiber layer atrophy as an indicator of glaucomatous optic nerve damage. *Arch Ophthalmol.* 1980;98:1564-1571.

14. Sommer A, Miller N, Pollack I, Maumenee A, George T. The nerve fiber layer in the diagnosis of glaucoma. *Arch Ophthalmol.* 1977;95:2149-2156.

15. Airaksinen P, Drance S. Neuroretinal rim area and retinal nerve fiber layer in glaucoma. *Arch Ophthalmol.* 1985;103:203-204.

16. Tuulonen A, Airaksinen P. Initial glaucomatous optic disc and retinal nerve fiber layer abnormalities and their progression. *Am J Ophthalmol.* 1991;111:485-490.

17. Varma R, Quigley H, Pease M. Changes in optic disk characteristics and the number of nerve givers in experimental glaucoma. *Am J Ophthalmol.* 1992;114:554-559.

18. Airaksinen P, Drance S, Douglas F, Schulzer M, Wijsman K. Visual field and retinal nerve fiber layer comparisons in glaucoma. *Arch Ophthalmol.* 1985;103:205-207.

19. Sommer A, Katz J, Quigley H, et al. Clinically detectable nerve fiber atrophy precedes the onset of glaucomatous field loss. *Arch Ophthalmol.* 1991;109:77-83.

20. Quigley H, Katz J, Derick R, Gilbert D, Sommer A. An evaluation of optic disc and nerve fiber layer examinations in monitoring progression of early glaucoma damage. *Ophthalmology.* 1992;99:19-28.

21. Diehl D, Quigley H, Miller N, Sommer A, Burney E. Prevalence and significance of optic disc hemorrhage in a longitudinal study of glaucoma. *Arch Ophthalmol.* 1990;108:545-550.

22. Airaksinen P, Tuulonen A. In: Varma R, Spaeth G, eds. *The Optic Nerve in Glaucoma.* Philadelphia, Pa: JB Lippincott Co; 1993.

23. Airaksinen PJ, Nieminen H. Retinal nerve fiber layer photography in glaucoma. *Ophthalmology.* 1985;92:877-879.

24. Jonas J, Nguyen N, Naumann G. The retinal nerve fiber layer in normal eyes. *Ophthalmology.* 1989;96:627-632.

25. Quigley H, Addicks E, Green W. Optic nerve damage in human glaucoma. III. Quantitative correlation of nerve fiber loss and visual field defect in glaucoma, ischemic neuropathy, papilledema, and tox neuropathy. *Arch Ophthalmol.* 1982;100:135-146.

26. Quigley HA, Reacher M, Katz J, Strahlman E, Gilbert D, Scott R. Quantitative grading of nerve fiber layer photographs. *Ophthalmology.* 1993;100:1800-1807.

27. Jonas J, Fernandez M, Naumann G. Glaucomatous optic nerve atrophy in small discs with low cup-to-disc ratios. *Ophthalmology.* 1990;97:1211-1215.

# Scanning Laser Polarimetry to Assess the Nerve Fiber Layer

*Marcia de Souza Lima, MD, Linda Zangwill, PhD,
Robert N. Weinreb, MD*


Defects in the retinal nerve fiber layer (RNFL) may be an early sign of glaucoma, preceding changes in the optic nerve head (ONH)[1] and visual field.[2-4] Although retinal ganglion cell atrophy cannot be visualized with clinical examinations, it can be detected indirectly as diffuse and/or wedge-shaped RNFL defects. In the former case, retinal vessels (which are embedded within the RNFL) may become clearer as retinal ganglion cells drop-out diffusely with progressive glaucoma. In the latter case, a RNFL defect may become wider, as retinal ganglion cell drop-out increases focally with progressive glaucoma. Alternatively, new defects may occur in eyes with pre-existing diffuse or wedge-shaped defects.

In studies reporting that RNFL defects precede the onset of standard visual field loss by as much as 6 years, such structural damage is evident for 60% of the subjects.[3] Hence, it is possible that current techniques are not sensitive enough to detect structural change before measurable field loss in some patients. Delineation of the earliest structural change in the peripapillary retinal nerve fibers might facilitate the diagnosis of glaucoma and improve the monitoring of progressive glaucomatous damage.

## BACKGROUND

Scanning laser polarimetry is a method that provides in vivo quantitative assessment of the peripapillary RNFL. This method is based on the assumption that the nerve fiber layer (NFL) is birefringent. The birefringence causes a change in the state of polarization of an illuminating laser beam. This change in the state of polarization, also known as retardation, can be quantitated by determining the phase shift between the extraordinary and ordinary beams, and is linearly related to the thickness and optical properties of the RNFL.[5]

Recent research has shown that the scanning laser polarimeter provides reproducible[6,7] measures of the RNFL in normal subjects which are similar to that expected from several known properties of the RNFL. These properties include:

- Peripapillary NFL is thickest in the superior and inferior arcuate regions.
- Peripapillary NFL thins with increasing distance from the ONH.
- The number of peripapillary nerve fibers decreases with increasing age.[8-10]
- Major arterioles and venules are embedded in the NFL and, hence, the NFL is thinner above blood vessels than adjacent areas.

In addition to the distribution of retardation measurements resembling several known properties of the normal NFL, differences in retardation between normal subjects and glaucoma patients[6] and normal subjects and age-matched ocular hypertensive patients[11] have been reported. Mean retardation is significantly higher in normal subjects than glaucoma and ocular hypertensive patients in the inferior and superior regions.[6,11]

## INSTRUMENTATION

The scanning laser polarimeter Nerve Fiber Analyzer ([NFA] Laser Diagnostic Technologies, San Diego, Calif) is a confocal scanning laser ophthalmoscope (CSLO) with a polarization modulator, a cornea polarization compensator, and a polarization detection unit.[12] The light source, a polarization modulated laser beam (wavelength 780 nm), is focused onto one point of the retina by the optical media of the eye. Due to the predominance of parallelism of the neurotubules of the retinal nerve fibers, the RNFL shows birefringent polarization properties that change the state of polarization (retardation) of light passing through it. The polarized light penetrates the birefringent NFL and is partially reflected from deeper layers of the retina. The light emerging from

**Figure 6-1a.** Case 1, OD. Disc photograph demonstrates RNFL defect (between arrows).

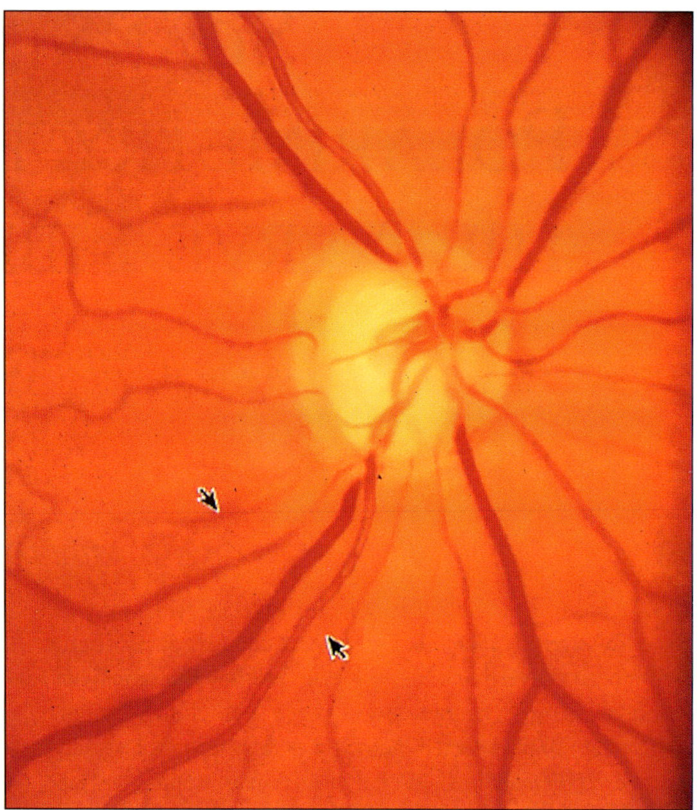

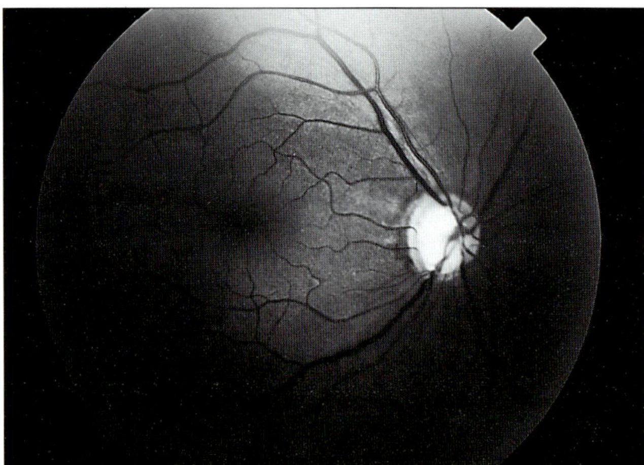

**Figure 6-1b.** NFL photograph confirms inferotemporal RNFL defect.

positions (pixels). For clinical use, we employ a field of view of approximately 15°. The time to acquire these 65,536 data sets is 0.7 seconds. During that time, a proprietary compensation device neutralizes anterior segment to isolate polarization measurements of the retina.[13] This device uses several rotating retarders constituting a variable retarder which can introduce polarization changes to the illuminating laser beam. Polarization changes are introduced such that they cancel out the polarization effects introduced by the anterior segment of the eye. In order to ascertain that the anterior segment polarization has been canceled, the specular reflection component of the light returning from the retina is maximized.

## DATA ANALYSIS

Immediately after acquiring the data, a computer algorithm calculates the amount of retardation at each measured retinal position. A retardation map describes the change in the state of polarization (retardation) at each location within the field of view. Processing time is approximately 15 seconds. The map consists of 256 by 256 pixels, and the value of each pixel represents the amount of retardation. For qualitative comparison, each pixel is color coded with yellow and white as high retardation and dark blue as low retardation. In clinical practice, we obtain three images of each eye and create a baseline image. Each case study is illustrated using the mean values of the baseline image.

the eye and collected by the instrument is separated from the illuminating light beam by a non-polarizing beamsplitter. Consequently, the polarization state of the light is analyzed by the polarization detection unit. The electrical outputs of the polarization detection unit are digitized and stored in the memory of a personal computer for later evaluation.

A scan unit deflects the illuminating laser beam to an adjacent retinal position where the above procedure is repeated. A complete scan consists of 256 by 256 individual retinal

Retardation information is obtained at user-defined distances from the disc margin and concentric with it. This disc margin is established by an operator who outlines a circle or ellipse placed around the inner margin of the peripapillary scleral ring. Retardation values along the concentric circle/ellipse are shown in an adjacent polar coordinate plot; coordinates in this plot that are further away from the circle represent higher retardation. Mean retardation along each circle is recorded in 16 equal sectors at 22.5° intervals, and transferred to an external computer for further analysis.

The following case studies describe the clinical application of RNFL assessment with the scanning laser polarimeter. They highlight both benefits and limitations of the instrument, and areas for future development and research.

## CASE STUDIES

### Case 1

A 74-year-old black female was first examined in 1987. There was no family history of glaucoma. Intraocular pressure (IOP) was uncontrolled despite maximum tolerated medical treatment. Argon laser trabeculoplasty was performed in the right eye (December 1993) and left eye (January 1994). In November 1995, her best corrected visual acuity was OD 20/25 (-0.25 +1.25 x 20) and OS 20/25 (-1.25 +3.50 x 170). IOPs were 17 mmHg in both eyes. She had open angles, grade 4 pigment in the trabecular meshwork, bilateral Krukenberg spindles, and no iris transillumination defects. Optic discs were excavated with undermining superiorly and inferiorly. There was a thin neuroretinal rim temporally in both eyes. In

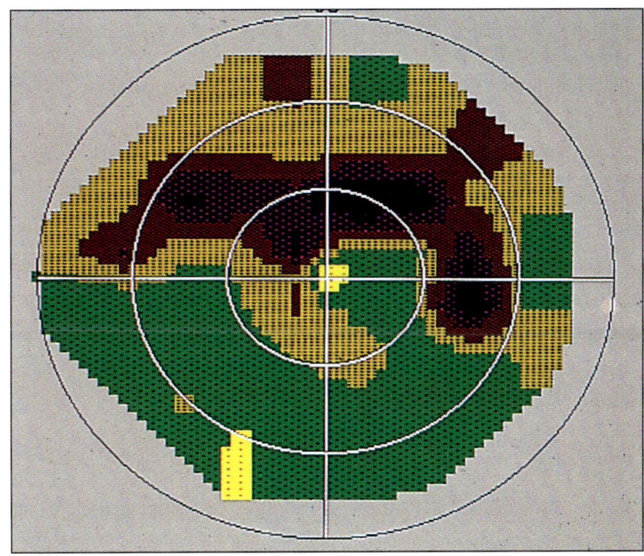

**Figure 6-1c.** Computerized visual field demonstrates superior arcuate defect.

the right eye, there was an inferotemporal NFL defect visible in the disc photograph (Figure 6-1a) and RNFL photograph (Figure 6-1b) corresponding to a superior arcuate defect in the visual field (Figure 6-1c). Scanning laser polarimetry also showed the defect clearly; in the retardation map and linear polar cross-section diagram (Figure 6-1d), the NFL defect was noted.

Comment: Qualitative and quantitative evaluation of retardation maps can identify wedge-shaped RNFL defects.

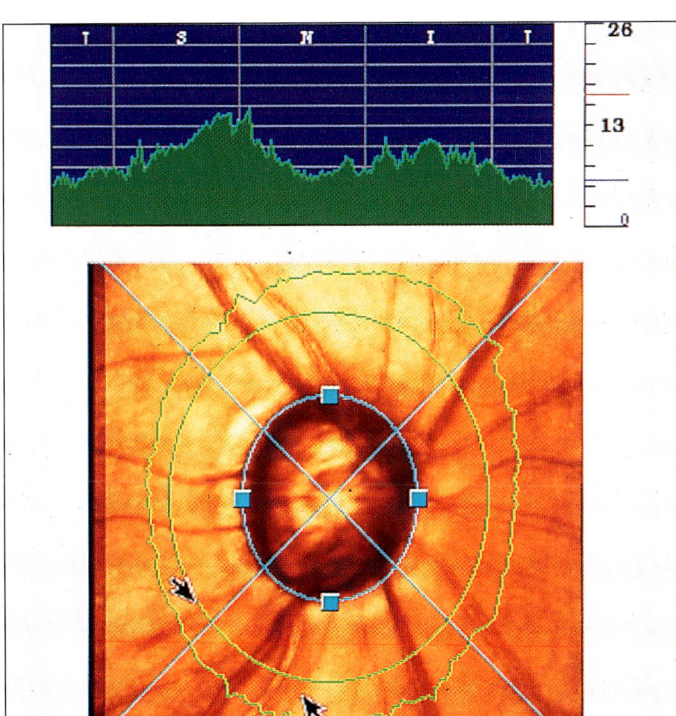

**Figure 6-1d.** Retardation in the inferior region of the linear polar cross-section diagram was lower than the superior region indicating thinning of this area. The qualitative retardation map (NFA II) documented the NFL defect (arrow). The circle diameter is 1.80 disc diameters and concentric with the disc margin. Retardation values along these points are shown in the adjacent polar coordinate plot; coordinates further away from the circle represent higher retardation.

## Case 2

A 42-year-old Japanese female with normal tension glaucoma was referred for evaluation in February 1996. Best corrected visual acuity was OD 20/20 (-4.25 +0.50 x 50) and OS 20/20 (-3.25 +1.00 x 79). Angles were wide open. IOPs were OD 15 mmHg and OS 16 mmHg in the early morning and slit lamp examination of both eyes was within normal limits. Optic discs of both eyes were tilted, excavated with almost no rim temporally and inferiorly. The right eye had an optic disc hemorrhage corresponding to an inferotemporal wedge-shaped RNFL defect (Figure 6-2a). Scanning laser polarimetry of the right eye showed inferior wedge-shaped RNFL defect and low retardation inferiorly, as emphasized by the polar cross-section diagram (Figure 6-2b).

Comment: This case illustrates the use of quantitative measurements to identify regional low retardation. The wedge-shaped RNFL defect is visible on the disc photograph and scanning laser polarimetry retardation map. The defect on the retardation map is not contiguous with the optic disc margin as it is on the disc photograph. This may be due to peripapillary atrophy with visible sclera in the inferior region and/or the RNFL hemorrhage. The sclera is brightly reflecting and may cause local artifacts in the retardation map.

## Case 3

A 39-year-old white female with a prominent family history of glaucoma was diagnosed with primary open-angle glaucoma approximately 19 years prior to her evaluation in August 1993. Visual acuity was OD 20/20 (-5.50 sph) and OS 20/20 (-6.50 +1.25 x 180). Gonioscopy showed wide open angles and IOPs were OD 26 mmHg and OS 31 mmHg on maximum tolerated medication. Slit lamp examination was within normal limits for both eyes. Discs appeared excavated with temporal thinning of rim and no notching or hemorrhages (Figure 6-3a). Visual fields (December 1993) showed OD inferior arcuate defect (Figure 6-3b) (values represent sensitivity loss compared to normal age-matched subjects) and OS large inferior and small superior arcuate defects. Scanning laser polarimetry (Figure 6-3c) of the right eye detected a normal-looking retardation map with higher retardation superiorly and inferiorly. A NFL photograph showed diffuse and focal (inferior greater than superior) thinning (Figure 6-3d). The patient underwent laser trabeculoplasty OS on January and July 1994. In January 1995, IOPs were OD 42 mmHg and OS 24 mmHg. There was progression of disc excavation and rim thinning in OD compared with 1993 (Figure 6-3e) and a general reduction in visual field sensitivity (Figure 6-3f). The 1995 retardation map showed reduced retardation compared to 1993 (Figure 6-3g). Comparison between the two diagrams indicated thinning of NFL in the superior region (sectors 40 to 130) and inferior region (sectors 230 to 300) (Figure 6-3h).

Comment: Changes in the optic nerve with corresponding progression in the visual fields can be detected as reduced retardation with scanning laser polarimetry.

## Case 4

A 19-year-old female developed glaucomatous optic neuropathy after steroid treatment for papillary conjunctivitis. In July 1995, visual acuity was OD 20/40 (-6.25 +1.00 x 180) and OS 20/20 (-6.25 +1.00 x 105). Her angles were wide open and IOPs were OD 30 mmHg and OS 32 mmHg on acetazolamide, timolol, and pilocarpine. Slit lamp examination of both eyes was within normal limits. Optic discs were excavated with temporal thinning of rim and peripapillary atrophy (Figure 6-4a). Visual fields had OD superior and inferior nasal depression (Figure 6-4b) and OS superonasal depression with indices and glaucoma hemifield test outside normal limits. One month later, at baseline, retardation appeared as a depressed double-hump pattern which indicated the possibility of diffuse loss in the superior and inferior regions (Figure 6-4c). High IOP persisted and, despite maximum tolerated medication, progressive visual field loss was observed. She underwent laser trabeculoplasty in October and trabeculotomy OS in December 1995. In February 1996, IOPs were OD 43 mmHg and OS 12 mmHg; photographs (Figure 6-4d) showed progressive excavation with thinning of the rim in the disc of the right eye. NFL photograph was consistent with diffuse loss (Figure 6-4e). Visual fields were progressively worse in the right eye, with larger and deeper superior and inferior arcuate defects (Figure 6-4f). Scanning laser polarimetry showed decreased retardation indicating thinning of the NFL (Figure 6-4g). The comparison graph of retardation ratio between the two polar cross-section diagrams indicated NFL loss (Figure 6-4h). The patient underwent trabeculotomy on OD 1 week later.

Comment: Scanning laser polarimeter detected change over a period of 6 months. It is not possible at this time to assess whether the visual field, stereophotograph, or retardation map showed the progression first. In addition, the ability to differentiate a normal-looking retardation map, as seen at the initial visit, from diffuse loss is not possible yet. A normative database is under development which may help identify RNFL loss from retardation maps.

## DISCUSSION

The scanning laser polarimeter employs a CSLO to detect, digitize, and display as a video image light reflected from the retina at each point of a two-dimensional scan with an illuminating laser beam. In the described glaucoma cases, thinning of the RNFL was detected using the retardation maps obtained with the scanning laser polarimeter. Cases 1

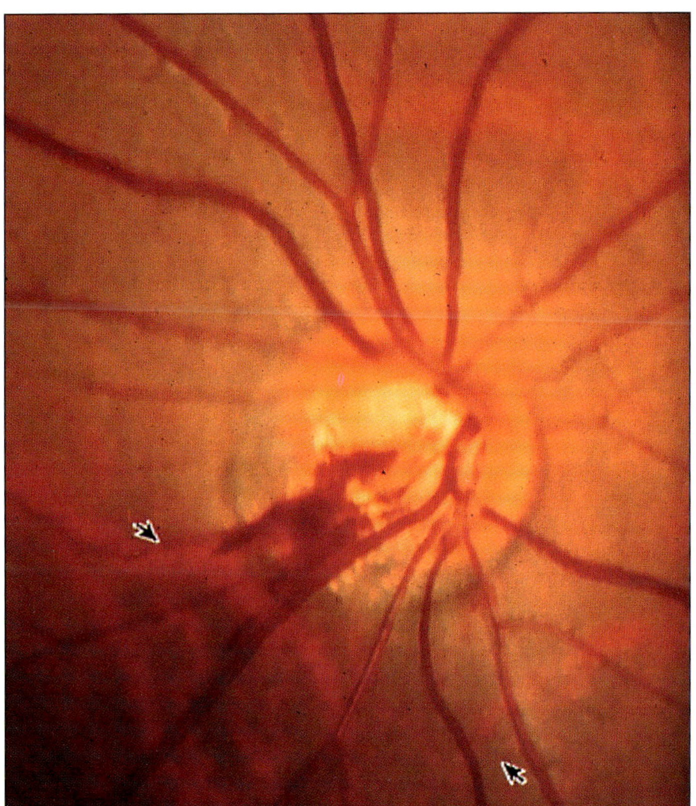

**Figure 6-2a.** Case 2, OD. Fundus photograph demonstrates an optic disc hemorrhage corresponding to the RNFL defect (between arrows).

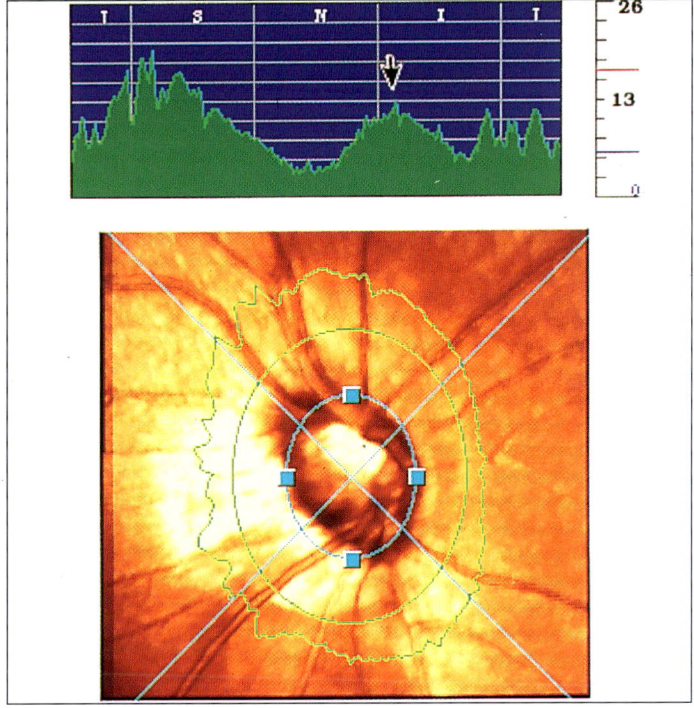

**Figure 6-2b.** An inferior wedge-shaped defect was detected in the retardation map and linear polar cross-section diagram (arrow) (NFA II). The RNFL defect could not be traced to the disc margin probably because of the high reflectivity of the peripapillary atrophy area.

and 2 illustrate that RNFL defects detected with photography also are visible qualitatively and quantitatively with polarimetry. The ability of this technique to detect change over time was illustrated with Cases 3 and 4.

In order for a new instrument to be accepted and imple-mented into clinical practice, it must be superior to existing instruments in clinically relevant ways. One advantage of the scanning laser polarimeter is that it provides real-time measures of the RNFL with reduced need for pupil dilation and clear media. Unlike photography, which requires an oph-

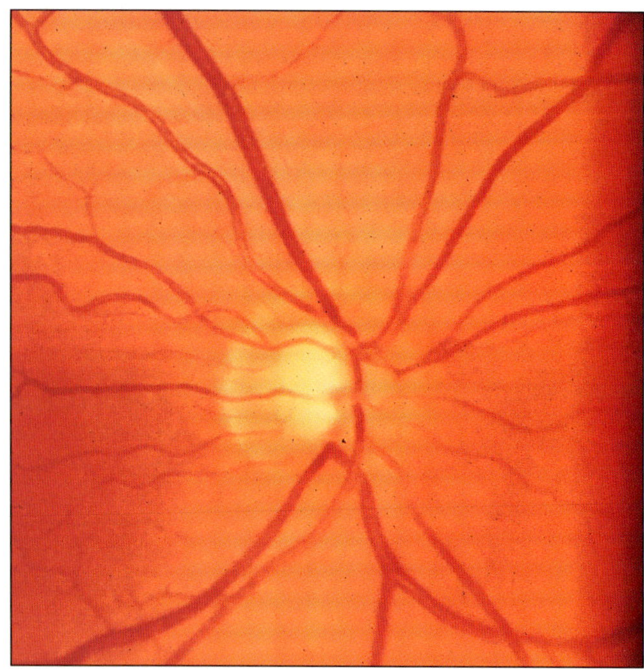

**Figure 6-3a.** Case 3. Fundus photograph demonstrates optic disc excavation and temporal thinning of rim (1993).

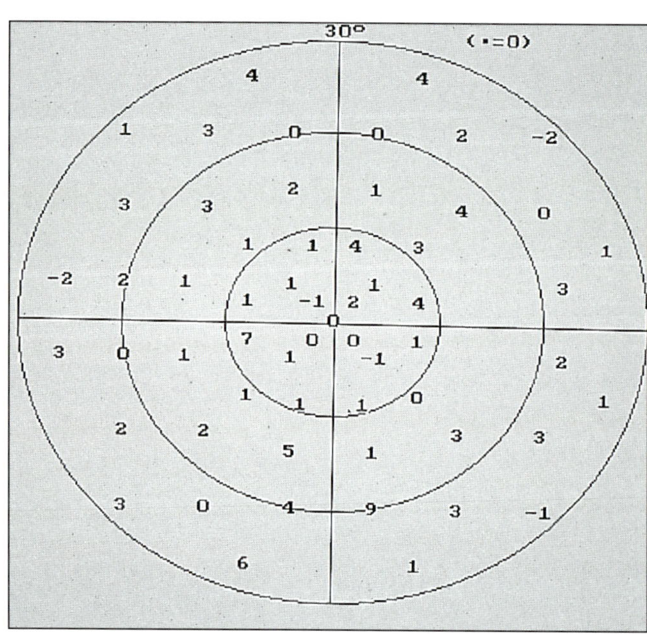

**Figure 6-3b.** Computerized visual field indicates inferior arcuate defect (1993) (values represent sensitivity loss compared to age-matched normal subjects).

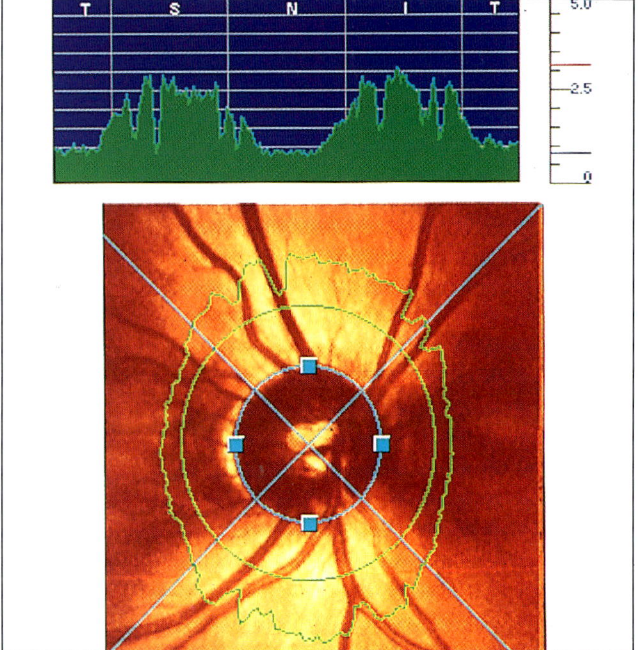

**Figure 6-3c.** Qualitative retardation map and linear polar cross-section diagram do not demonstrate a detectable defect (1993).

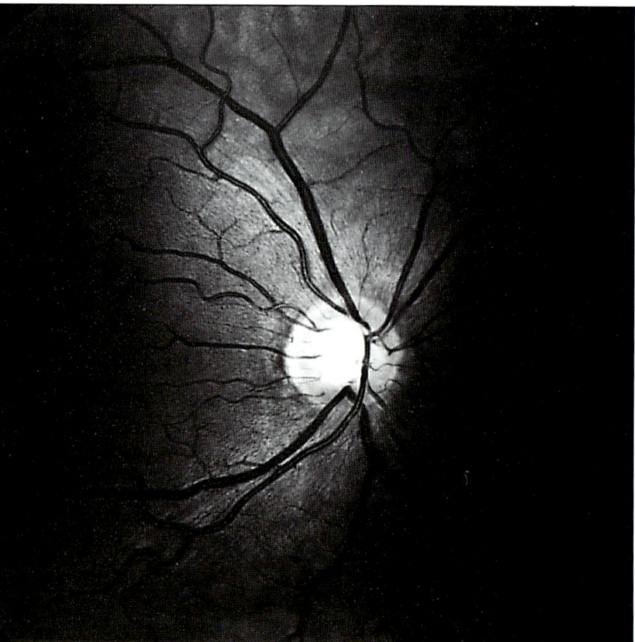

**Figure 6-3d.** NFL photograph demonstrates diffuse and focal loss of nerve fibers (1993).

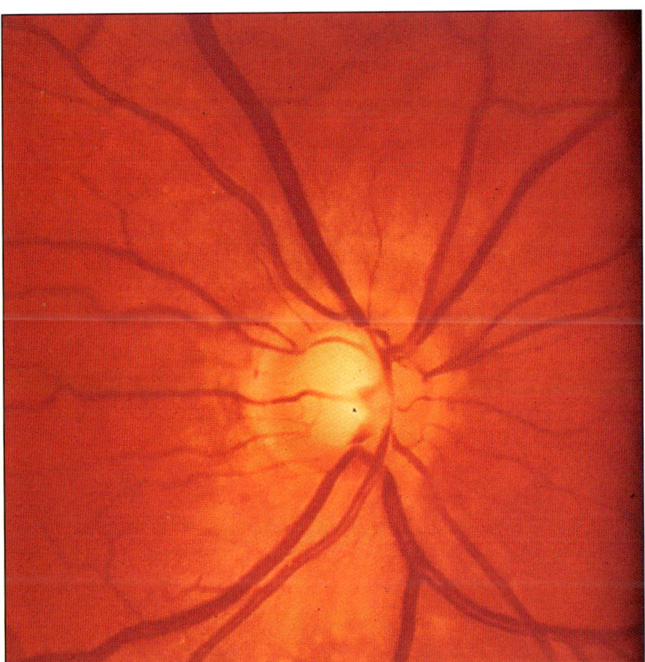

**Figure 6-3e.** Optic disc photograph demonstrates progression of excavation and rim thinning (1995).

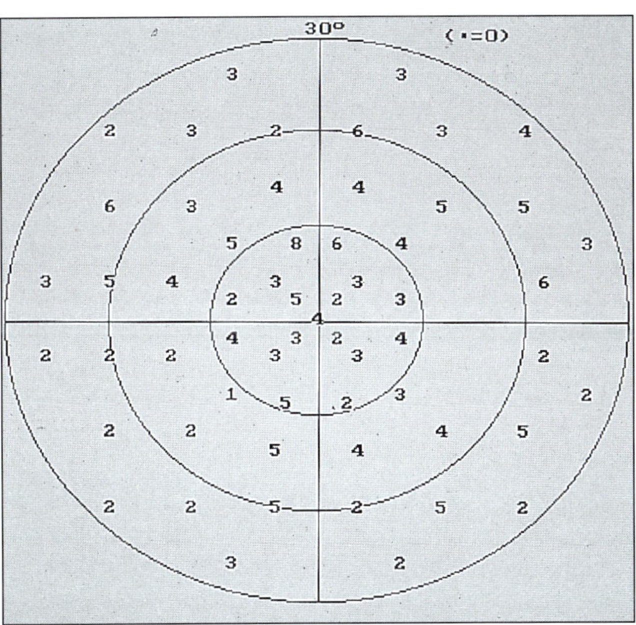

**Figure 6-3f.** Computerized visual field indicates general reduction of sensitivity (1995).

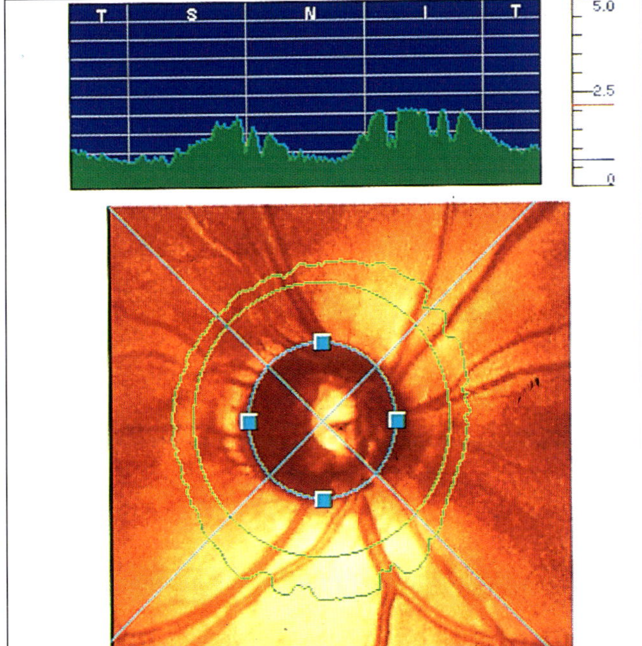

**Figure 6-3g.** A depressed double-hump pattern in the 1995 linear polar cross-section diagram (NFA I) indicates progression from that of 1993. The polar coordinate plot also shows decrease in NFL thickness.

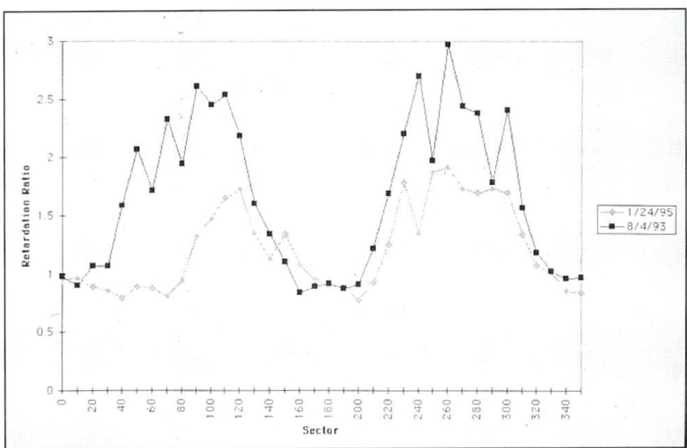

**Figure 6-3h.** In the comparison graph of retardation ratio, difference between the two polar cross-section diagrams indicates NFL loss between 1993 and 1995. With 0° as temporal, with thicker NFL superiorly (approximately 90°) and inferiorly (approximately 180°). Retardation is measured in degrees within a 10-pixel-width ring concentric with the disc margin and at 1.75 disc diameters. The ratio of mean global and regional (superior or inferior) retardation in a segment from 350° to 356° is calculated between 1.5 to 2.0 disc diameters with the existing software (version 2.1.03 of NFA I). The retardation ratio is used in this case to standardize the measures and reduce the influence of optic disc size and operator input.

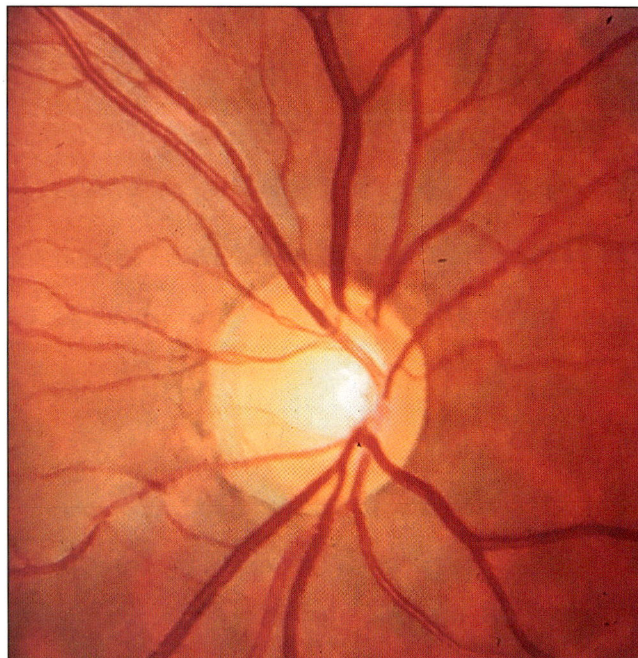

**Figure 6-4a.** Case 4. Fundus photograph shows disc excavation, temporal thinning of rim, and peripapillary atrophy (1995).

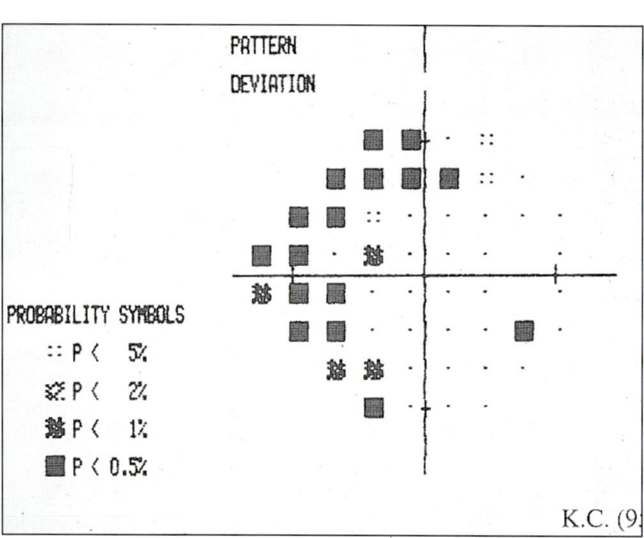


**Figure 6-4b.** Computerized visual field demonstrates superior and inferior nasal depression (1995).

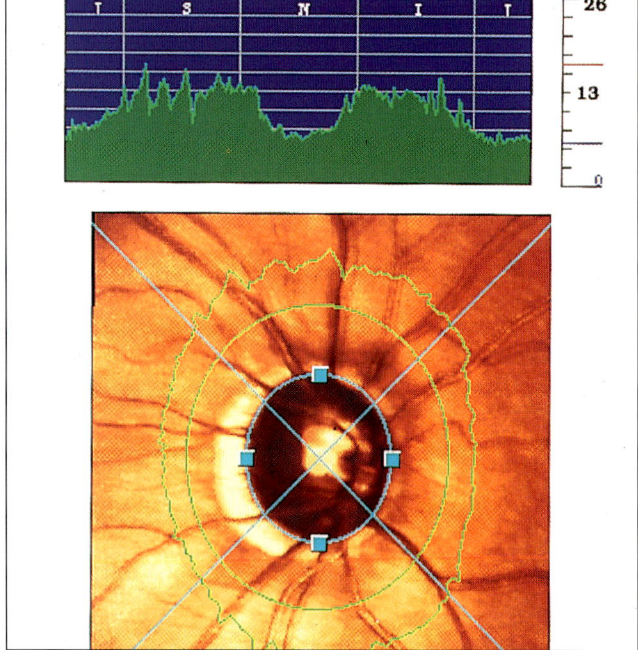


**Figure 6-4c.** Retardation (NFA II) appears as a double-hump pattern with the possibility of diffuse loss (1995).

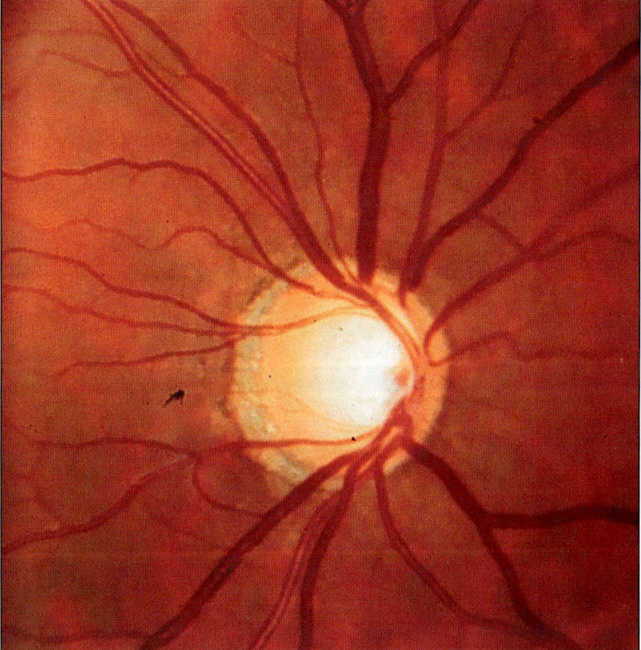

**Figure 6-4d.** The optic disc is more excavated with rim thinning (1996).

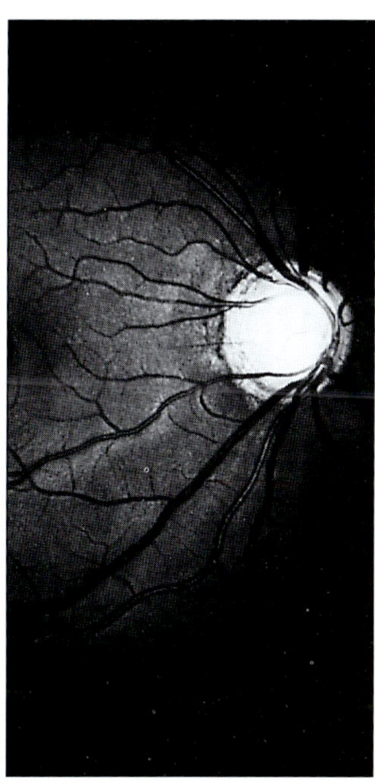

**Figure 6-4e.** NFL photograph consistent with diffuse loss (1996).

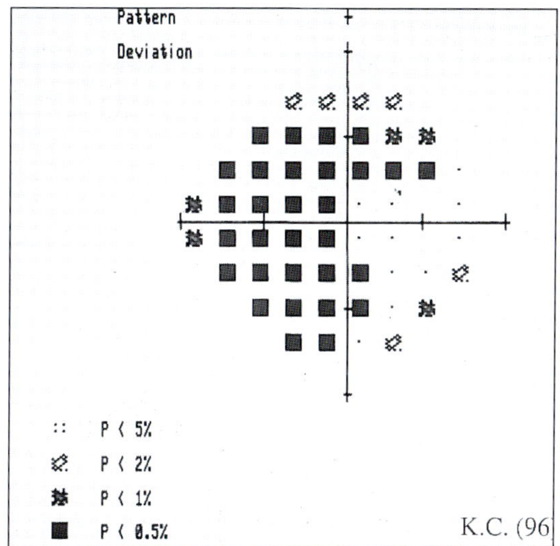


**Figure 6-4f.** Computerized visual field demonstrates larger and deeper superior and inferior arcuate defects.

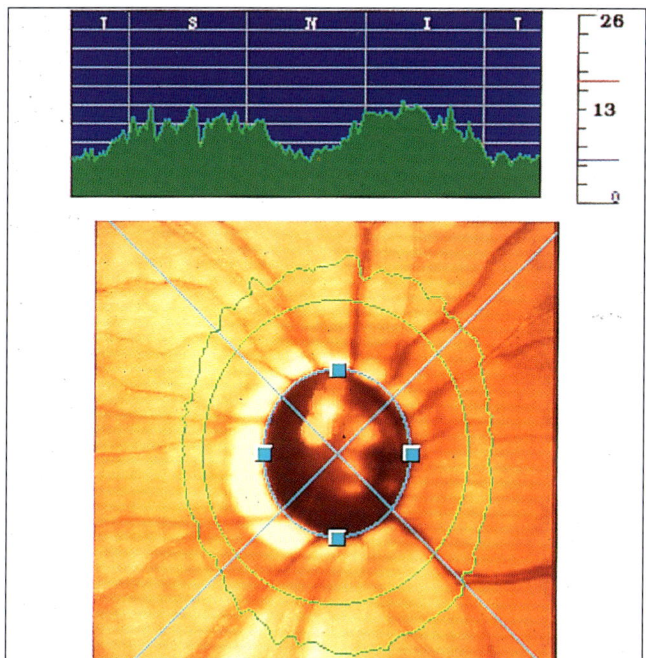

**Figure 6-4g.** Decrease in the double-hump retardation pattern indicates loss of nerve fibers (1996). The polar coordinate plot also shows progression from the previous one.

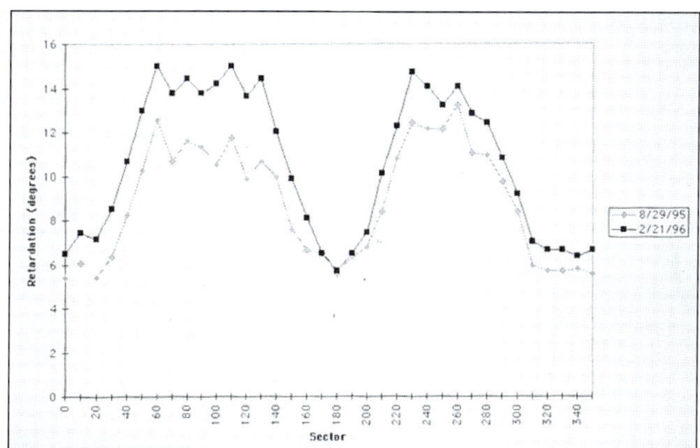


**Figure 6-4h.** Comparison between the two retardation diagrams indicates thinning of NFL from 1995 to 1996. With 0° as temporal, higher retardation is seen superiorly and inferiorly.

thalmic photographer, film, and processing time, the scanning laser polarimeter allows assessment of the retinal nerve layer during the clinic visit. Compared with other methods for indirectly evaluating the NFL, measurement of retardation has other advantages. First, it is not based on optical imaging principles; therefore, the resulting measurements do not have magnification errors. Second, a reference plane is not required. It should be noted that retardation is a measure of relative, not absolute, NFL thickness. Although this instrument shows promise, longitudinal studies are needed to determine whether these quantitative measurements will improve our ability to detect glaucoma and monitor its progression.

The basis for describing our measurements in retardation units rather than microns relates to an earlier study in which we validated the technique. Another device, a retinal ellipsometer, was implemented to measure retardation.[14] In two monkey retinas from hemisected eyes in which the cornea and lens were removed, there was an excellent correlation between retardation and the histopathologic measurement of RNFL thickness.[14] It is unclear whether correlation between retardation and histopathologic measurement will be as strong in clinical use with the current scanning laser polarimeter. In addition, since accuracy and completeness of compensation for anterior segment birefringence directly influences retardation measurements, information is needed on how cataract, lens implants, and corneal changes effect these measurements. Histopathologic studies also are needed to determine how well retardation values obtained with the scanning laser polarimeter correlate directly with RNFL thickness. Hence, we present our results in units of retardation rather than microns. Regardless, these measures often appear to be clinically relevant for monitoring change in RNFL over time.

These cases highlight other issues that need to be addressed before this technique can be fully implemented into clinical practice. Spurious measurements of retardation are observed in some eyes, particularly in areas of peripapillary atrophy with visible sclera in which retardation is uniformly high.[6] Similar high values also have been observed in areas of chorioretinal scars in which sclera is visible. We speculate that such values are artifacts and are related to the high reflectivity of the sclera in these locations. The NFA II includes changes to minimize these artifacts, but Cases 3 and 4 indicate that high retardation values are visible still in areas of peripapillary atrophy of some eyes. Also, retardation artifacts appear to be present immediately adjacent to the disk margin. We speculate that these may be related to the sloping course of the nerve fibers around the disk margin which caus-

es reflected light to be scattered away from the incident beam. These artifacts near the disc margin may limit the ability to qualitatively detect a wedge-shaped RNFL defect that fans out from the disc margin. All quantitative measurements, however, are routinely obtained in the peripapillary retina, where these artifacts are uncommon.

Glaucomatous damage results in retinal ganglion cell axonal loss with thinning of the RNFL. With scanning laser polarimetry, it may be possible to improve our ability to detect NFL change to monitor glaucomatous progression.

## REFERENCES

1. Airaksinen PJ, Alanko HI. Effect of retinal nerve fiber loss on the optic nerve head configuration in early glaucoma. *Graefes Arch Clin Exp Ophthalmol.* 1983;220:193-196.

2. Tuulonen A, Lehtola J, Airaksinen PJ. Nerve fiber layer defects with normal visual fields. Do normal optic disc and normal visual field indicate absence of glaucomatous abnormality? *Ophthalmology.* 1993;109:77-83.

3. Sommer A, Katz J, Quigley HA, et al. Clinical detectable nerve fiber atrophy precedes the onset of glaucomatous field loss. *Arch Ophthalmol.* 1991;109:77-83.

4. Quigley HA, Enger C, Katz J, et al. Risk factors for the development of glaucomatous visual field loss in ocular hypertension. *Arch Ophthalmol.* 1994;112:644-649.

5. Dreher AW, Reiter K, Weinreb RN. Spatially resolved birefringence of the retinal nerve fiber layer assessed with a retinal laser ellipsometer. *Applied Optics.* 1992;31:3730-3735.

6. Weinreb RN, Shakiba S, Zangwill L. Scanning laser polarimetry to measure the nerve fiber layer of normal and glaucomatous eyes. *Am J Ophthalmol.* 1995;119:627-636.

7. Chi Q, Tomita G, Inazumi K, Hayakawa T, Tadayoshi I, Kitazawa Y. Evaluation of the effect of aging on the retinal nerve fiber layer thickness using scanning laser polarimetry. *J Glaucoma.* 1995;4:406-413.

8. Mikelberg FS, Drance SM, Schulzer M, Yidegiligne HM, Weis MM. The normal human optic nerve. Axon count and axon diameter distribution. *Ophthalmology.* 1989;96:1325-1328.

9. Mikelberg FS, Yidegiligne HM, White VA, Schulzer M. Relation between optic nerve axon number and axon diameter to scleral canal area. *Ophthalmology.* 1991;98:60-63.

10. Jonas JB, Schmidt AM, Muller-Bergh JA, Schlotzer-Schrehardt UM, Naumann GO. Human optic nerve fiber count and optic disc size. *Invest Ophthalmol Vis Sci.* 1992;33:2012-2018.

11. Anton A, Zangwill L, Emdadi A, Weinreb RN. Nerve fiber layer measurements with scanning laser polarimetry in ocular hypertension. *Arch Ophthalmol.* In press.

12. Dreher AW, Reiter K. Scanning laser polarimetry of the retina nerve fiber layer. *SPIE Proceedings.* 1992;1746:34-38.

13. Dreher AW, Reiter KR. Retinal laser ellipsometry: a new method for measuring the retinal nerve fiber layer thickness distribution. *Clin Vision Sci.* 1992;7:481-488.

14. Weinreb RN, Dreher AW, Coleman A, Quigley H, Shaw B, Reiter K. Histopathologic validation of Fourier-ellipsometry measurements of retinal nerve fiber layer thickness. *Arch Ophthalmol.* 1990;108:557-560.

# Optical Coherence Tomography for Imaging and Quantitation of Nerve Fiber Layer Thickness

*Joel S. Schuman, MD*

## INTRODUCTION

Optical Coherence Tomography (OCT) is a new technology that permits high resolution cross-sectional imaging of biological tissue using light. OCT utilizes interferometry and near infrared, low coherence light to achieve a resolution of approximately 10 microns in the eye.[1-10] OCT enables non-contact and non-invasive imaging of the optic nerve head (ONH) and nerve fiber layer (NFL).[1-5] Like CT scanning, which uses X-rays, magnetic resonance imaging (MRI), which uses electron spin resonance, and ultrasound B mode imaging, which uses soundwaves, OCT produces cross-sectional images of tissue, but unlike the above technologies, OCT uses light to perform optical ranging and imaging, and thereby achieves a significantly higher resolution than CT, MRI, or ultrasound. A transverse sequence of longitudinal optical ranging measurements is used to construct a false color tomographic image of tissue microstructure, which appears remarkably similar to histologic section.

In the evaluation of glaucoma, OCT is used to create cylindrical sections of the retina around the optic nerve. A circle diameter of 3.4 mm is scanned for this purpose; the circular scan results in the cylindrical retinal cross-section. This circle size was chosen after studies revealed that a 3.4-mm circle produced reproducible data,[11] with most of the retina composed of NFL at this distance from the ONH, but that the circle diameter was large enough to avoid the edge of the ONH and peripapillary atrophy in nearly all discs.[4] This cylinder is unfolded, analogous to a Mercator projection of the Earth, to allow analysis of the cross-sectional data.

OCT is therefore a means of both imaging the NFL and directly quantitating NFL thickness.[4,11] The cross-sectional image of the retina is examined for focal NFL defects, localized regions of NFL attenuation, and diffuse NFL atrophy. NFL thickness is quantitated by an automated computer algorithm that identifies the anterior and posterior borders of the NFL, and the data are summarized by clock hour, quadrant, and overall.

This chapter describes the technology of OCT, the correlation between OCT and conventional clinical parameters, the reproducibility of OCT measurements, the results of a longitudinal study of experimental glaucoma in monkeys tracked with OCT, and the current and potential clinical applications of the device in glaucoma.

## TECHNOLOGY

The OCT device is manufactured by Humphrey Instruments (San Leandro, Calif); however, the images in this chapter and the studies described herein were performed prior to the introduction of the Humphrey instrument with a prototype system which has been described previously.[1-13] The development of this system is the result of a collaborative effort between basic scientists and clinicians at New England Eye Center, Massachusetts Institute of Technology, and Lincoln Laboratories.

The prototype device (Figure 7-1) is a fiberoptic delivery system which couples the OCT unit with a slit lamp biomicroscope for in vivo tomography of the retina. Computer-driven galvanometric scanners permit manipulation of the beam

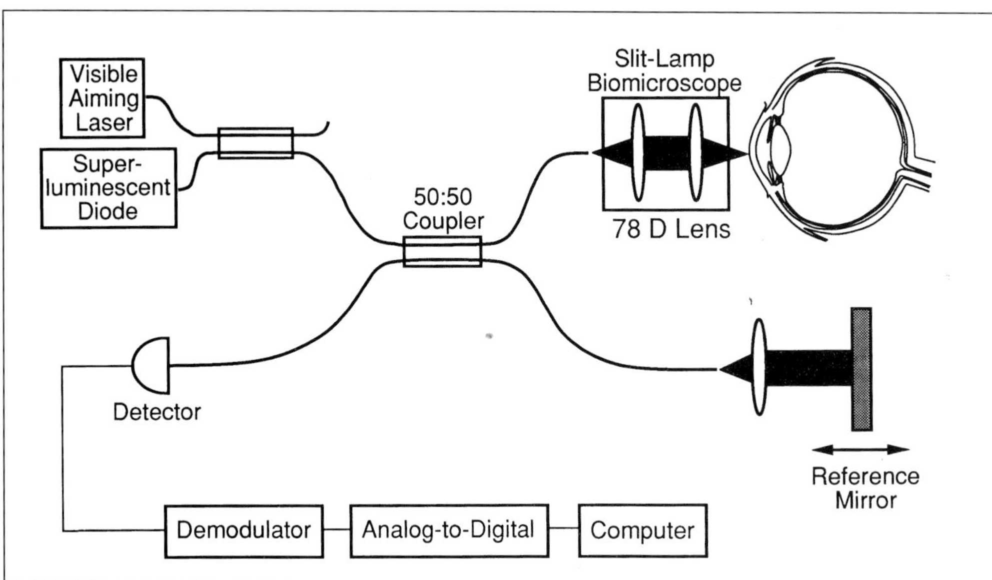



**Figure 7-1.** Schematic diagram of the high-speed, fiberoptic OCT scanner. Axial profiles of backscattering within biological tissue were measured by translating the reference mirror and recording the interferometric signal. The axial resolution was determined by the coherence length of the superluminescent diode (SLD) source and was 10 microns (FWHM) inside the eye. Reprinted from Schuman JS, Hee MR, Puliafito CA, et al. Quantification of nerve fiber layer thickness in normal and glaucomatous eyes using optical coherence tomography: a pilot study. *Arch Ophthalmol.* 1995;113:586-596. Copyrighted 1995, American Medical Association.

directed into the eye. The beam passes through a 78 D Volk lens for indirect imaging, and the beam focus is coincident with the slit lamp image plane, which allows visualization of the eye with a near-infrared CCD camera while scanning. The tomogram is displayed in real time on a computer monitor, and the video image is similarly shown on a separate video display.

The prototype OCT system acquires a typical 3-mm deep by 100 axial scan wide image in under 2.5 seconds. The commercial system will capture the same image in under 1 second. The axial resolution of the OCT system was experimentally shown to be 14 microns in air by measurement of the full width at half maximum (FWHM) of the reflection obtained by imaging a mirror placed in the image plane of the slit lamp biomicroscope. This measurement predicts a FWHM resolution of 10 microns in the retina due to the difference in refractive index between air and tissue. The actual ability of the instrument to distinguish between two closely spaced structures might be expected to be better than this figure when locating structures with high contrast (eg, the vitreoretinal interface), or worse when identifying closely placed structures with similar reflectivities (eg, the retinal pigment epithelium [RPE] and the choriocapillaris). The lateral resolution is determined by the larger of the beam waist diameter in the retina, or the sampling distance between adjacent transverse pixels in the tomogram. The beam spot diameter in the retina employed for glaucoma investigations with this prototype instrument is approximately 13 microns as computed

from the Gullstrand reduced schematic eye. A typical 3.4-mm diameter circular tomogram contains 100 axial scans spaced approximately 110 microns apart.

Images are corrected for artifacts due to involuntary subject motion during data acquisition using a standard image processing technique of cross-correlation scan registration.[5] An image processing computer program was written to quantitate total retinal thickness and retinal nerve fiber layer (RNFL) thickness for the cylindrical OCT sections obtained by circular scanning around the ONH. After subject motion in the longitudinal direction is corrected with the cross-correlation scan registration technique, a digital filter is applied to smooth the tomograms and reduce image speckle noise. Smoothing is accomplished by first applying a median filter to remove extreme values of reflectivity in the image. Two-dimensional linear convolution with a center-weighted kernel is then employed to reduce remaining speckle variations.

Retinal thickness is quantitated by computer for each axial scan in the image as the distance between the first reflection at the vitreoretinal interface and the anterior boundary of the red, reflective layer corresponding to the RPE and choriocapillaris. NFL thickness is also automatically determined by computer. The NFL is assumed to be correlated with the extent of the red, highly reflective layer at the vitreoretinal interface. Boundaries are located by searching for the first points on each scan where the reflectivities exceed a certain threshold. For example, the inner limiting membrane is located by starting anteriorly and searching posteriorly in the image. The posterior margin of the NFL is located by starting within the photoreceptor layer (posteriorly) and searching anteriorly in the image. The RPE is similarly located by starting within the photoreceptor layer and searching posteriorly in the image. The location of the photoreceptor layer is assumed to lie at the position of minimum reflectivity within the neurosensory retina.

Thresholds are separately determined by the computer for each axial scan in the image as two thirds of the maximum reflectivity in each smoothed axial scan evaluated on a logarithmic scale. Linear interpolation is performed to remove gaps in the boundaries resulting from shadowing due to blood vessels. The boundaries chosen by the computer are then overlaid on a false color display of each image. The NFL and RPE boundaries are highlighted with a blue line, and the superficial surface of the retina is denoted with a white line.

Retinal and NFL thicknesses are reported as averages over each quadrant (superior, inferior, temporal, nasal), as averages for each clock hour, and as averages over the entire cylindrical section. Thicknesses can be displayed individually for each axial scan as well.[11]

## CORRELATION BETWEEN OCT AND CONVENTIONAL CLINICAL PARAMETERS

Quantitative measurements made with OCT of NFL thickness correlate well with clinical parameters such as visual fields[4] and NFL appearance.[14] In a normal eye, as shown in Figures 7-2 through 7-3b, the NFL is thickest superiorly and inferiorly, and the thicker areas are shifted slightly temporally. In a glaucomatous eye, NFL is thinner in areas corresponding to visual field loss and cupping.[4] In an eye with a superior arcuate scotoma, as illustrated in Figures 7-4a through 7-4c, the NFL is thinned inferiorly. This NFL attenuation is seen on the OCT image, and is quantitated both by quadrant and by clock hour.

Focal NFL defects can be demonstrated by OCT, and also correspond to areas of visual field loss. Figures 7-5a through 7-5d show an individual with an inferior temporal focal arcuate NFL defect and a superior paracentral scotoma on Humphrey visual field testing. The OCT demonstrates an area of focal NFL thinning in the region of the clinically apparent NFL defect.

Figures 7-6a through 7-6d illustrate an individual with two focal NFL defects, one inferiorly and a denser NFL defect superiorly. These can be seen on the NFL photograph, and match areas of abnormality on the Humphrey visual field. There is a dense inferonasal step, extending to an inferior paracentral scotoma, and a superior arcuate scotoma as well. On OCT, the NFL defects appear as localized areas of

NFL attenuation. These images are reproducible, and can be followed for change over time.

Figures 7-7a through 7-7h exhibit an individual whose glaucoma progressed over time. In the initial study, this patient had significantly less visual field loss than on follow-up, but his stereoscopic ONH photographs and NFL photographs appear similar. OCT reveals thinning of the NFL over time. OCT of the ONH also demonstrates thinning of the neuroretinal rim, but this was found to be a much less sensitive parameter for glaucoma evaluation than NFL thickness.[4]

Figures 7-8a through 7-8c show a patient with end-stage glaucoma. There is almost total cupping of the ONH, with only a small, central island of visual field remaining. Dramatic global attenuation of the NFL is evident on OCT.

OCT shows a statistically significant difference in NFL thickness between normal and glaucomatous eyes, particularly in the inferior quadrant (Figure 7-9).[4] While there is substantial overlap between the two groups, this may be due to the small number of normal eyes in this pilot study or to the fact that the groups were not matched for age.[4] This is relevant in that NFL thickness, measured by both OCT[4] and polarimetry,[15] decreases with aging (Figures 7-10a through 7-10c), but there is no significant change in cup-to-disc ratio or neuroretinal rim area with age.[4,16-18] OCT supports the findings of Hoyt and Newman,[19] Quigley,[20] and Sommer[21,22] that NFL thickness has a closer relationship to glaucoma status and visual function than does the appearance of the ONH.

The clinically important finding with regard to OCT measurements of NFL thickness in these eyes is that OCT may be able to differentiate between normal and glaucomatous eyes, once a normative database is developed, similar to the way in which automated perimetry is capable of separating normal from glaucoma with the use of computerized statistical programming; however, OCT would be expected to have much higher sensitivity and specificity than perimetry. In the future, we may use OCT to determine structurally, quantitatively, and objectively whether or not glaucoma is present or has progressed, even without functional testing (eg, visual fields). At the present, however, OCT remains a tremendously useful adjunct in the assessment of glaucoma.

## REPRODUCIBILITY

An important test for any new diagnostic technology is whether or not its measurements can be made reproducibly. Such studies of OCT portray the fact that NFL can be reproducibly measured using this device.[11] A series of measurements were made on 21 eyes of 21 subjects, 10 with glaucoma and 11 normals. Each subject had five repetitions of a series of scans on five separate occasions within a 1-month period. Each series consisted of three circular scans around

**Figure 7-2.** Stereoscopic ONH photograph (Nidek $3D_x$, Nidek Technologies, Inc, Pasadena, Calif) from a normal eye.

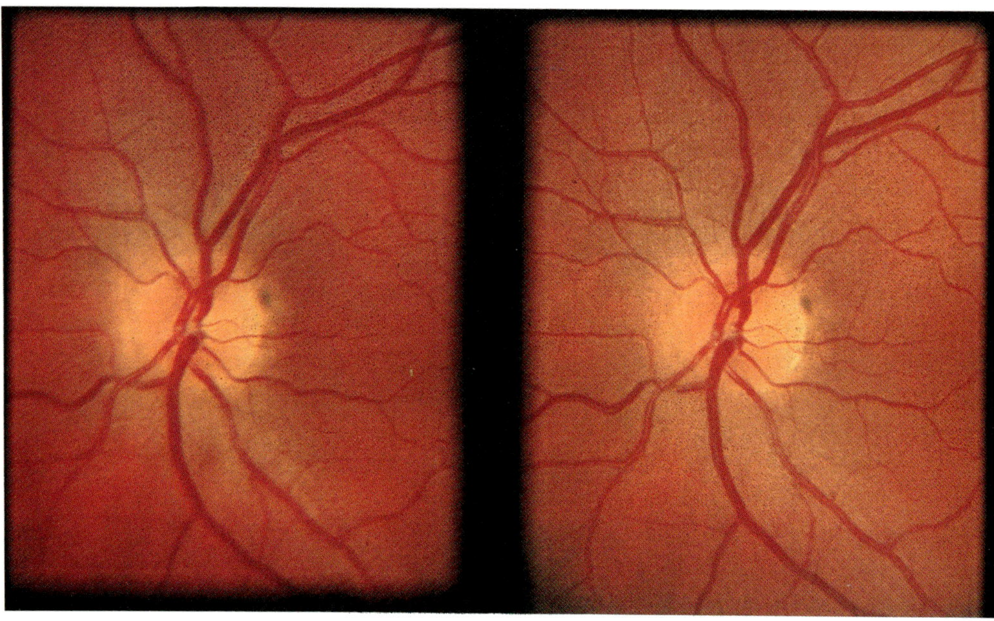

the ONH (circle diameters were 2.9, 3.4, and 4.5 mm). Each series was performed using internal and external fixation techniques. Internal fixation meant that the eye being studied fixated on an internal beam that could be offset a measured transverse distance from the scanning circle. This offset was recorded in the subject's computer log, and was then recalled for each subsequent scan. External fixation meant that the slit lamp fixation target was used for fixation with the contralateral eye. The eye studied and the sequence of testing were randomly assigned.[11]

Internal fixation provides a slightly higher degree of reproducibility than external fixation.[11] This may be due to the fact that the offset between the fixation target and the scanning circle was exactly the same for each scan with internal fixation, while external fixation required operator placement of the scanning circle centered on the ONH for each scan.

Reproducibility is better in a given eye on a given visit than from visit to visit.[11] While the difference between intervisit variability and intravisit variability is small, it is statistically significant. There is little practical clinical application to this finding, except that while a measurement made one day can be very closely reproduced on a subsequent visit, it can be reproduced even more closely on the same visit.

Reproducibility is higher with circle diameter 3.4 mm than with either 2.9 or 4.5 mm.[11] Because of this finding, and the fact that internal fixation provided slightly more reproducible results than external fixation, even given a skilled technician, OCT is now routinely performed using internal fixation at a circle diameter of 3.4 mm.

One way of measuring reproducibility is by examining the standard deviation of measurements. The standard deviation of OCT NFL thickness measurements is on the order of 10 to 20 microns for mean overall NFL thickness, 15 to 30 microns for each clock hour.[11] Another method is to use the intraclass correlation coefficient, which is over 0.50 for nearly all circle diameters, using internal fixation.[11]

## EXPERIMENTAL GLAUCOMA

To determine whether or not OCT could track NFL thickness changes over time, we created an accelerated model of glaucoma by elevating intraocular pressure (IOP) in one eye of each of seven cynomolgus monkeys after establishment of stable baseline IOP. This model was initially described by Gaasterland and Kupfer[23] and Quigley and Holman.[24] We then followed both eyes of each monkey, examining them at least weekly, for a mean of 14 weeks, measuring IOP, performing slit lamp biomicroscopy, taking NFL and stereoscopic ONH photographs, and obtaining OCT.[25,26] Five of seven treated eyes developed a sustained IOP elevation.[26]

At baseline, the ONH and NFL in both treated and control eyes appeared healthy. At termination, the control ONH and NFL continued to look well, while the treated eyes clinically had severe cupping and NFL loss. While the baseline IOPs were the same in both groups, the final pressures were highly statistically different, with the laser treated eyes having a mean IOP of $31\pm1$ mmHg, and the control eyes $17\pm1$ mmHg.[25,26]

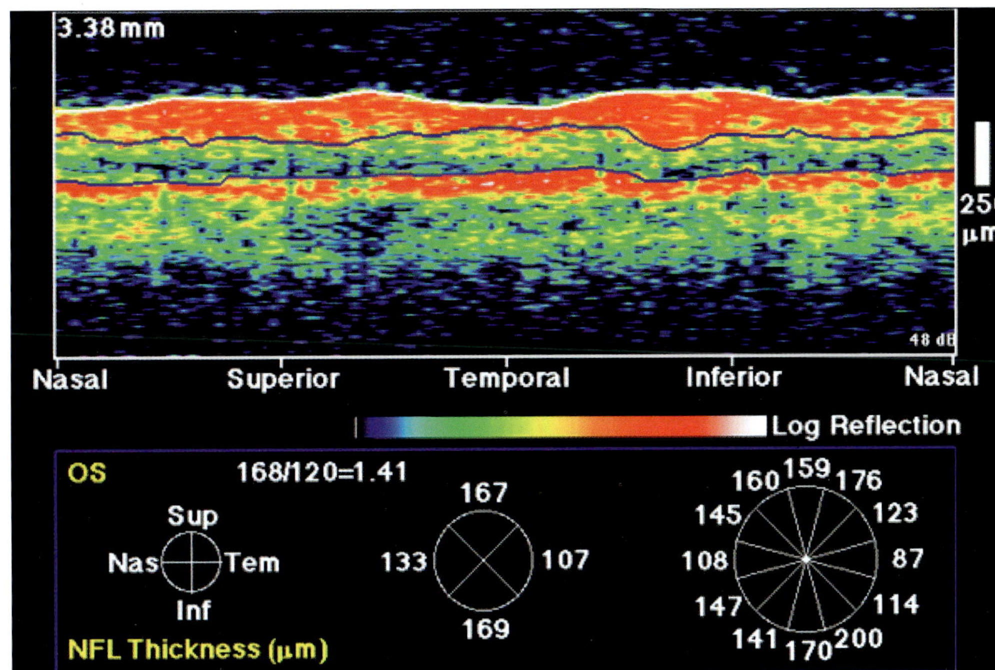


**Figure 7-3a.** Circular OCT tomographs in normal eye taken in cylindrical section of tissue surrounding the ONH, with scan at 3.37-mm diameter, centered on ONH. The vertical scale has been expanded by a factor of three to accentuate axial depth information. Note thicker NFL, the anteriormost red reflection in the false color image, superiorly and inferiorly. A number of layers may be distinguished in the OCT, including the NFL, the inner and outer plexiform layers (yellow), the photoreceptor layer (dark on OCT), and a red reflection of the retinal pigment epithelium, choroid, and sclera.

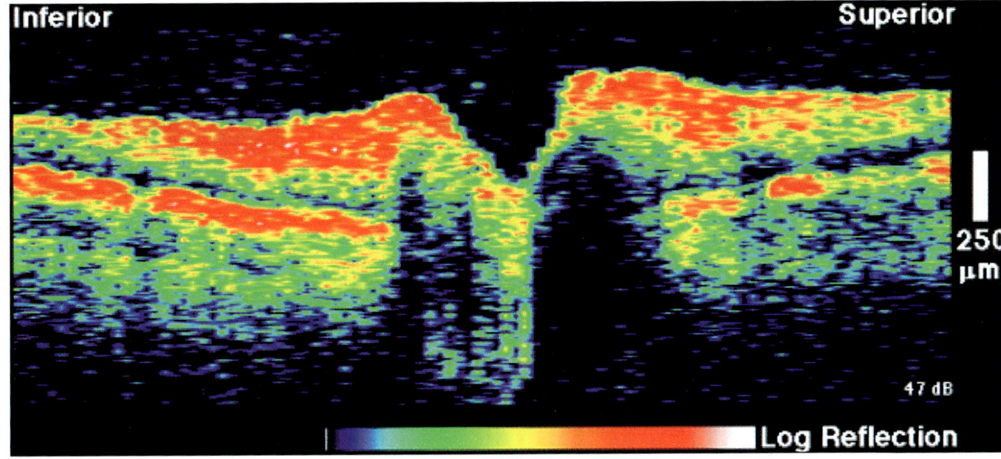


**Figure 7-3b.** Radial OCT tomograph.

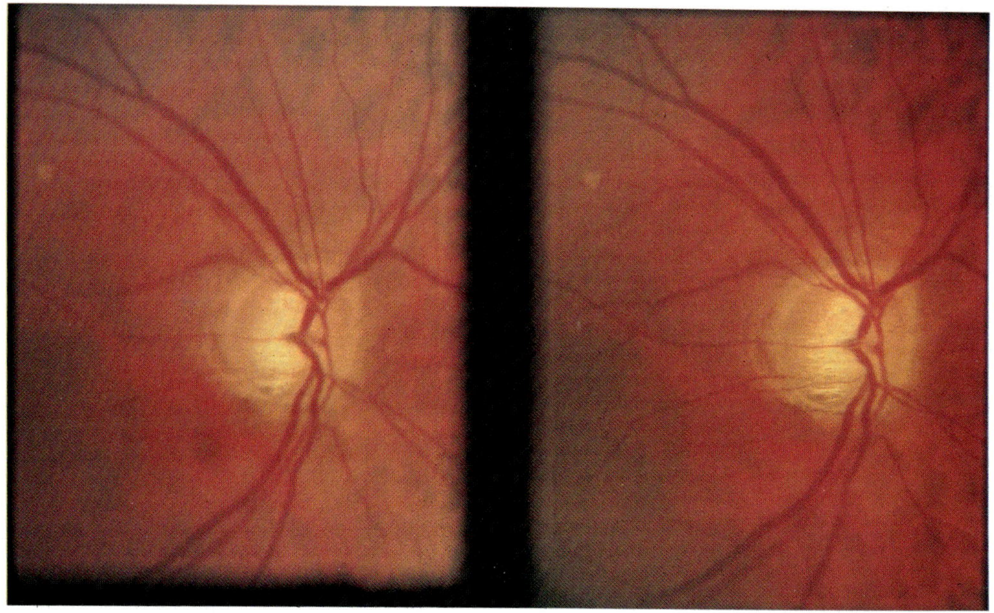

**Figure 7-4a.** Stereo optic disc photograph of subject with glaucoma. Moderate to marked cupping of the ONH is seen, particularly inferiorly.

**Figure 7-4b.** Humphrey 24-2 visual field. Subject has dense superior arcuate scotoma.

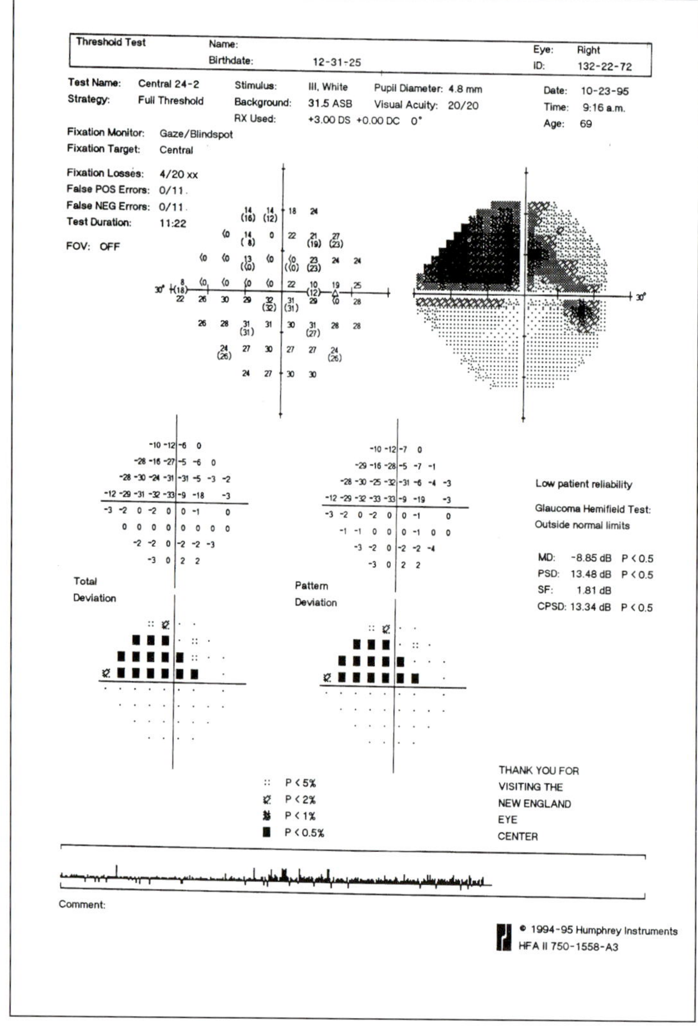

Threshold Test  Name:  Eye: Right
Birthdate: 12-31-25  ID: 132-22-72

Test Name: Central 24-2  Stimulus: III, White  Pupil Diameter: 4.8 mm  Date: 10-23-95
Strategy: Full Threshold  Background: 31.5 ASB  Visual Acuity: 20/20  Time: 9:16 a.m.
RX Used: +3.00 DS +0.00 DC 0°  Age: 69

Fixation Monitor: Gaze/Blindspot
Fixation Target: Central

Fixation Losses: 4/20 xx
False POS Errors: 0/11
False NEG Errors: 0/11
Test Duration: 11:22

FOV: OFF

Total Deviation

Pattern Deviation

:: P < 5%
P < 2%
P < 1%
P < 0.5%

Low patient reliability

Glaucoma Hemifield Test:
Outside normal limits

MD: -8.85 dB  P < 0.5
PSD: 13.48 dB  P < 0.5
SF: 1.81 dB
CPSD: 13.34 dB  P < 0.5

THANK YOU FOR
VISITING THE
NEW ENGLAND
EYE
CENTER

Comment:

© 1994-95 Humphrey Instruments
HFA II 750-1558-A3

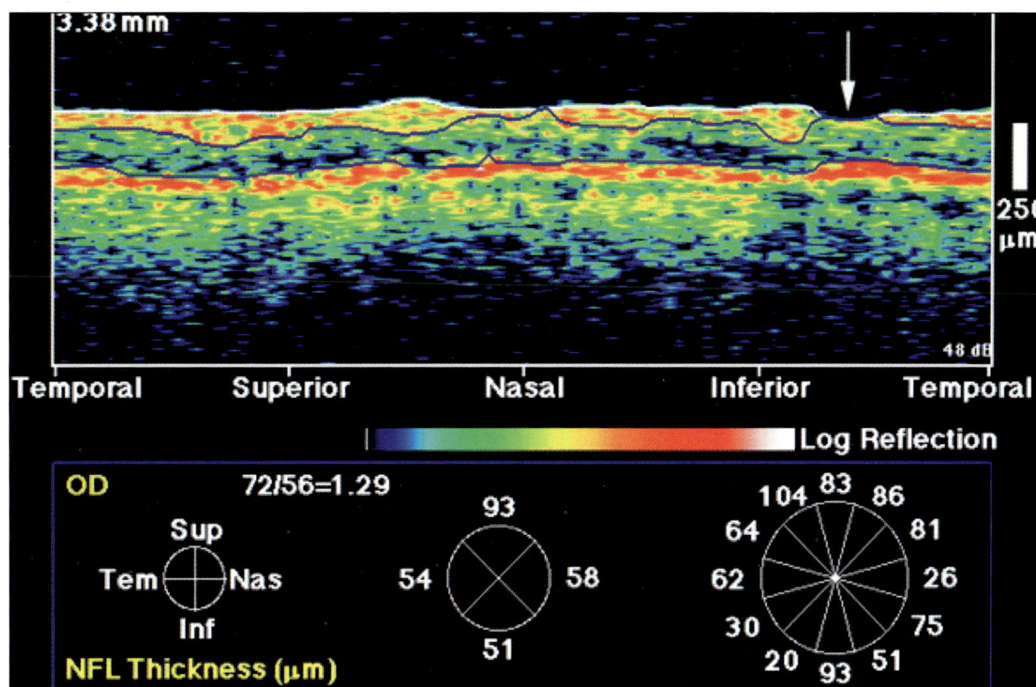



**Figure 7-4c.** OCT shows thinning of NFL inferiorly, with an area of marked focal attenuation (arrow) corresponding to superior visual field loss.

As in our human studies, NFL thickness decreased with increasing distance from the ONH (p=0.000), NFL was thickest in the superior and inferior quadrants, and NFL thickness was lower in glaucomatous than normal eyes.[11,25,26] Also as in our human studies, reproducibility of OCT measurements in monkey eyes was 14 microns overall, 20 to 24 microns for each quadrant (SD).[26]

Most importantly, OCT demonstrated a nearly linear decay in NFL thickness over time in those eyes with elevated IOP, while the control eyes showed no change in NFL thickness during the follow-up period.[25,26]

Finally, histologic correlation between OCT performed in vivo and microscopic examination of the same eye revealed agreement of NFL thickness measurements within 10 microns.[13]

These pivotal experimental glaucoma studies demonstrate the ability of OCT to track changes in NFL thickness over time, and that measurements made with OCT correlate within 10 microns with those made histologically. They also confirm the findings of our human OCT studies with regard to the structure and distribution of the NFL.

## CURRENT AND POTENTIAL APPLICATIONS OF OCT

OCT has potential applications in many areas of medicine. In the eye, OCT can be used to measure thicknesses in the anterior and posterior segment, as well as reflectivities in those tissues and in the crystalline lens. In addition, there may be other possibilities for OCT applications beyond those of tissue thickness measurement.

For the purposes of this book, the glaucoma applications of OCT are explored. The preceding sections of this chapter provided the fundamental aspects of the technology, as well as the pivotal studies that support the application of OCT in glaucoma. The fact that OCT measurements correlate with clinical findings of structure and function, that these measurements are reproducible, that OCT can track changes in NFL thickness over time (in the glaucomatous monkey model), and that OCT measurements in vivo compare well with histologic measurement of the same tissue, all give credence to the clinical use of OCT in glaucoma diagnostics.

A note of caution, however, is necessary. OCT is a new technology that is still evolving. There is no normative database from which to decide if a given patient's OCT NFL thickness measurements are abnormal. These issues must be resolved before OCT can be accepted for widespread clinical use in glaucoma. Nevertheless, OCT has applicability, even now, in clinical patient care. The series of cases below illustrate this point.

Figures 7-11a through 7-11e show a 67-year-old woman with pseudoexfoliation. This patient has normal IOPs, but small ONHs with a suggestion of inferior extension of the cup. Visual fields repeatedly demonstrate superior arcuate scotomas; however, this patient has mild ptosis. OCT is extremely helpful in illustrating good NFL thickness both superiorly and inferiorly bilaterally, with no evidence of focal or sectoral thinning. **While there is no large scale normative database, our OCT findings to date indicate that NFL thickness greater than 125 to 130 microns in the superior and inferior quadrants appears to be in the normal**

**Figure 7-5a.** Stereo optic disc photograph of left eye of subject with a localized arcuate NFL defect inferotemporally. Note also the flame-shaped disc hemorrhage in the area of the NFL defect.

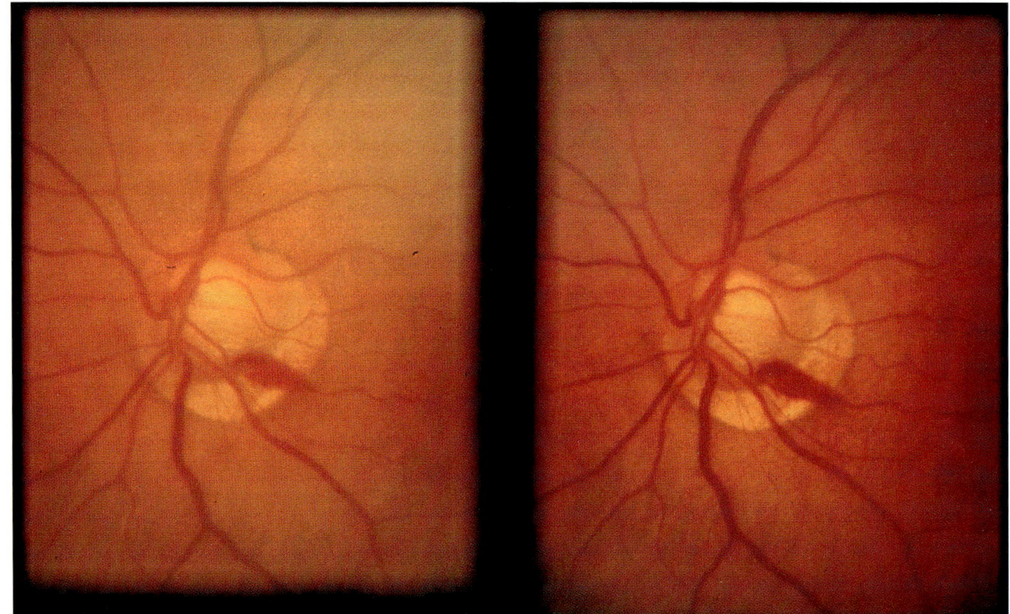

**Figure 7-5b.** Red-free NFL photograph demonstrates the localized arcuate NFL defect inferotemporally.

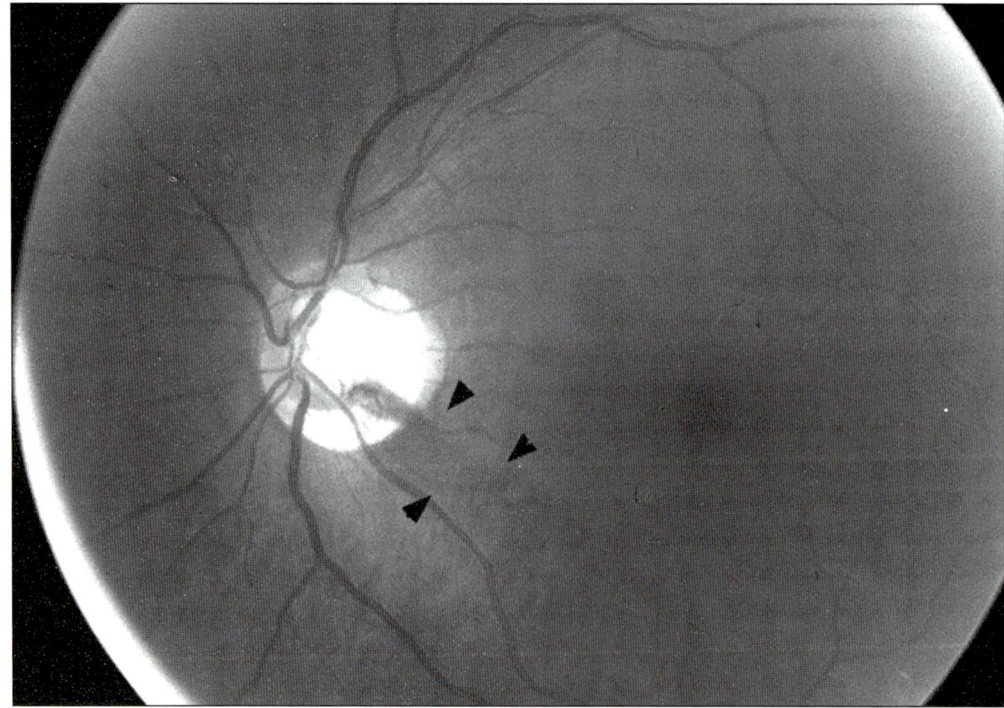

**range.**[4,11] The patient is followed for her pseudoexfoliation, but based on her OCT findings, the suspicion for glaucoma is extremely low.

Figures 7-12a through 7-12d demonstrate another patient with small ONHs, but with IOPs elevated to the mid-20s. This patient has a normal visual field, and the OCT shows good NFL thickness, again without focal or sectoral NFL thinning. The patient is followed yearly, and has shown no change in any clinical parameter, including OCT, which has been performed over the past three yearly visits.

Figures 7-13a through 7-13d show a patient with large ONHs and big cups, but with normal IOPs and normal visual fields. OCT again shows good NFL thickness and no localized abnormalities.

Figures 7-14a through 7-14h illustrate a patient with asymmetric cupping. The IOP and visual field is normal in both eyes. OCT demonstrates essentially equal NFL thickness bilaterally. The most likely explanation is asymmetric disc size, which is the case in this individual. This is a fairly common finding, and many patients followed for asymmetric cupping as glaucoma

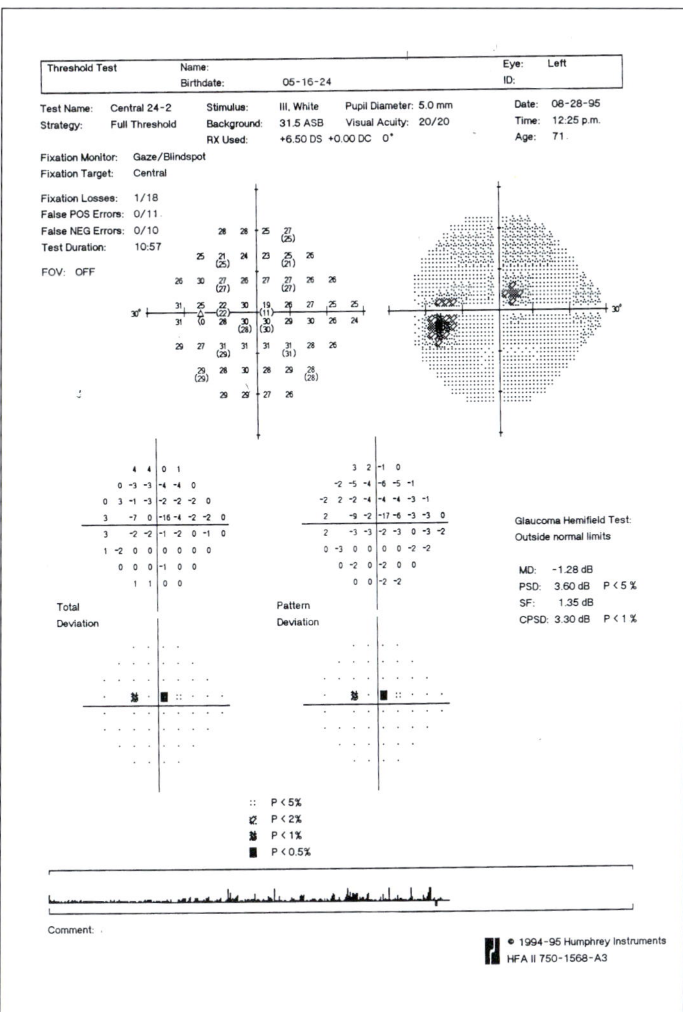

**Figure 7-5c.** Humphrey 24-2 visual field shows a superior paracentral scotoma corresponding to inferotemporal NFL defect.

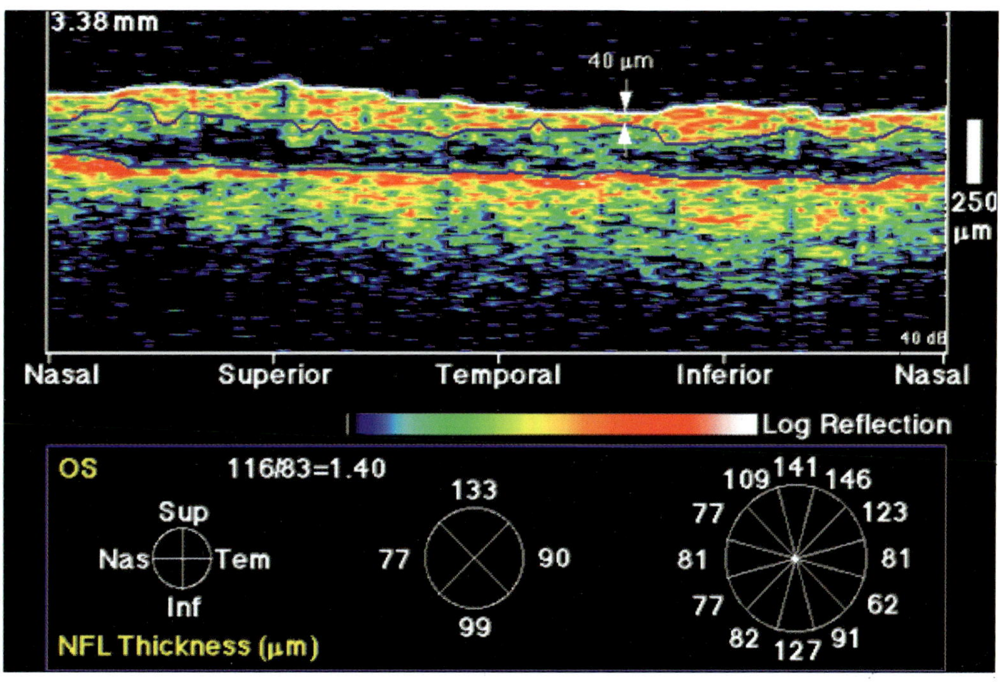



**Figure 7-5d.** OCT illustrates NFL defect inferotemporally in cross-section. Note especially thinning of the NFL in the region of the defect from below.

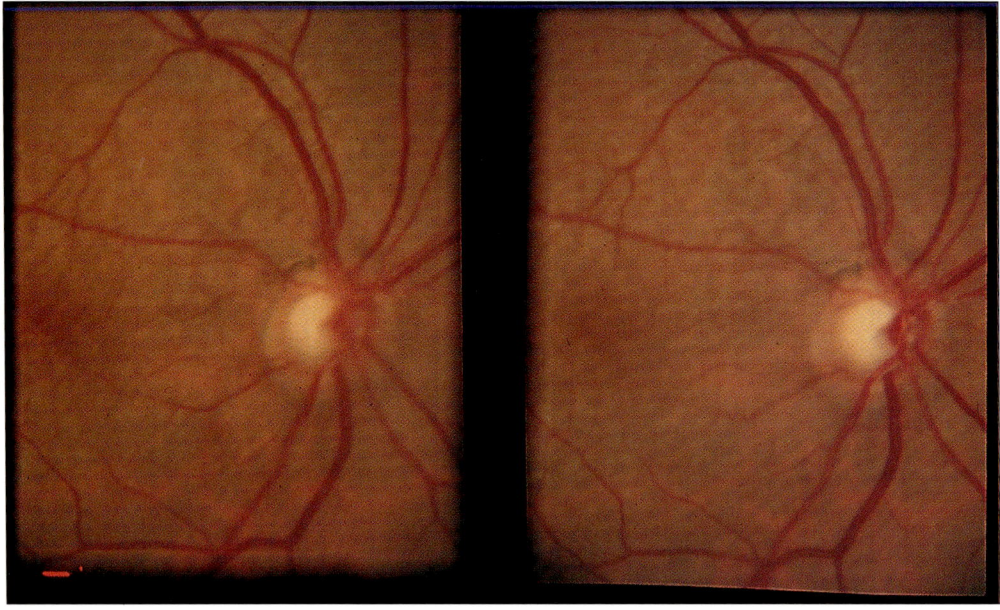

**Figure 7-6a.** Stereoscopic ONH photograph of right eye of subject with a two focal NFL defects: a defect inferiorly, and a broader, denser superior NFL defect.

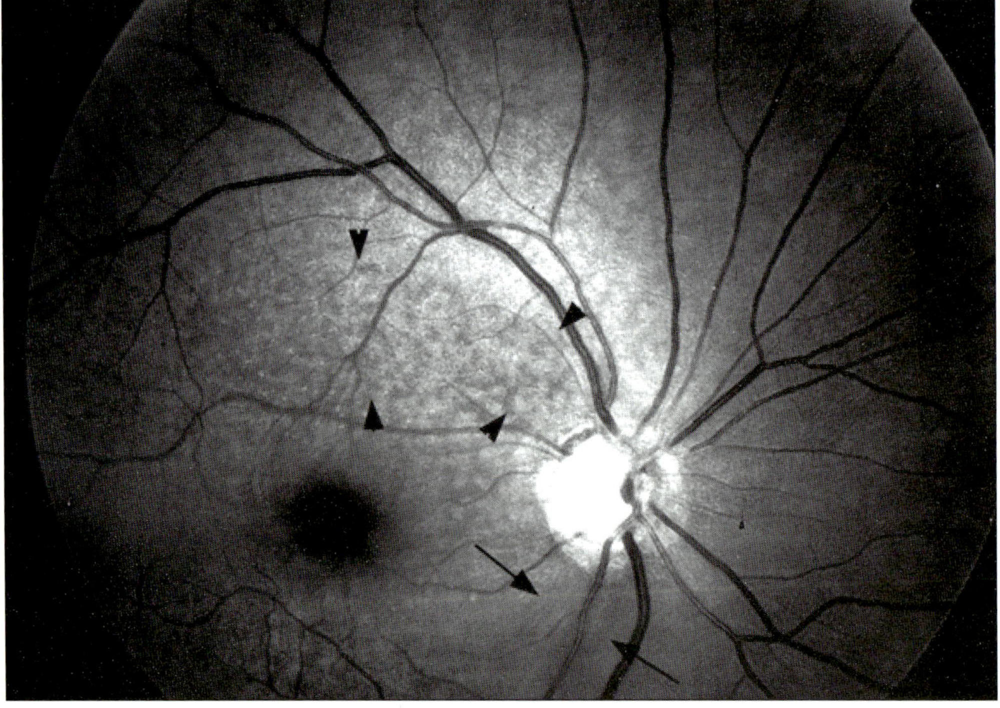

**Figure 7-6b.** Red-free NFL photograph highlights the superior and inferior NFL defects.

suspects may indeed simply have asymmetric disc size and equal NFL thickness in the two eyes, and may not require frequent follow-up visits on suspicion of glaucoma.[27]

Figures 7-15a through 7-15g picture a patient with asymmetric cupping as well. This patient has bilateral glaucoma with elevated IOP; however, the patient is treated in the right eye only for glaucoma when referred for evaluation.

OCT demonstrates marked thinning of the NFL bilaterally, as well as ONH drusen, which accounts for the fullness of the left ONH. Glaucoma therapy in both eyes is initiated.

Interestingly, optic nerve drusen alone can cause thinning of the NFL, and the more obvious the drusen, the more thinning tends to occur.[28] In eyes with glaucoma and ONH drusen, however, there is the additional complication, as

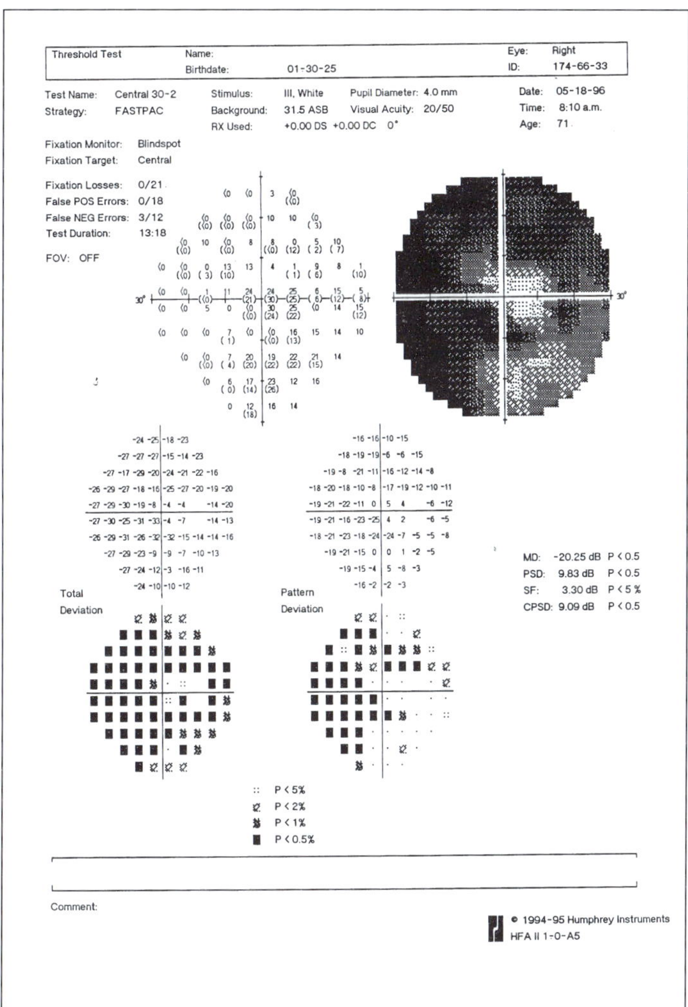

**Figure 7-6c.** Humphrey 24-2 visual field shows a superior arcuate scotoma with a much denser inferonasal step extending to an inferior paracentral scotoma, corresponding to inferotemporal and superotemporal NFL defects respectively.

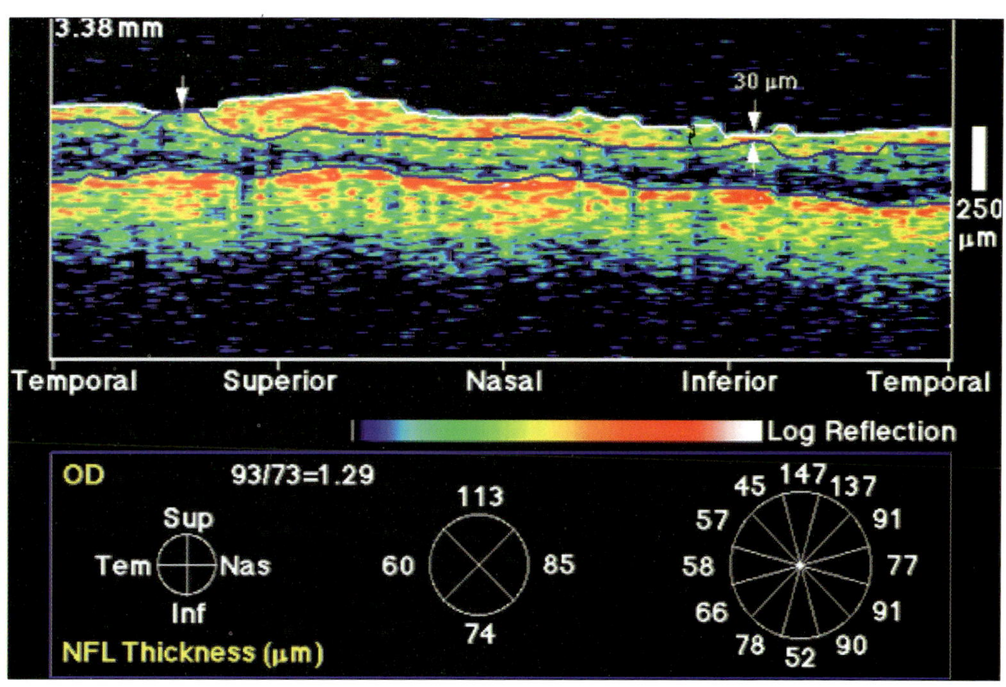


**Figure 7-6d.** OCT demonstrates the NFL defects both superotemporally and inferotemporally in cross-section as regions of localized thinning. Note that the superior defect is significantly thinner than the inferior one.

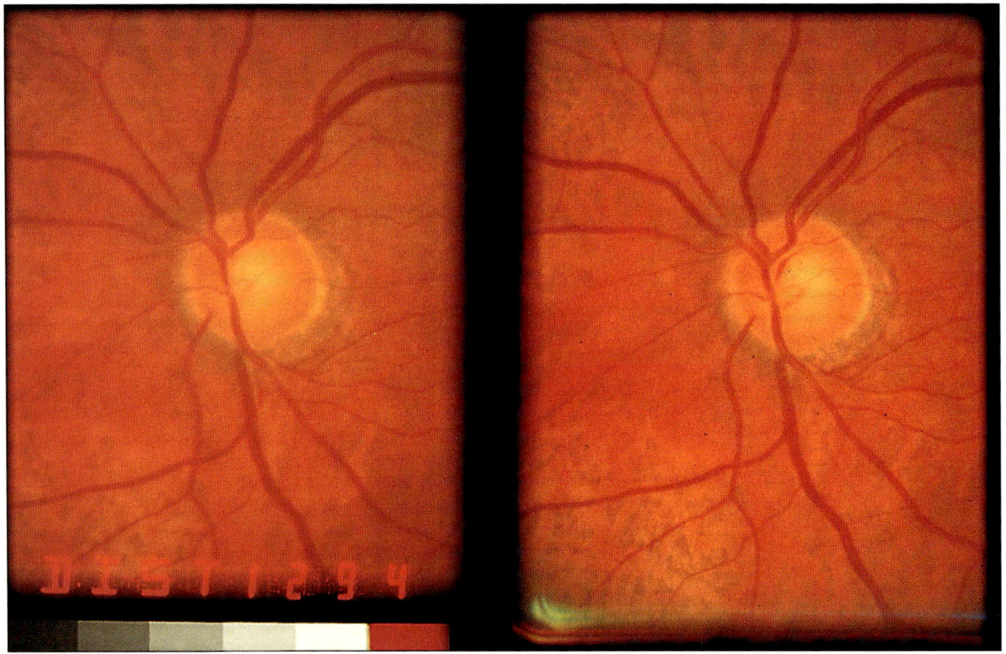

**Figure 7-7a.** Stereoscopic ONH photograph from January 1994.

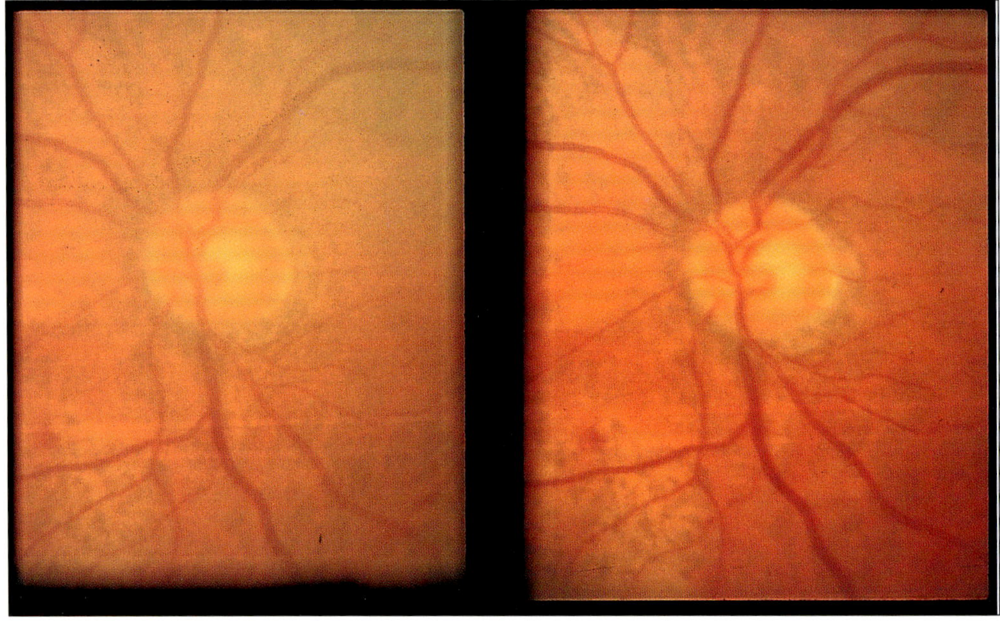

**Figure 7-7b.** Stereoscopic ONH photograph from March 1996. There is subtle detectable interval change.

illustrated by the patient in Figures 7-15a through 7-15g, that the drusen may mask ONH cupping, and delay the initiation of treatment for glaucoma.

Figures 7-16a through 7-16e show an 18-year-old woman with a Krukenberg spindle in the left eye only. She has 4+ black pigment in the trabecular meshwork in the left eye, and the angles are wide open bilaterally to ciliary body band. The IOP is elevated in the left eye only, to a level in the high 20s.

This patient is referred with the diagnosis of pigment dispersion glaucoma, which, while occasionally asymmetric, is not often completely monocular. The nature of the pigment in the trabecular meshwork suggests another process, and ultrasound biomicroscopy (UBM), discussed by Ritch, Liebmann, Iezzi, and Tello in Chapter 10, reveals a ciliary body mass, most likely an adenoma.

This patient has no visual field defect but does have somewhat more cupping of the ONH in the left than the right eye. OCT shows a slightly thinner NFL on the left than the right, and the patient is treated for her elevated IOP in the left eye. The IOP is reduced to the mid-teens on one medication.

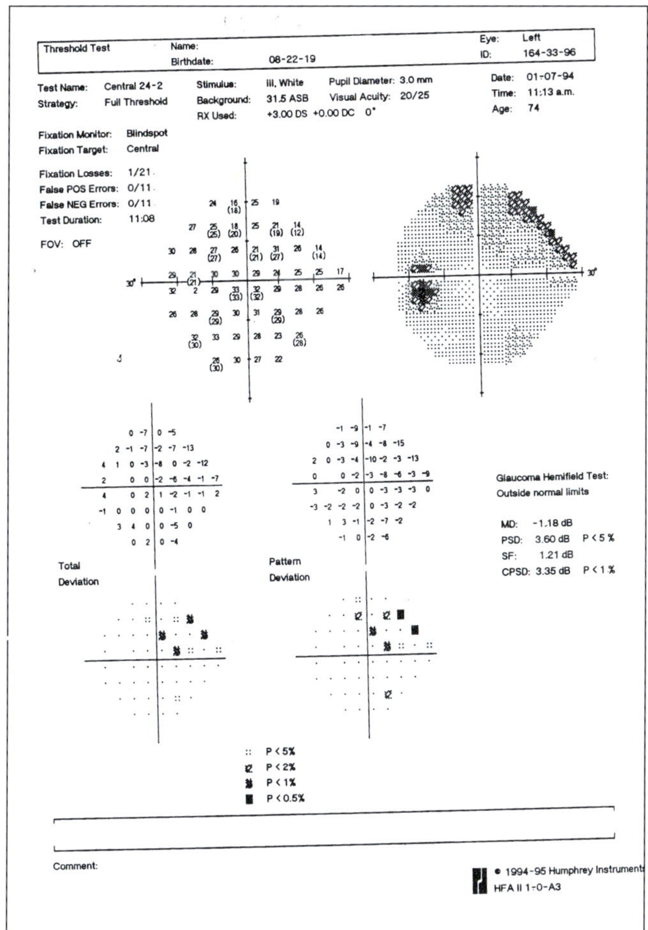

**Figure 7-7c.** Automated visual field from January 1994.

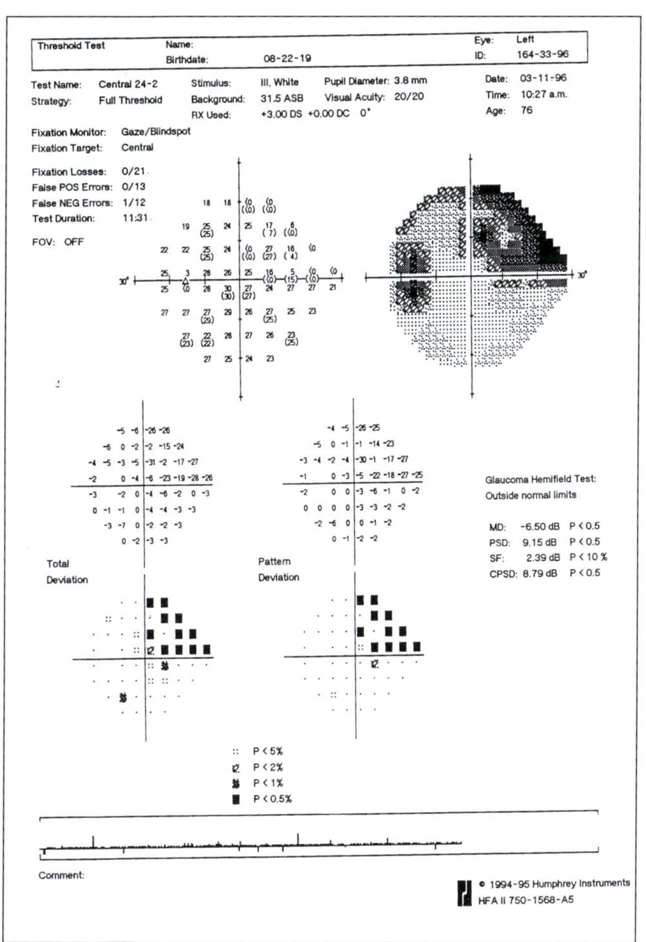

**Figure 7-7d.** Automated visual field from March 1996. Note progression of superior arcuate scotoma. This visual field change was reproducible.

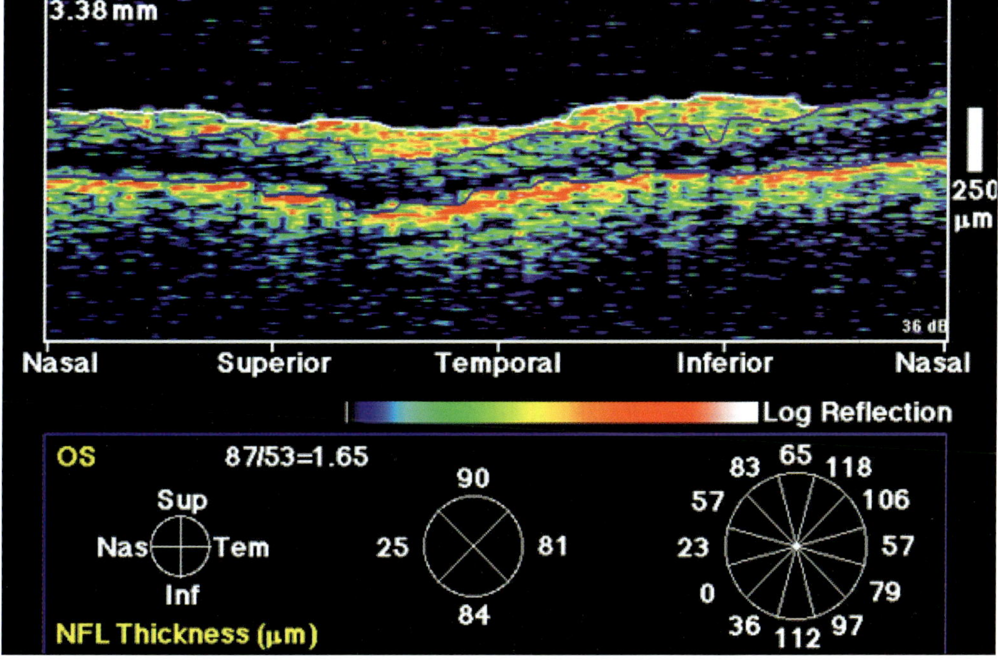


**Figure 7-7e.** Circular OCT scan from January 1994.

**Figure 7-7f.** Circular OCT scan from March 1996. There is a quantifiable loss of NFL tissue, more inferiorly than superiorly.

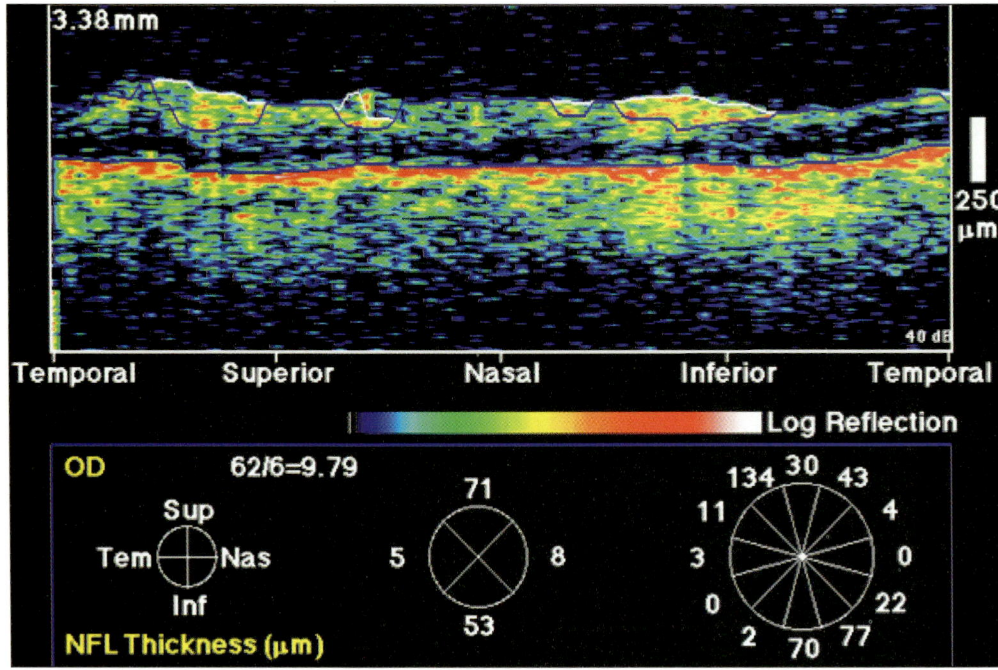


**Figure 7-7g.** Radial OCT scan through ONH from January 1994.

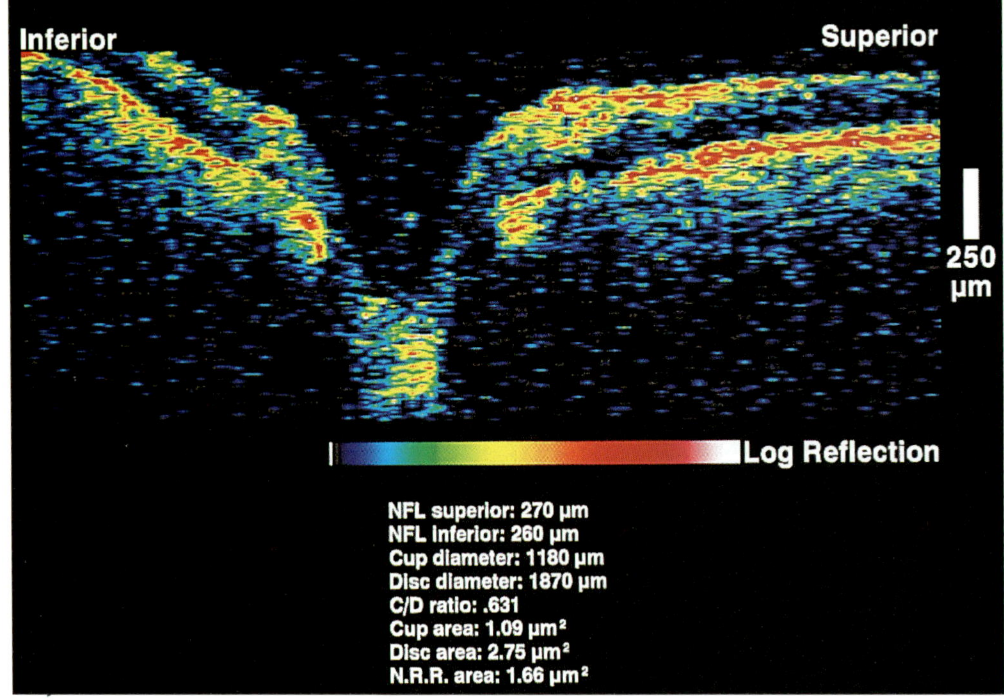


Repeat UBMs show no change in the size or nature of the ciliary body mass. OCT remains stable, as does ONH appearance and visual field.

## CONCLUSIONS

The potential utility of OCT as a glaucoma diagnostic tool is extremely high. Unlike polarimetry, OCT provides a cross-sectional image of the tissue being studied, in addition to quantitative, objective NFL thickness measurements. The OCT image allows the clinician to visually evaluate the NFL for areas of local abnormalities, such as focal defects or sectoral thinning, and provides a useful additional parameter to examine.

As noted, OCT is a new technology. This introduces both difficulties and opportunities. The lack of large scale normative data is perhaps the greatest issue in interpretation of OCT results at this point; however, adequate data exist with which to evaluate patients in conjunction with other clinical para-

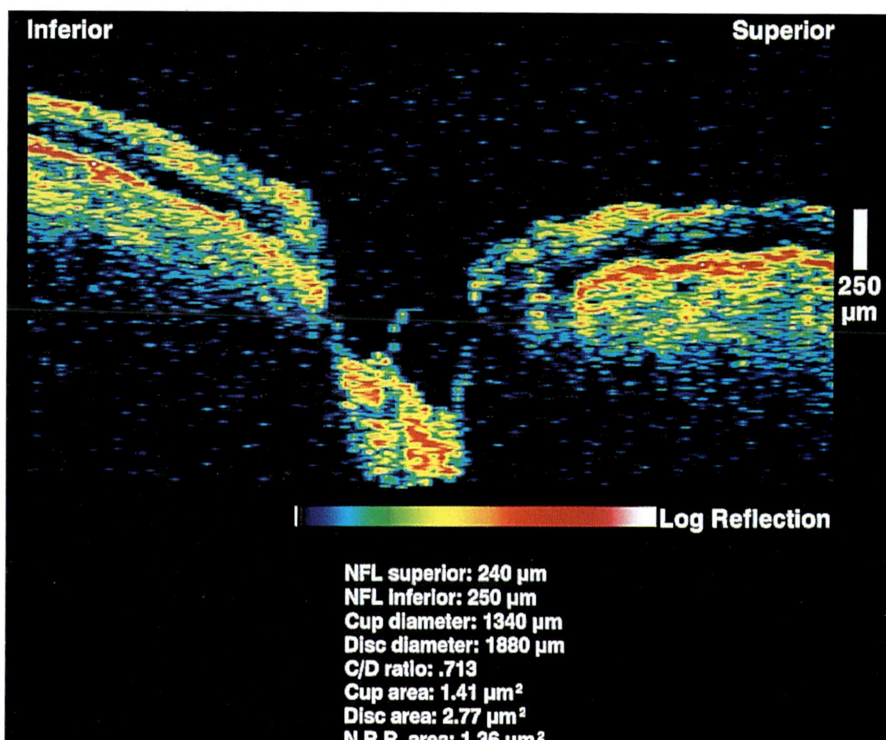


**Figure 7-7h.** Radial OCT scan through ONH from March 1996. A thinning of the neuroretinal rim and enlargement of the cup has occurred, while the disc diameter remains constant.

meters. Additionally, a given patient can be followed over time, using the patient as his or her own baseline. The two eyes of a patient can be compared for asymmetry, and a single eye can be examined for focal or sectoral NFL thinning.

The fact that OCT is new affords many opportunities. OCT opens a window on the examination of the NFL, retina, and even the ONH. There is much to learn about normal NFL anatomy in vivo, as well as how the normal NFL changes over time. Glaucoma evaluation with OCT is in its infancy. Longitudinal studies now underway will examine NFL loss in glaucomatous and normal eyes, as well as the patterns of NFL damage in glaucoma.

Even at this stage, OCT is an extraordinarily useful clinical tool in the assessment of glaucoma and other eye diseases. The potential future utility of OCT is limited only by our own creativity.

## ACKNOWLEDGMENTS

The author acknowledges the work of Tamar Pedut-Kloizman, MD, Ellen Hertzmark, MPH, Cynthia Mattox, MD, Liselotte Pieroth, MD, Wayne Scott, MD, Anthony Terraciano, MD, Farah K. Galaydh, MD, Jason R. Wilkins, BS, Jeffery G. Coker, BS, and Carmen A. Puliafito, MD, from the New England Eye Center, Tufts University School of Medicine, Boston, Massachusetts; Michael R. Hee, MS, Joseph A. Izatt, PhD, and James G. Fujimoto, PhD, from the Massachusetts Institute of Technology, Cambridge; Eric A. Swanson, MS, from the MIT-Lincoln Laboratory, Lexington, Massachusetts; and David Huang, MD, from the University of Southern California, Los Angeles, each of whom contributed to the development of OCT, and to the basic and clinical studies that form the basis of this chapter.

**Figure 7-8a.** Stereoscopic ONH photograph illustrates markedly excavated ONH with little or no remaining neural rim tissue in this individual with end-stage glaucoma. Visual acuity is 20/40.

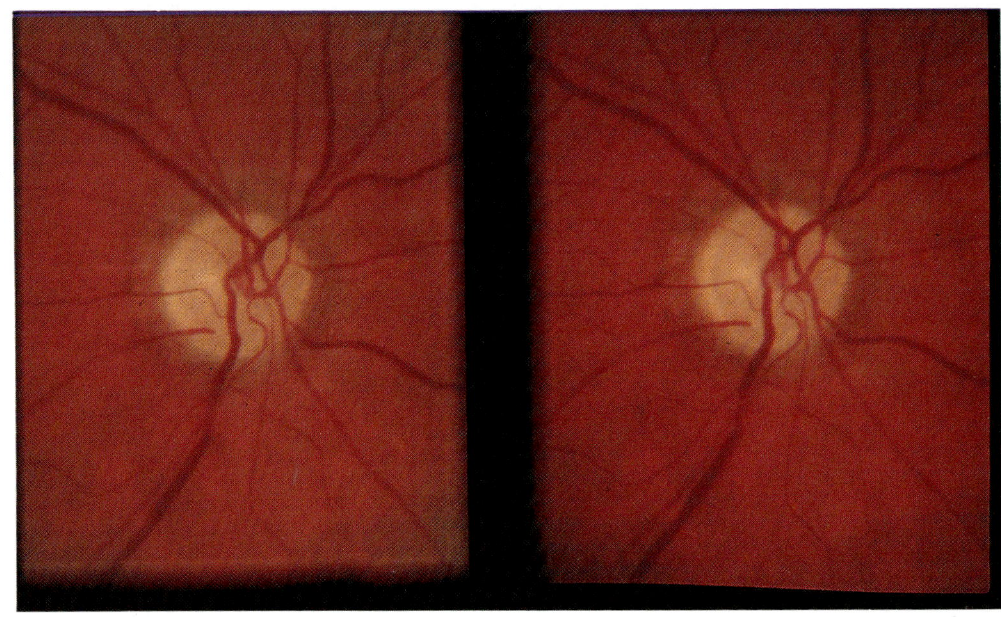

**Figure 7-8b.** Visual field shows only a central island remaining.

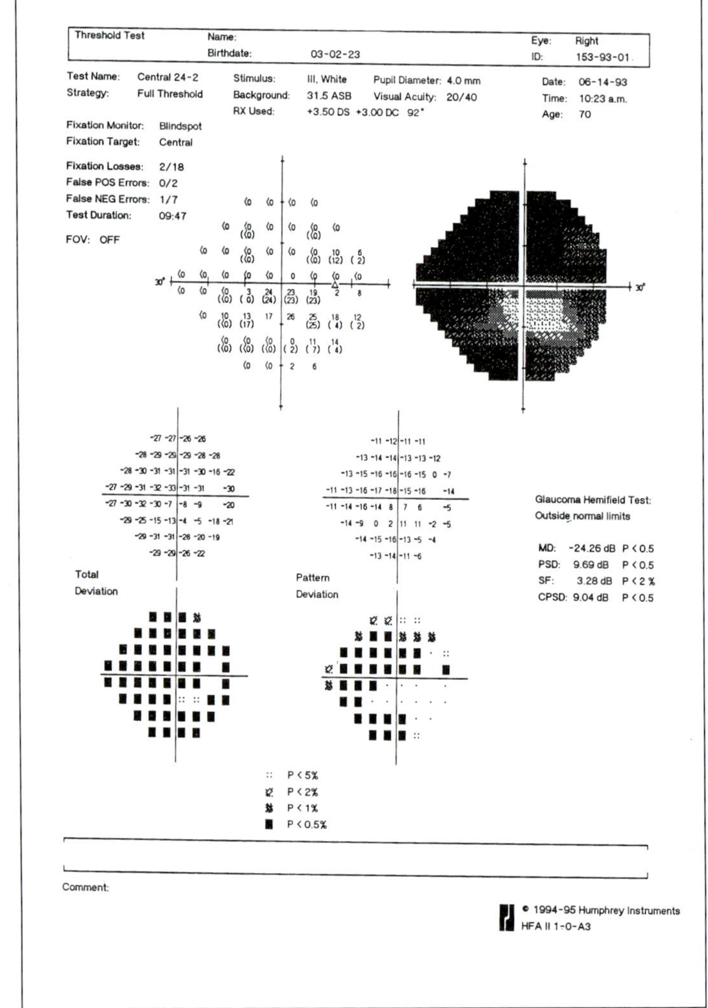

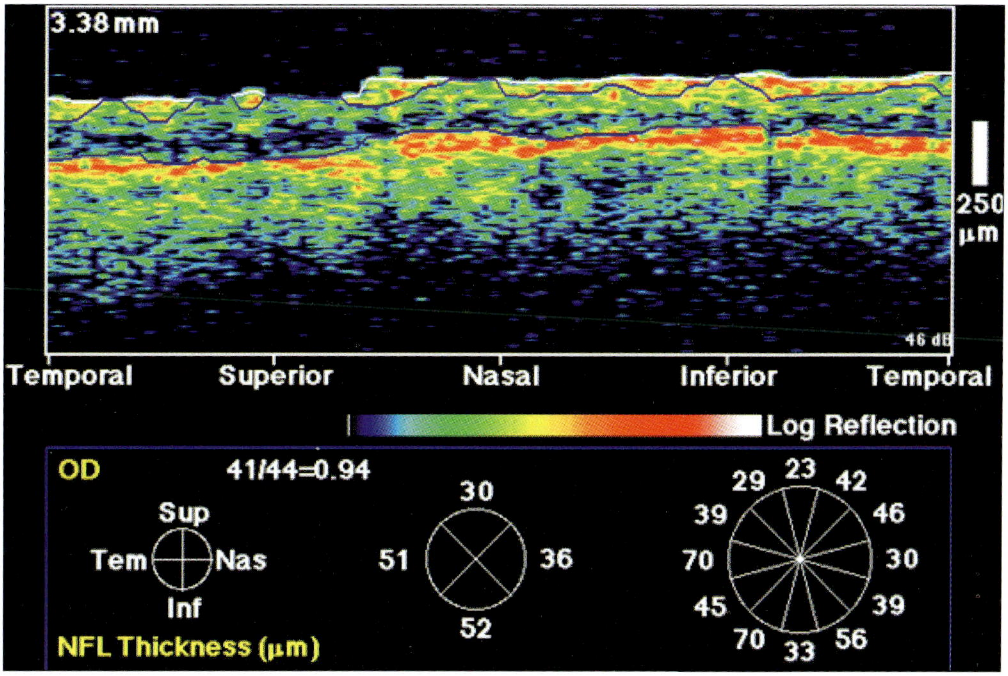

**Figure 7-8c.** OCT demonstrates marked attenuation of the NFL, with only a thin remnant of tissue remaining.

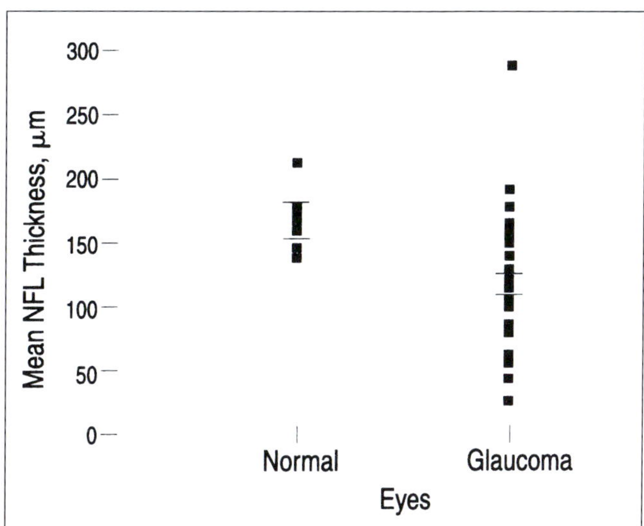

Figure 7-9. Mean inferior-quadrant NFL thickness in normal and glaucomatous eyes. Mean NFL thickness was 165.0±16.2 microns in normal eyes (n=7) and 125.7±6.4 microns in glaucomatous eyes (n=44) (p=0.04). The inferior quadrant (the 4:30 to 7:30 positions) proved most sensitive to the difference in NFL thickness between normal and glaucomatous eyes. Reprinted from Schuman JS, Hee MR, Puliafito CA, et al. Quantification of nerve fiber layer thickness in normal and glaucomatous eyes using optical coherence tomography: a pilot study. *Arch Ophthalmol.* 1995;113:586-596. Copyrighted 1995, American Medical Association.

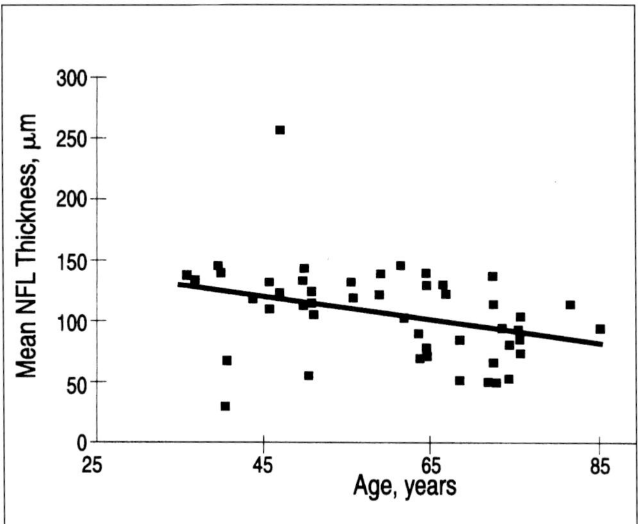

**Figure 7-10a.** The relationship between NFL thickness and age. There is a significant decrease in NFL thickness with aging (p=0.03), controlling for variables associated with glaucoma. Reprinted from Schuman JS, Hee MR, Puliafito CA, et al. Quantification of nerve fiber layer thickness in normal and glaucomatous eyes using optical coherence tomography: a pilot study. *Arch Ophthalmol.* 1995;113:586-596. Copyrighted 1995, American Medical Association. Copyrighted 1995, American Medical Association.

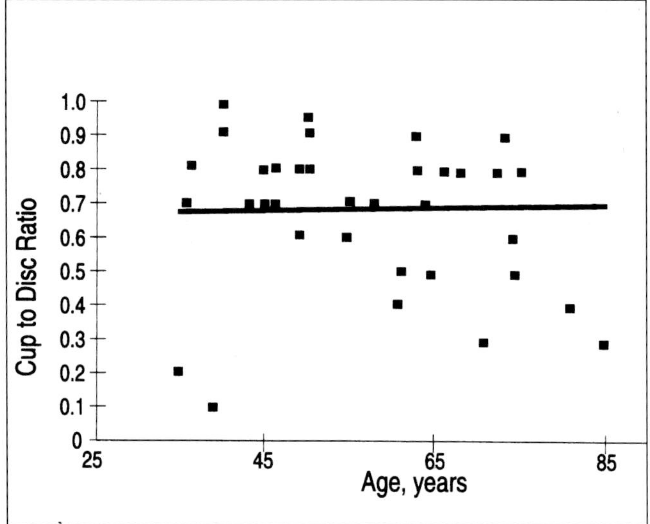

**Figure 7-10b.** There is no relationship between cup-to-disc ratio and aging. Copyrighted 1995, American Medical Association. Reprinted from Schuman JS, Hee MR, Puliafito CA, et al. Quantification of nerve fiber layer thickness in normal and glaucomatous eyes using optical coherence tomography: a pilot study. *Arch Ophthalmol.* 1995;113:586-596. Copyrighted 1995, American Medical Association.

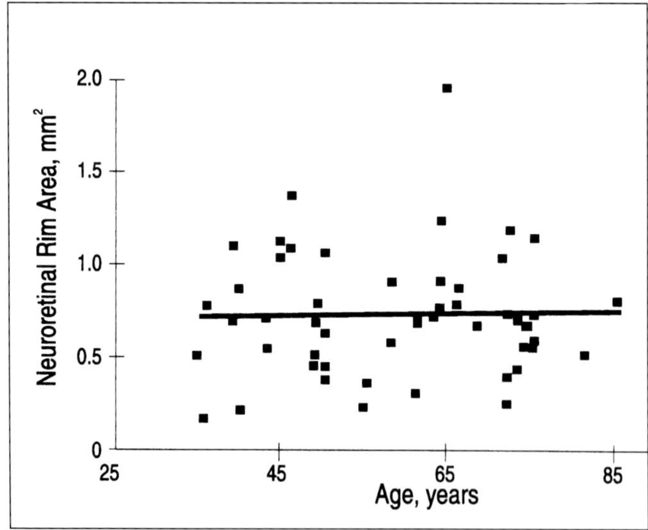

**Figure 7-10c.** There is no relationship between neuroretinal rim area and aging. Reprinted from Schuman JS, Hee MR, Puliafito CA, et al. Quantification of nerve fiber layer thickness in normal and glaucomatous eyes using optical coherence tomography: a pilot study. *Arch Ophthalmol.* 1995;113:586-596. Copyrighted 1995, American Medical Association.

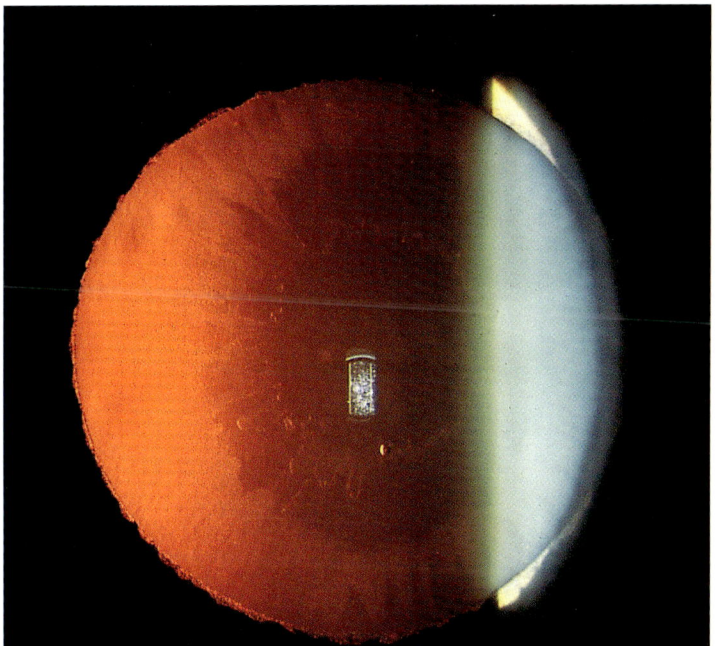

**Figure 7-11a.** Pseudoexfoliation material on the anterior lens capsule of a 67-year-old woman.

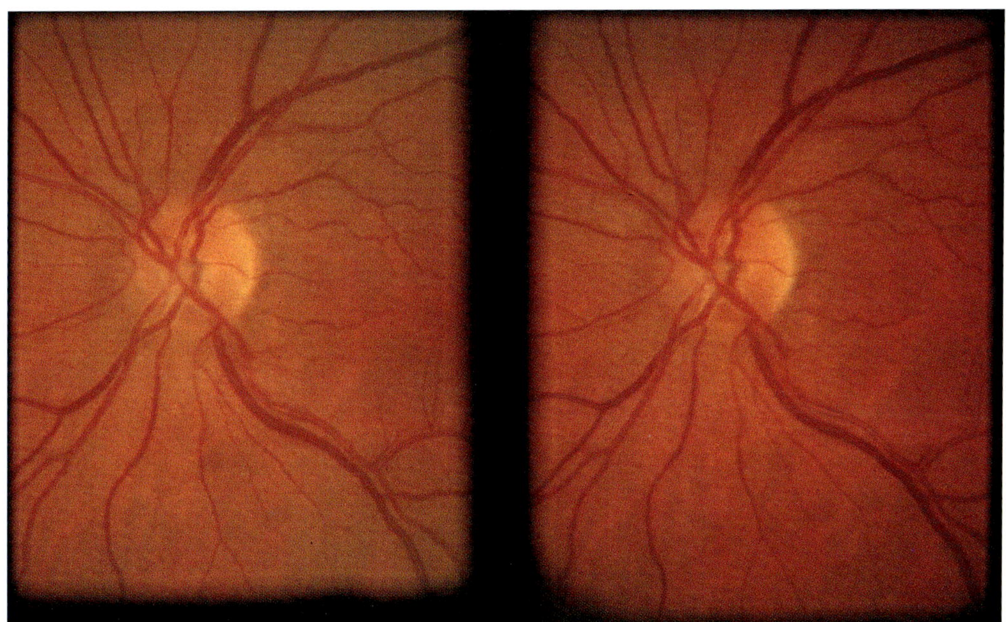

**Figure 7-11b.** Stereoscopic ONH photographs show small ONH with small cup. There is a suggestion of inferior extension of the cup.

**Figure 7-11c.** The NFL appears normal photographically.

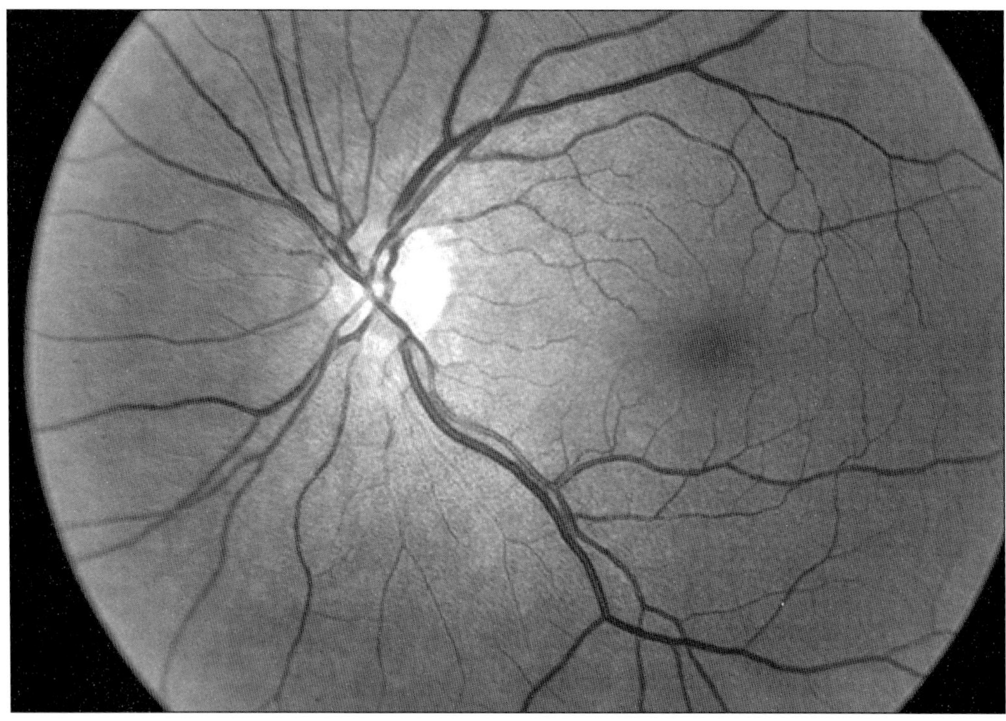

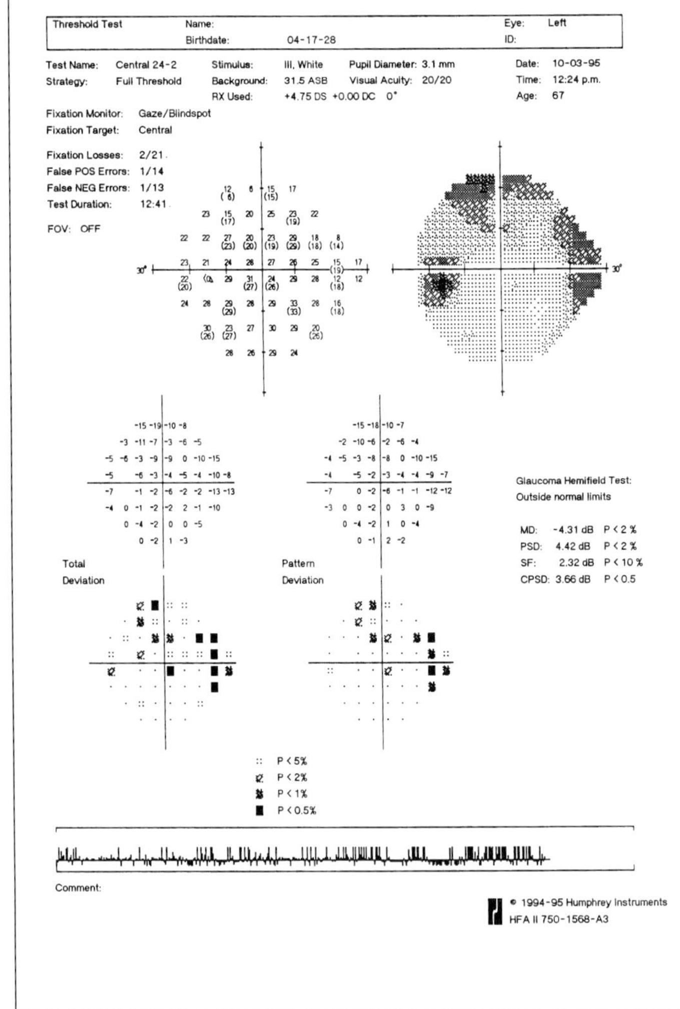

**Figure 7-11d.** A superior arcuate scotoma is revealed by Humphrey visual field. This defect persists on repeated testing. The patient has mild ptosis, but the visual field was performed with the eyelid taped out of the pupillary axis.

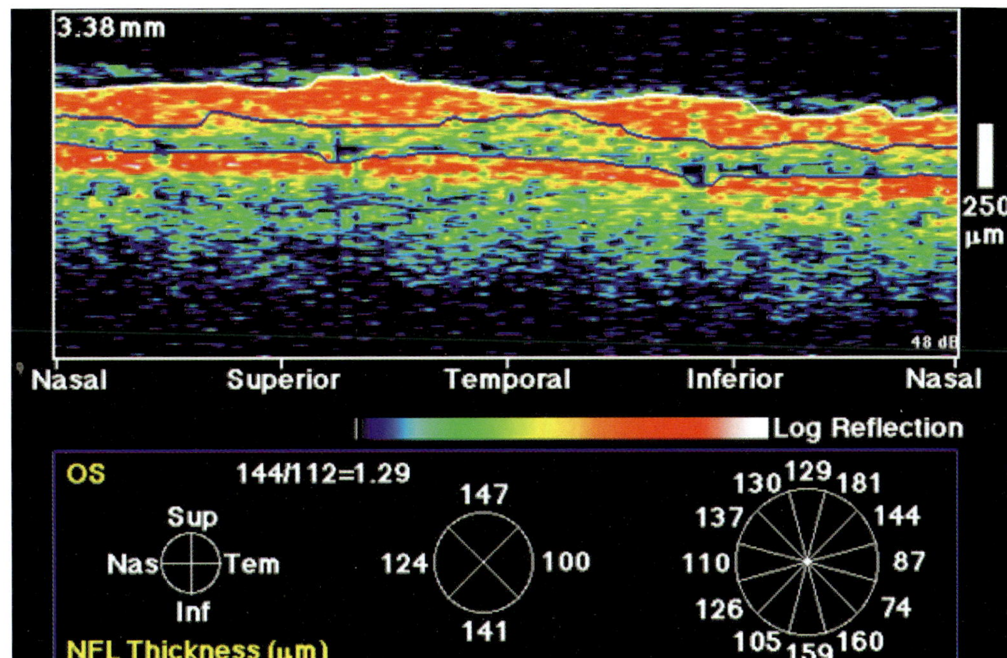


**Figure 7-11e.** OCT demonstrates good NFL thickness, with no evidence of focal or sectoral defects.

**Figure 7-12a.** Stereoscopic ONH photograph of right eye of subject with small ONHs and an IOP in the mid-20s.

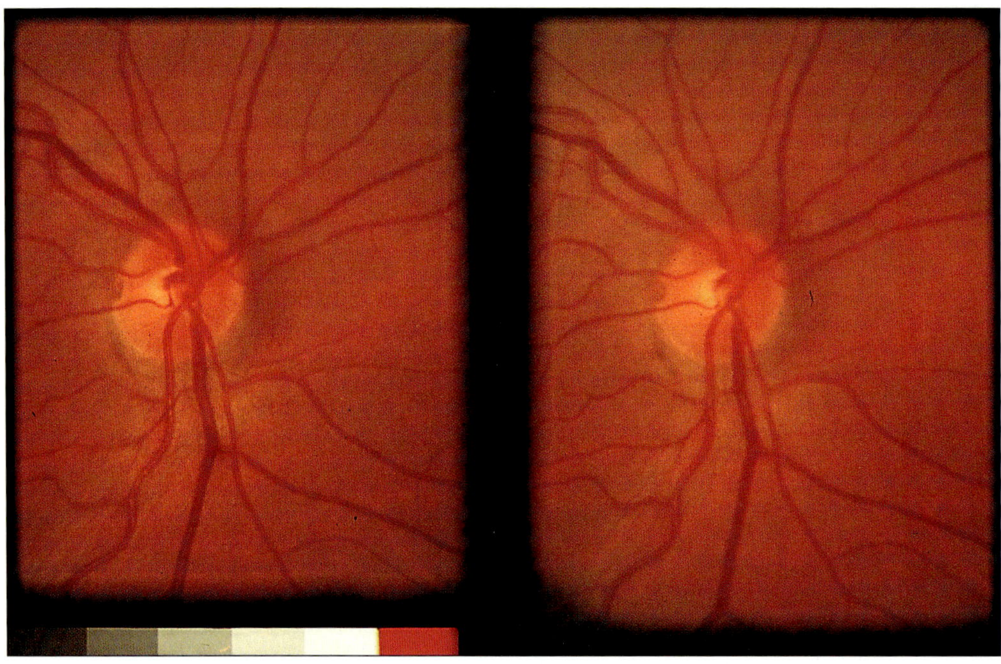

**Figure 7-12b.** Red-free NFL photograph appears normal.

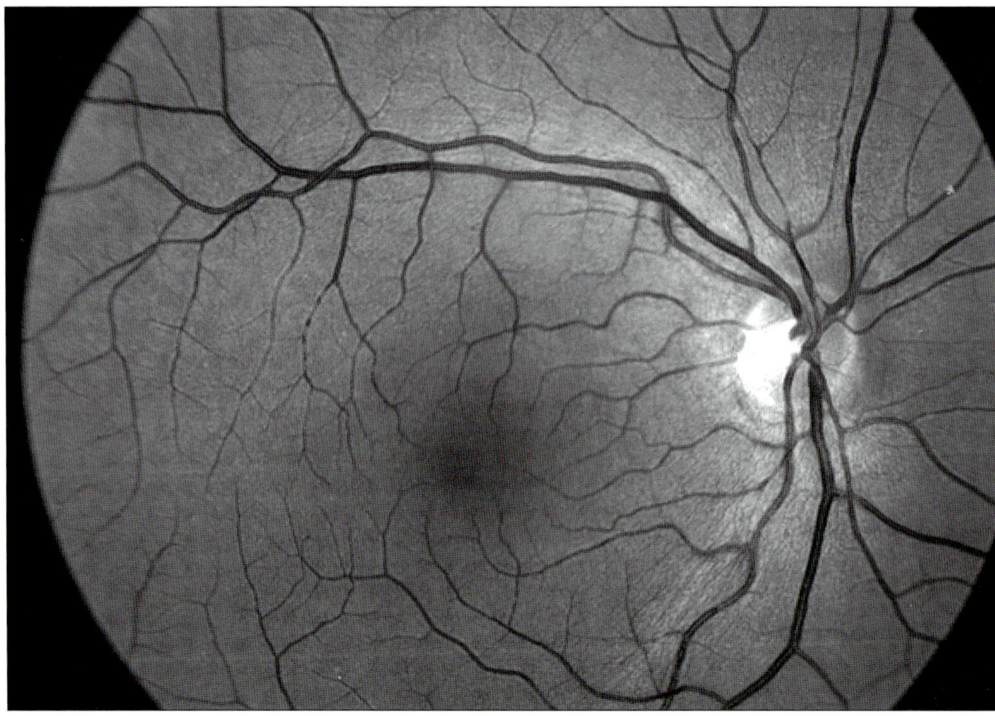

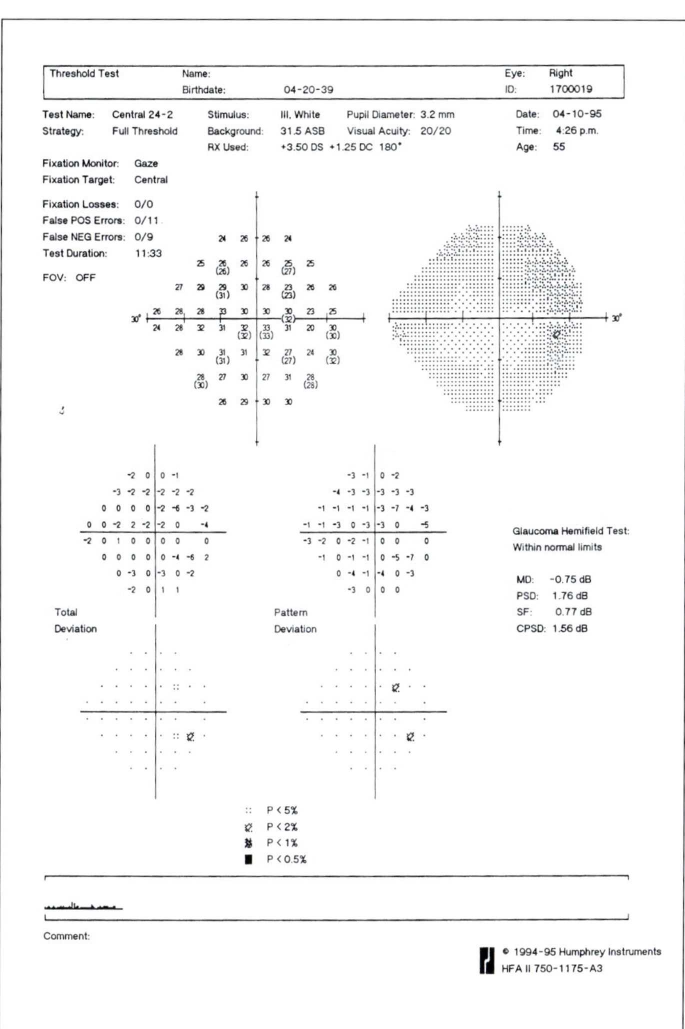

| Threshold Test | Name: | | | Eye: | Right |
| --- | --- | --- | --- | --- | --- |
| | Birthdate: | 04-20-39 | | ID: | 1700019 |

| | | | | | |
| --- | --- | --- | --- | --- | --- |
| Test Name: | Central 24-2 | Stimulus: | III, White | Pupil Diameter: 3.2 mm | Date: 04-10-95 |
| Strategy: | Full Threshold | Background: | 31.5 ASB | Visual Acuity: 20/20 | Time: 4:26 p.m. |
| | | RX Used: | +3.50 DS +1.25 DC 180° | | Age: 55 |

Fixation Monitor: Gaze
Fixation Target: Central

Fixation Losses: 0/0
False POS Errors: 0/11
False NEG Errors: 0/9
Test Duration: 11:33

FOV: OFF

Total Deviation

Pattern Deviation

Glaucoma Hemifield Test:
Within normal limits

MD: −0.75 dB
PSD: 1.76 dB
SF: 0.77 dB
CPSD: 1.56 dB

:: P < 5%
P < 2%
P < 1%
■ P < 0.5%

Comment:

© 1994-95 Humphrey Instruments
HFA II 750-1175-A3

**Figure 7-12c.** Humphrey 24-2 visual field is full.

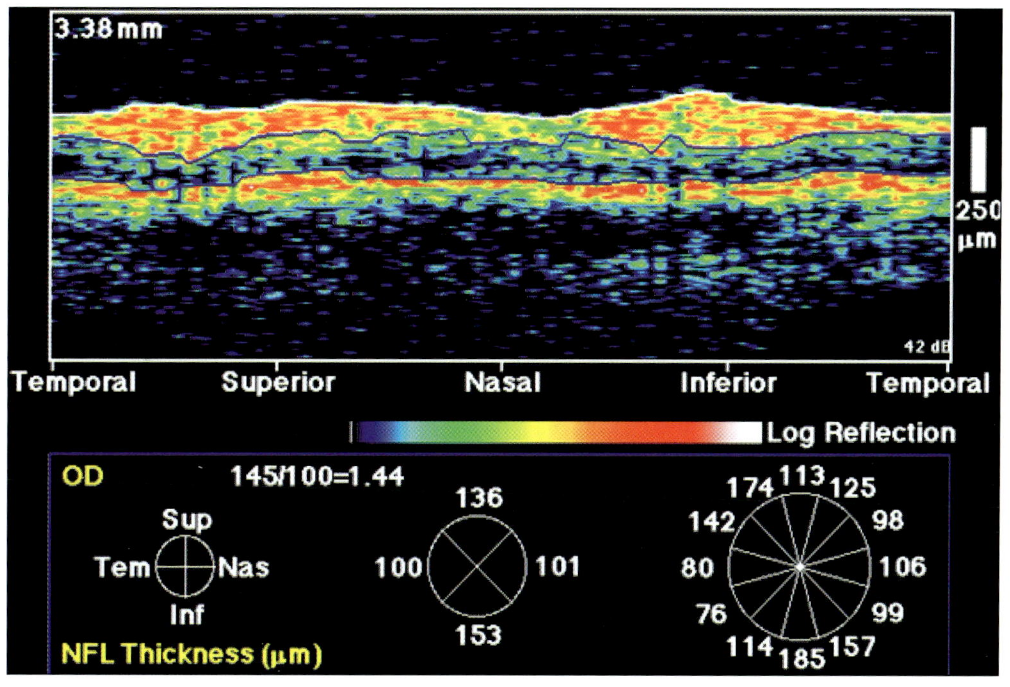


**Figure 7-12d.** OCT illustrates good NFL thickness.

**Figure 7-13a.** Stereoscopic ONH photograph of right eye of subject with large cups and large ONHs and normal IOP.

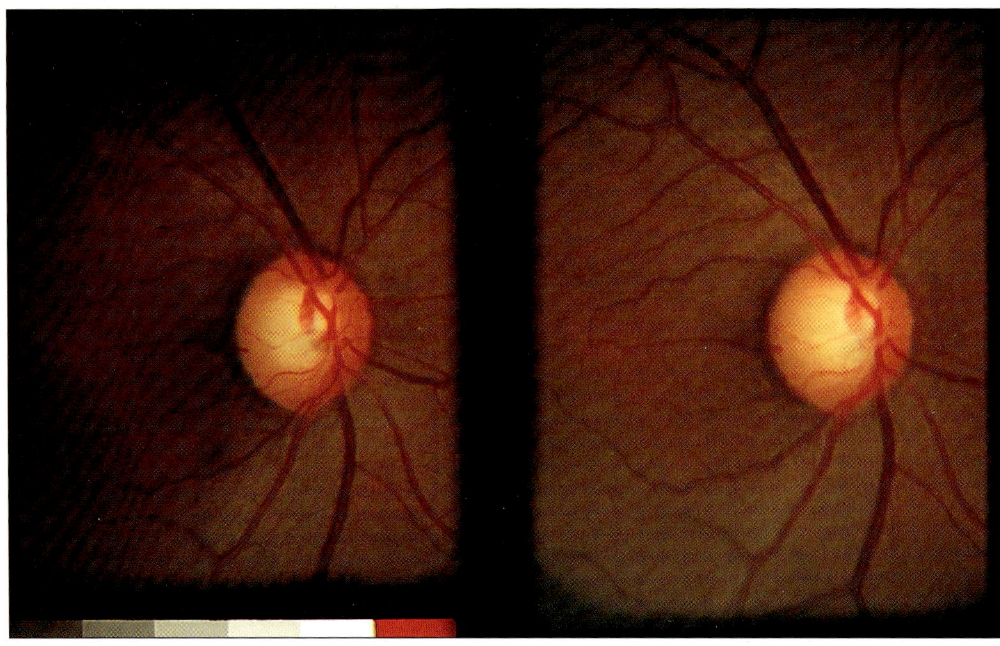

**Figure 7-13b.** Red-free NFL photograph appears normal.

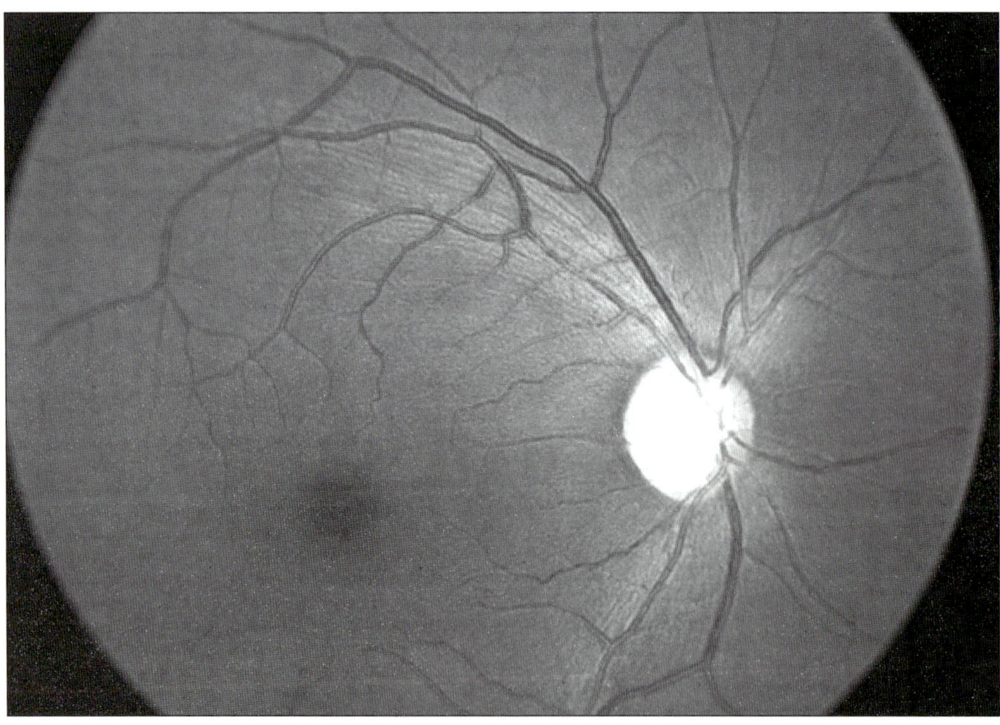

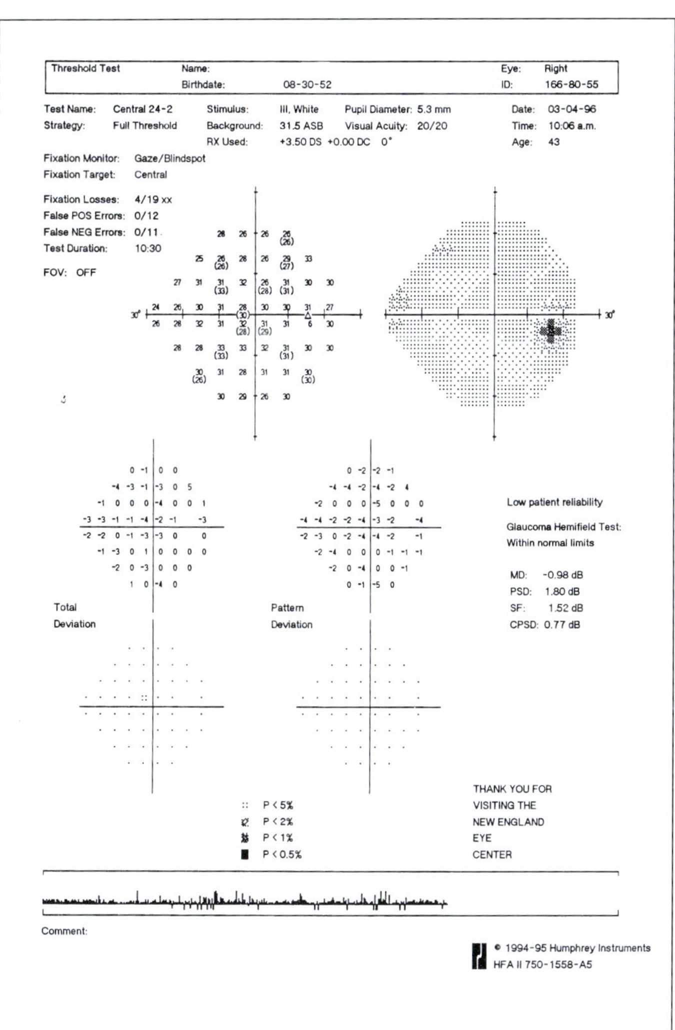

**Figure 7-13c.** Humphrey 24-2 visual field is full.

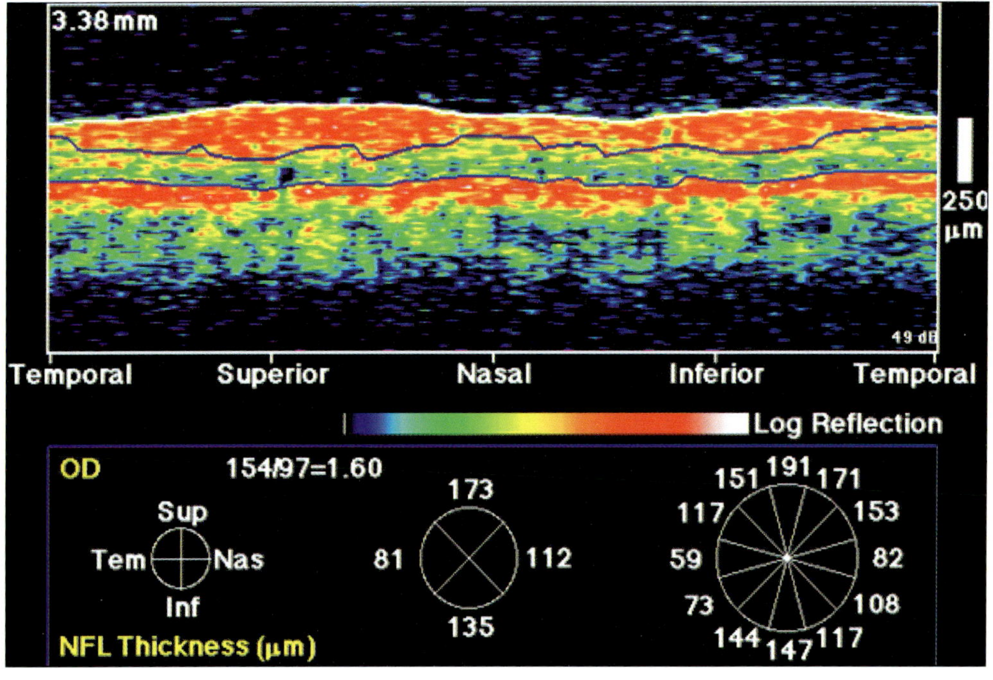



**Figure 7-13d.** OCT shows good NFL thickness.

**Figure 7-14a.** Stereoscopic ONH photograph of right eye of subject with asymmetric cupping and normal IOP.

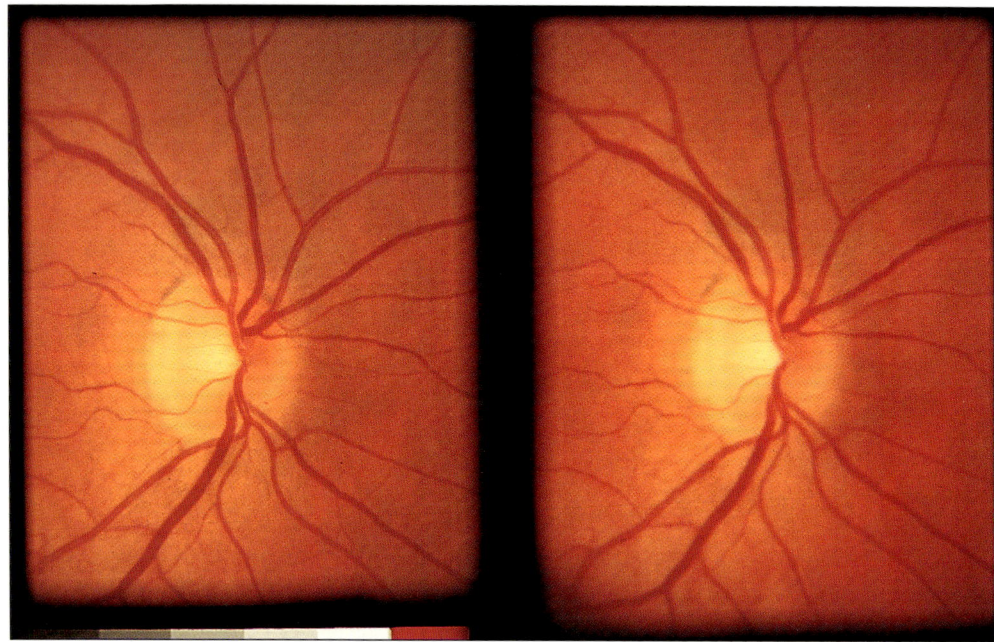

**Figure 7-14b.** Stereoscopic ONH photograph of left eye of subject with asymmetric cupping and normal IOP.

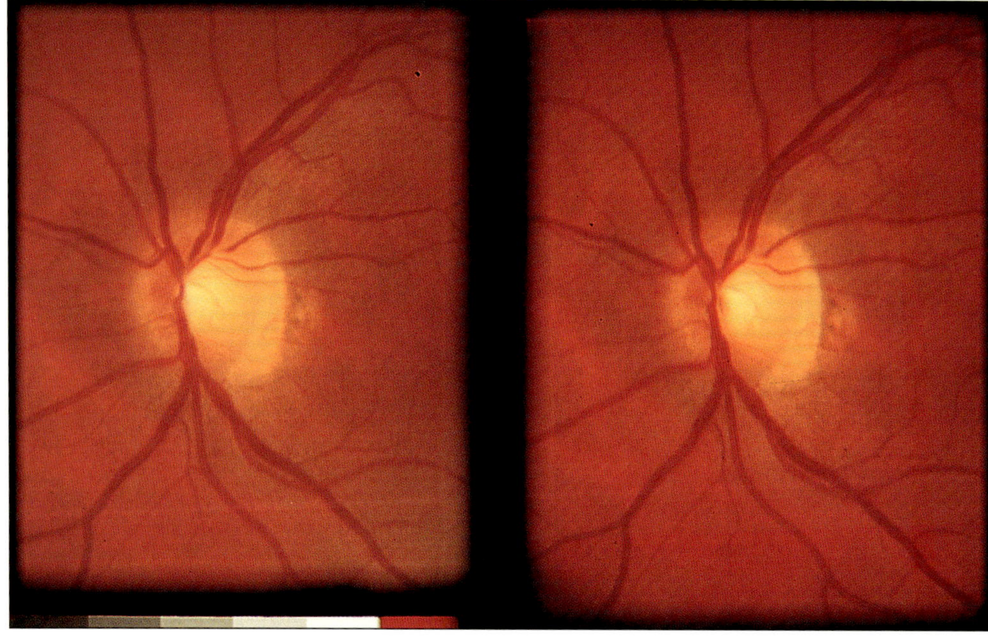

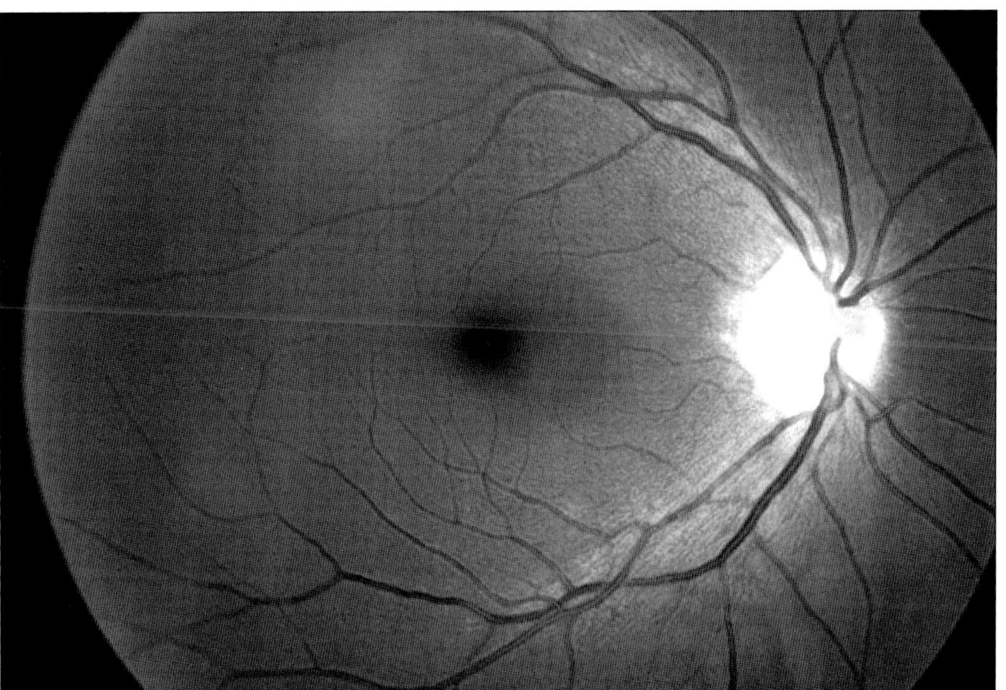

**Figure 7-14c.** Right eye red-free NFL photograph appears normal.

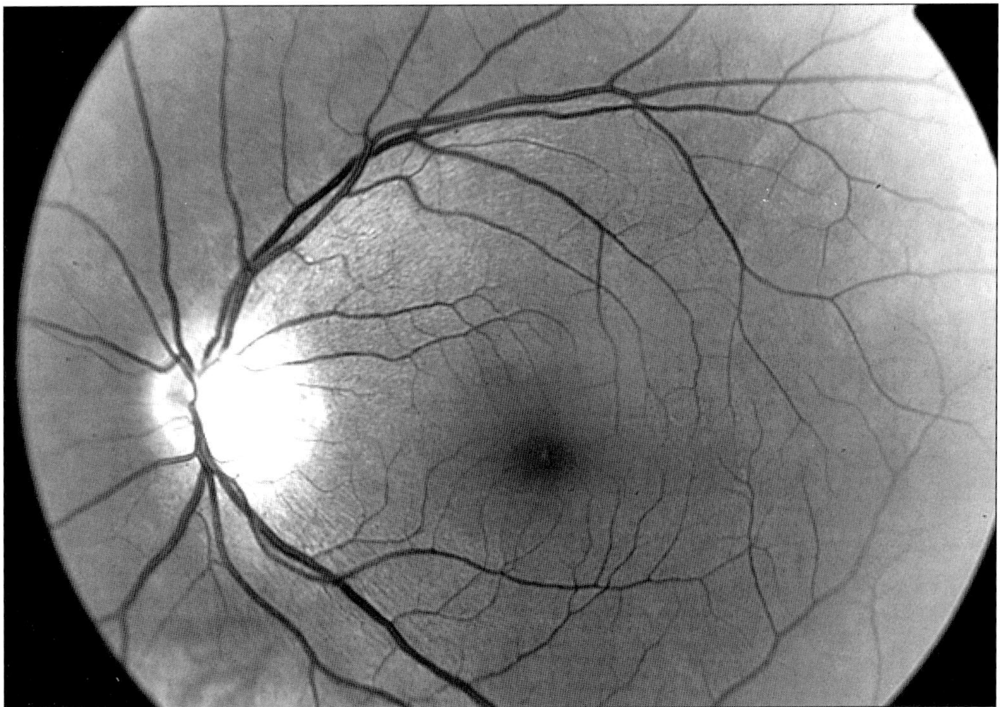

**Figure 7-14d.** Left eye red-free NFL photograph appears normal.

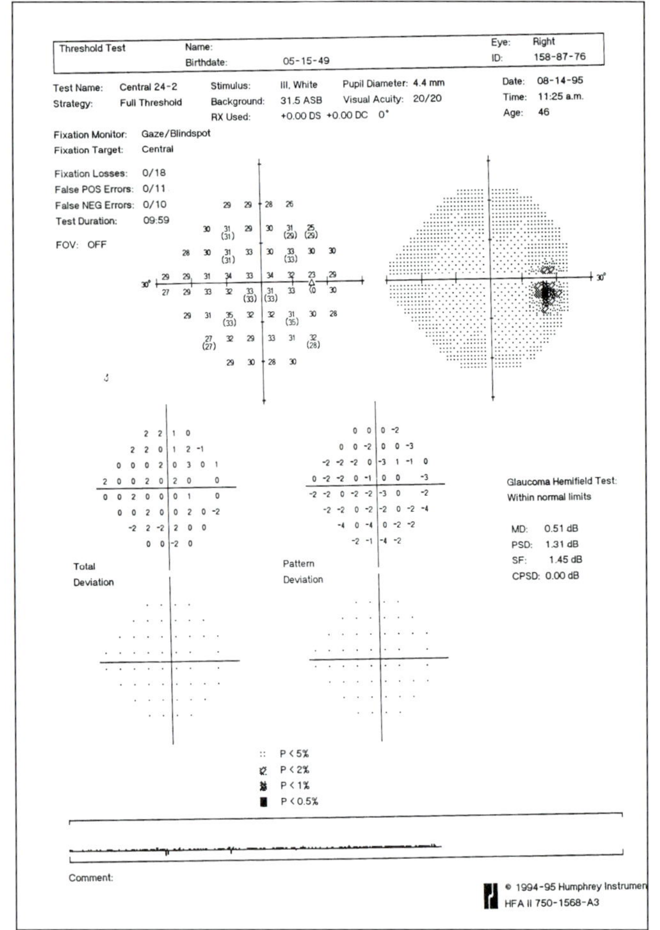

**Figure 7-14e.** Right eye Humphrey 24-2 visual field is full.

**Figure 7-14f.** Left eye Humphrey 24-2 visual field is full.

**Figure 7-14g.** Right OCT demonstrates good NFL thickness.

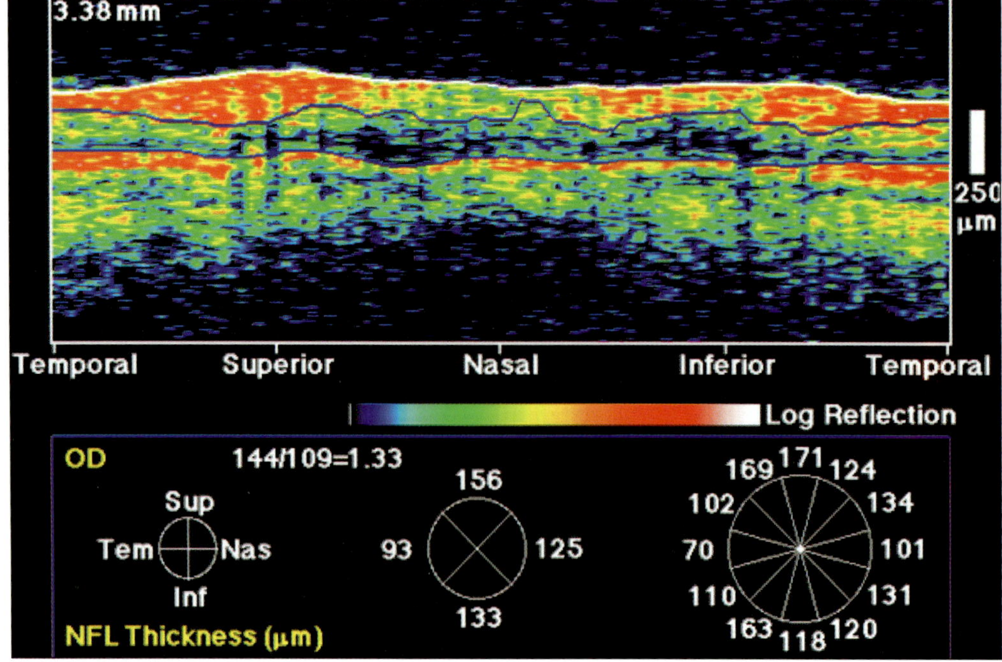

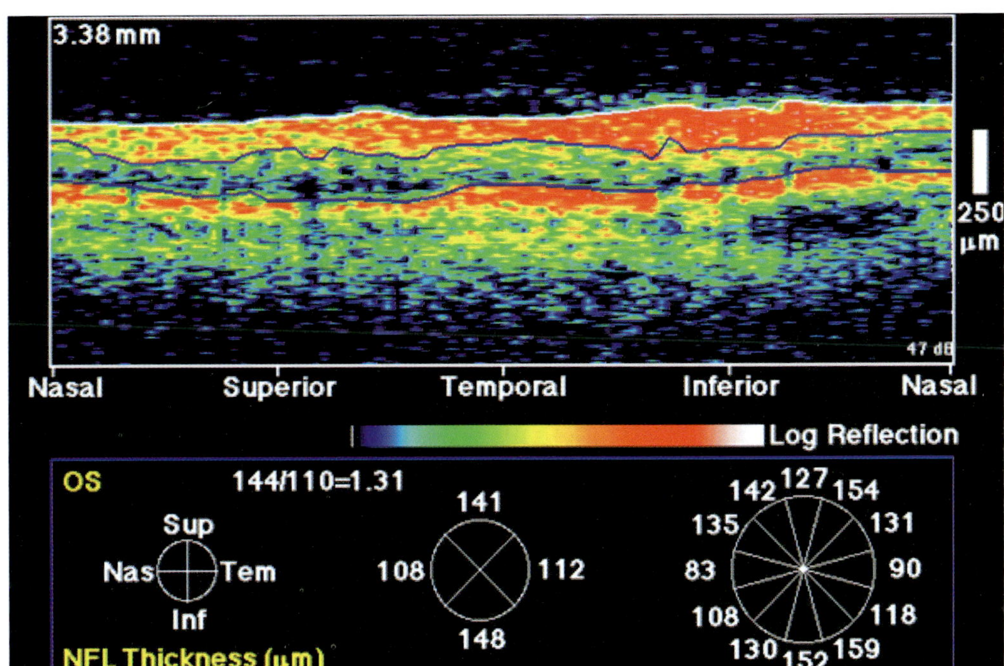


**Figure 7-14h.** Left eye OCT demonstrates good NFL thickness.

**Figure 7-15a.** Stereoscopic ONH photograph of right eye of subject with asymmetric cupping and elevated IOP.

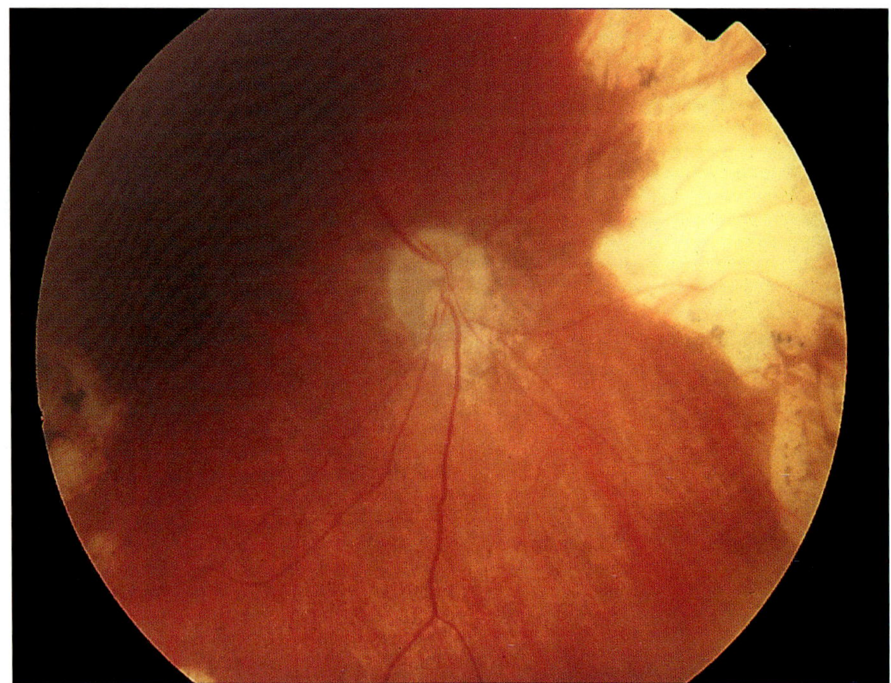

**Figure 7-15b.** Stereoscopic ONH photograph of left eye of subject with asymmetric cupping and elevated IOP.

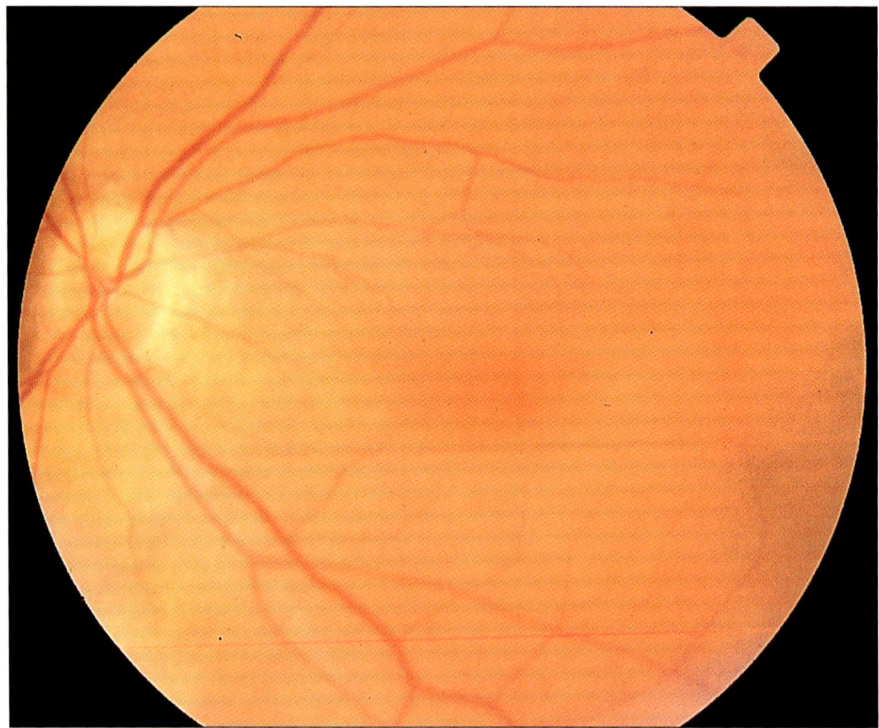

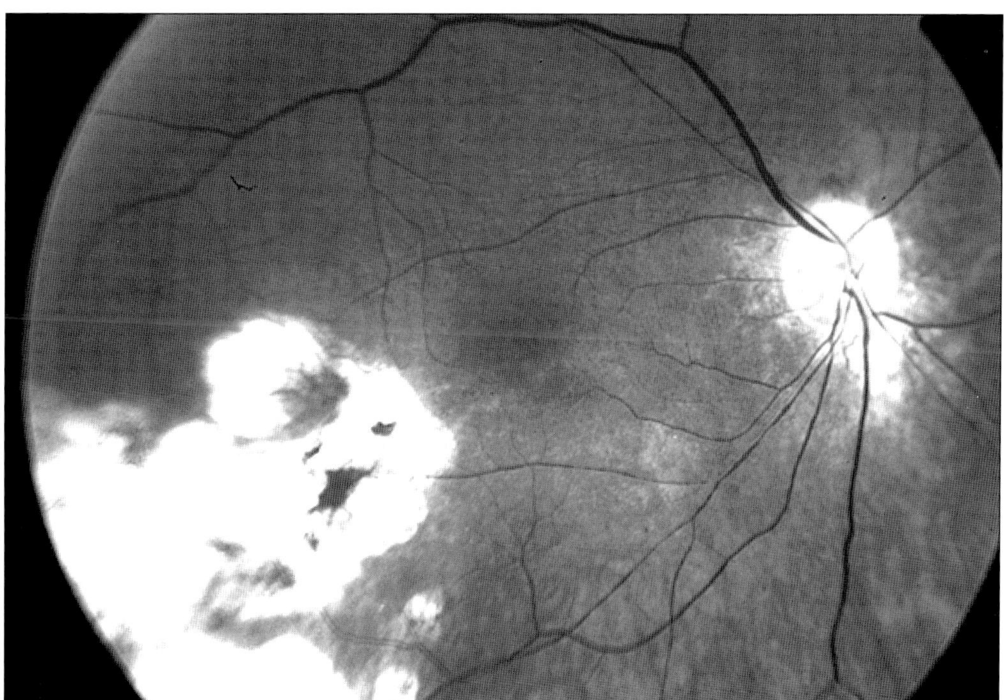

**Figure 7-15c.** Right eye red-free NFL photograph shows diffuse NFL atrophy.

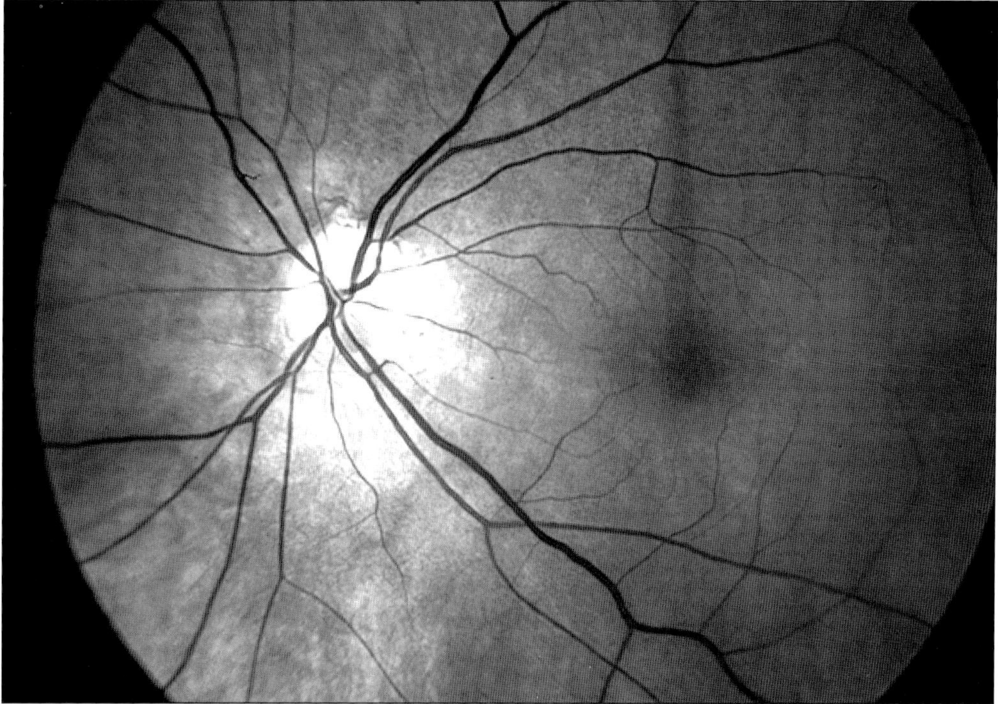

**Figure 7-15d.** Left eye red-free NFL photograph shows diffuse NFL atrophy.

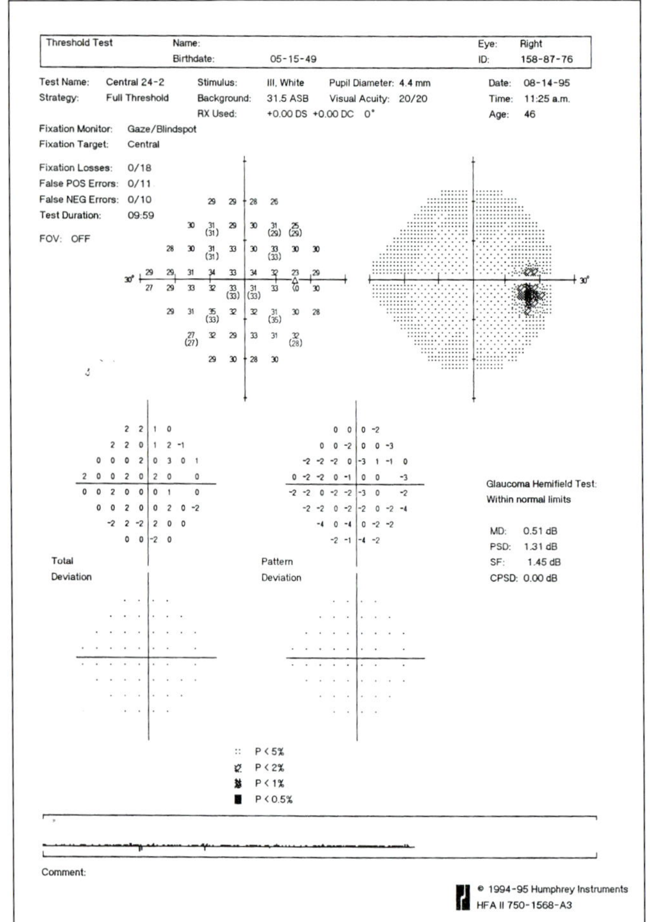

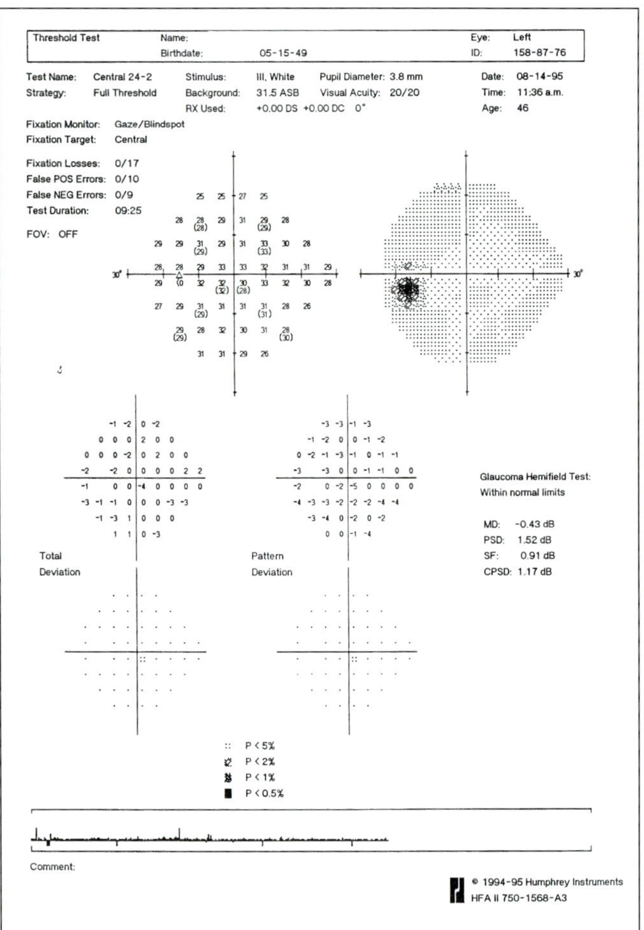

**Figure 7-15e.** Left eye Humphrey 24-2 visual field is abnormal (poor vision in right eye precludes visual field testing).

**Figure 7-14f.** Left eye Humphrey 24-2 visual field is full.

**Figure 7-15f.** Right eye OCT illustrates bilateral attenuation of NFL, more on the right than the left.

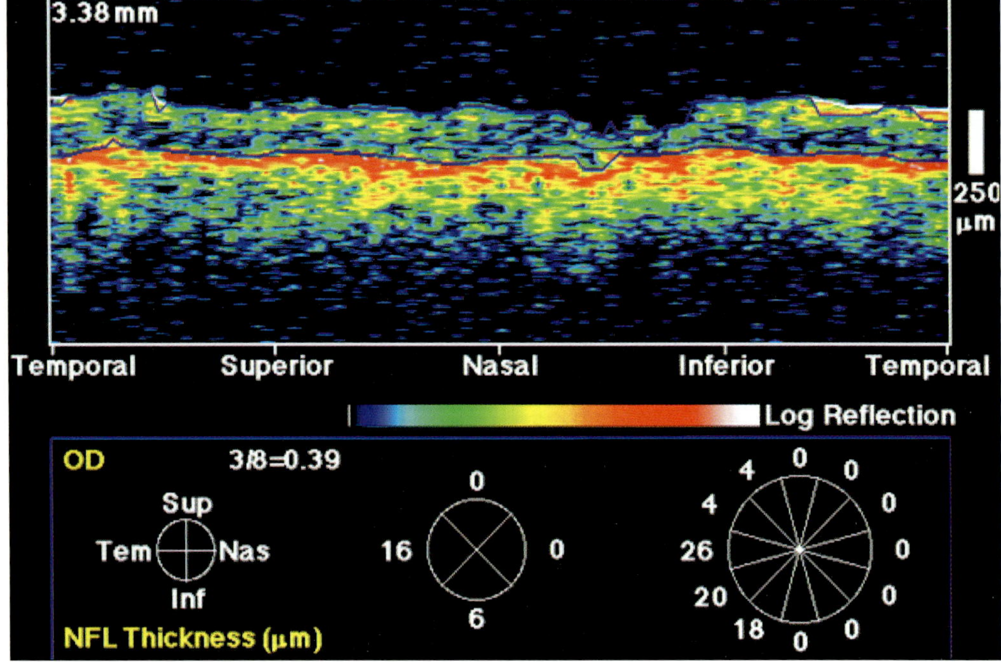

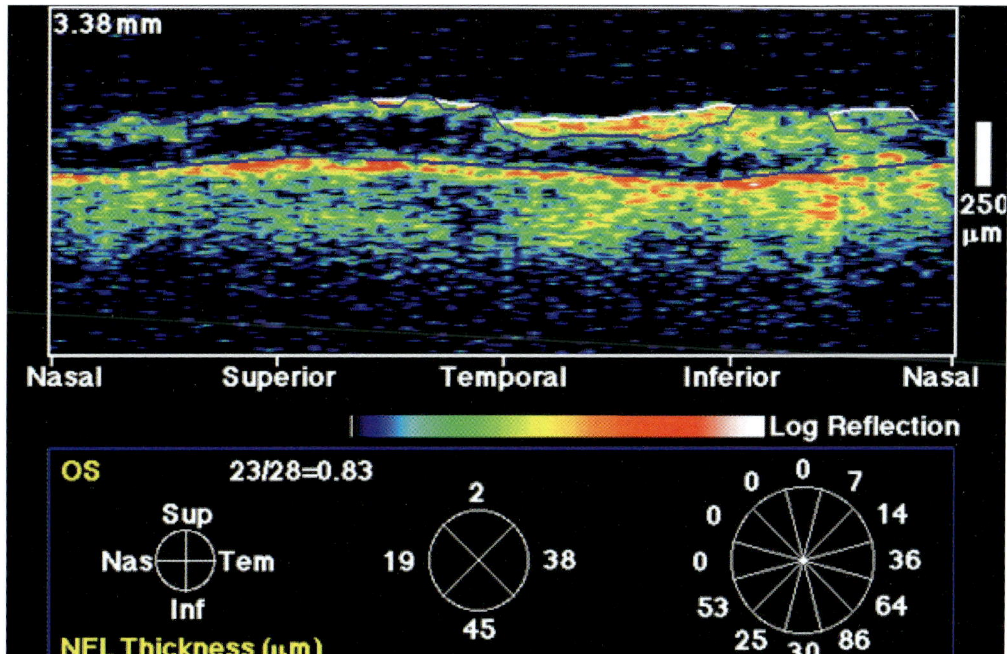


**Figure 7-15g.** Left eye OCT illustrates bilateral attenuation of NFL, more on the right than the left.

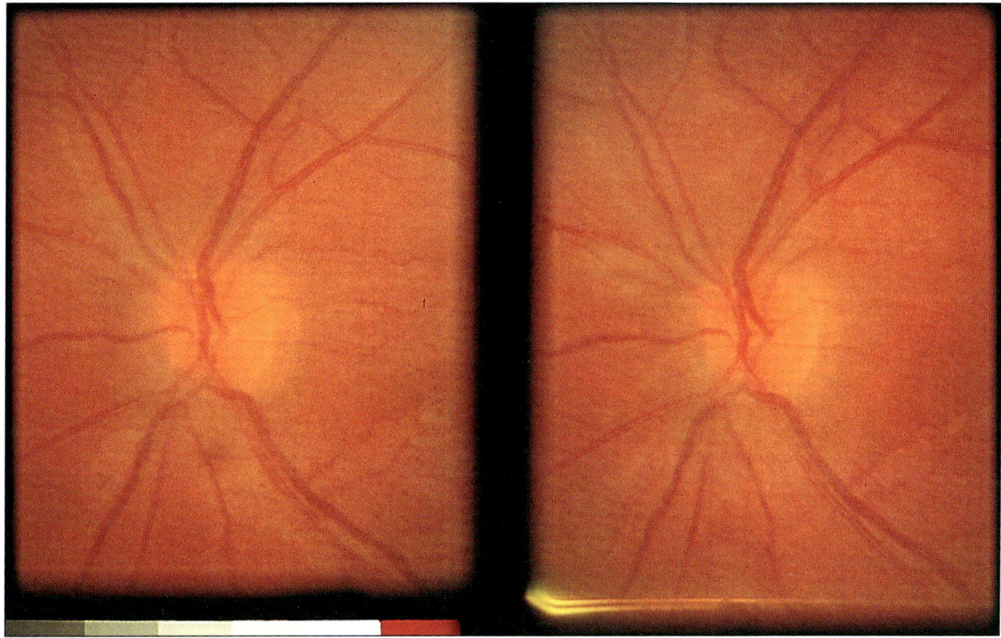

**Figure 7-16a.** Stereoscopic ONH photograph of left eye of subject with pigment dispersion due to a ciliary body mass, with elevated IOP.

**Figure 7-16b.** Ultrasound biomicroscopy demonstrates the ciliary body lesion.

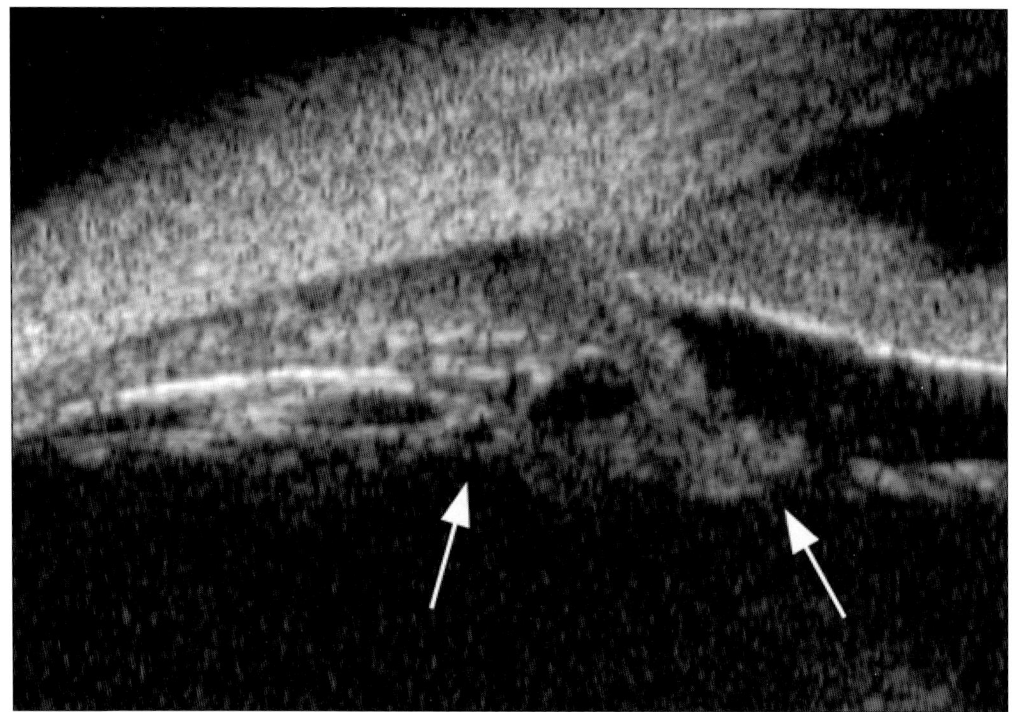

**Figure 7-16c.** Red-free NFL photograph appears normal.

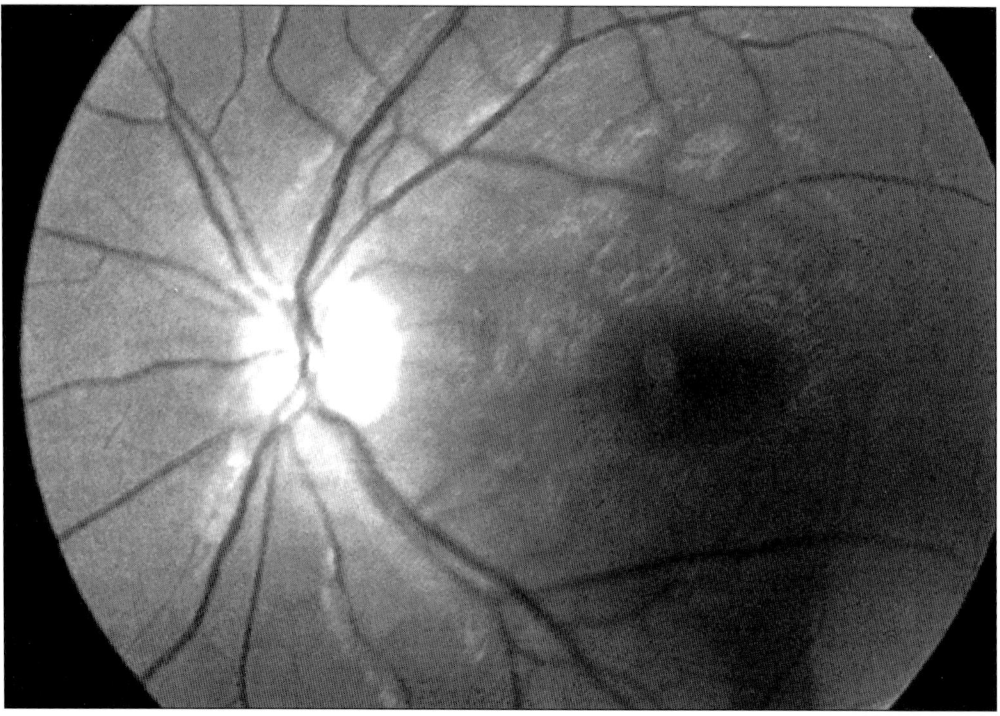

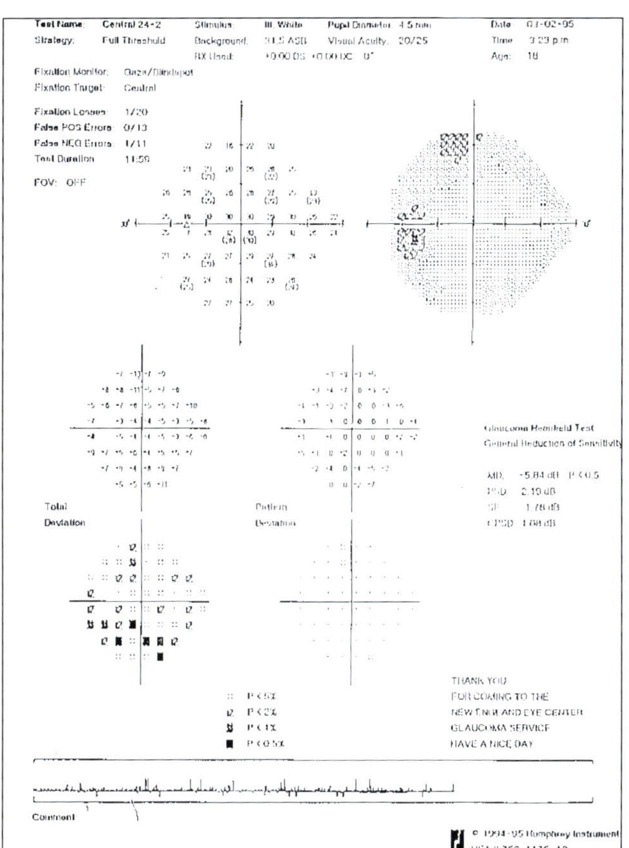

**Figure 7-16d.** Humphrey 24-2 visual field is full, with just the hint of the beginning of a superior defect.

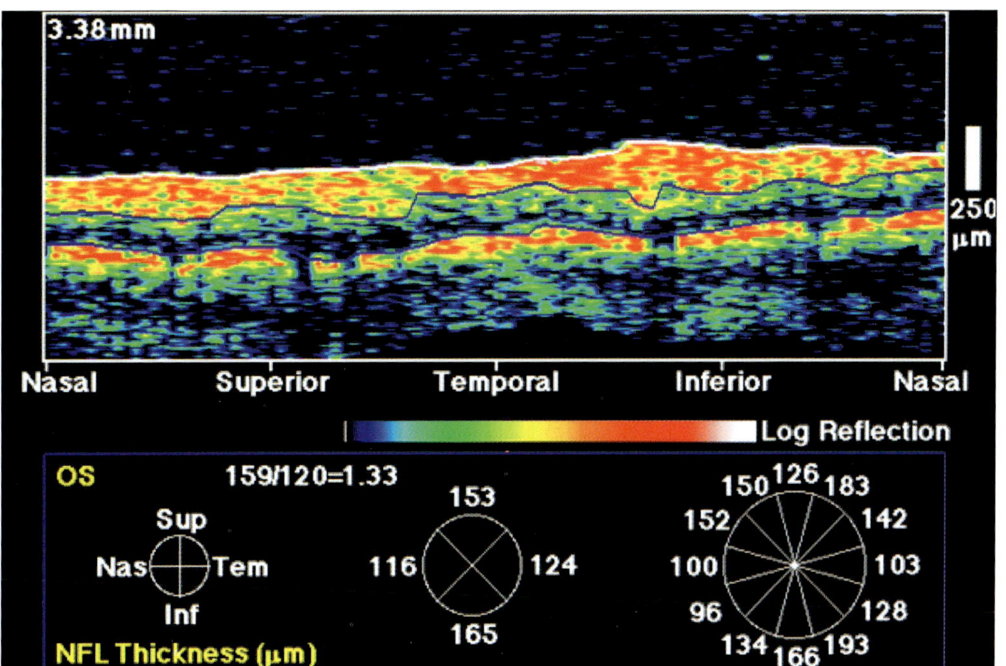


**Figure 7-16e.** OCT shows good NFL thickness, but values are slightly lower on the left than the right.

## REFERENCES

1. Hee MR, Izatt JA, Swanson EA, et al. Optical coherence tomography of the human retina. *Arch Ophthalmol.* 1995;113:325-332.
2. Huang D, Swanson EA, Lin CP, et al. Optical coherence tomography. *Science.* 1991;254:1178.
3. Izatt JA, Hee MR, Huang D, et al. Ophthalmic diagnostics using optical coherence tomography. In: Ren Q, Pavel JM, chairs/eds. Proceedings of Ophthalmic Technologies III. January 16-18, 1992, Los Angeles, Calif. Bellingham, Wash: SPIE, 1993; 136-44. (Progress in biomedical optics; Proceedings of SPIE; v.1877.)
4. Schuman JS, Hee MR, Puliafito CA, et al. Quantification of nerve fiber layer thickness in normal and glaucomatous eyes using optical coherence tomography: a pilot study. *Arch Ophthalmol.* 1995;113:586-596.
5. Swanson EA, Izatt JA, Hee MR, et al. In vivo retinal imaging using optical coherence tomography. *Opt Lett.* 1993;18:1864-1866.
6. Izatt JA, Hee MR, Swanson EA, et al. Micrometer-scale resolution imaging of the anterior eye in vivo with optical coherence tomography. *Arch Ophthalmol.* 1994;112:1584-1589.
7. Puliafito CA, Hee MR, Lin CP, et al. Imaging of macular diseases with optical coherence tomography. *Ophthalmology.* 1995;102:217-229.
8. Hee MR, Izatt JA, Swanson EA, et al. Optical coherence tomography for micron-resolution ophthalmic imaging. *IEEE Engineering in Medicine & Biology.* 1995;14(1):67-75.
9. Swanson EA, Huang D, Hee MR, et al. High-speed optical coherence domain reflectometry. *Opt Lett.* 1992;17:151-153.
10. Huang D, Stinson WG, Schuman JS, et al. High-resolution measurement of retinal thickness using optical coherence domain reflectometry. *Invest Ophthalmol Vis Sci.* 1991;32(Suppl):S1019.
11. Schuman JS, Pedut-Kloizman T, Hertzmark E, et al. Reproducibility of nerve fiber layer thickness measurements using optical coherence tomography. *Ophthalmology.* In press.
12. Hee MR, Puliafito CA, Wong C, et al. Optical coherence tomography of macular holes. *Ophthalmology.* 1995;102:748-756.
13. Schuman JS. Imaging optic nerve and nerve fiber layer: optical coherence tomography. In: Bucci MG, ed. *Glaucoma: Decision Making in Therapy.* Milan: Springer-Verlag. In press.
14. Pieroth L, Schuman JS, Hee MR, et al. Evaluation of focal defects in the nerve fiber layer using optical coherence tomography. *Invest Ophthalmol Vis Sci.* 1996;37(Suppl):S1094.
15. Chi Q, Tomita G, Inazumi K, Hayakawa T, Tadayoshi I, Kitazawa Y. Evaluation of the effect of aging on the retinal nerve fiber layer thickness using scanning laser polarimetry. *J Glaucoma.* 1995;4:406-413.
16. Varma R, Tielsch JM, Quigley HA. Race-, age-, gender-, and refractive error-related differences in the normal optic disc. *Arch Ophthalmol.* 1994;112:1068-1076.
17. Balazsi AG, Rootman J, Drance SM, et al. The effect of age on the nerve fiber population of the human optic nerve. *Am J Ophthalmol.* 1984;97:760-766.
18. Johnson BM, Miao M, Sadun AA. Age-related decline of human optic nerve axon populations. *Age.* 1987;10:5-9.
19. Hoyt WF, Newman NM. The earliest observable defect in glaucoma? *Lancet.* 1972;1:692-693.
20. Quigley HA, Addicks EM, Green WR. Optic nerve damage in human glaucoma. *Arch Ophthalmol.* 1982;100:135.
21. Sommer A, Miller NR, Pollack I, et al. The nerve fiber layer in the diagnosis of glaucoma. *Arch Ophthalmol.* 1977;95:2149-2156.
22. Sommer A, Katz J, Quigley HA, et al. Clinically detectable nerve fiber atrophy preceded the onset of glaucomatous field loss. *Arch Ophthalmol.* 1991;109:77.
23. Gaasterland D, Kupfer C. Experimental glaucoma in the rhesus monkey. *Invest Ophthalmol Vis Sci.* 1974;13:455-457.
24. Quigley HA, Holman RM. Laser energy levels for trabecular meshwork damage in the primate eye. *Invest Ophthalmol Vis Sci.* 1983;24:1305-1307.
25. Pedut-Kloizman T, Schuman JS, Hee MR, et al. Quantitative assessment of nerve fiber layer thickness in cynomolgus monkey eyes in vivo using optical coherence tomography. *Invest Ophthalmol Vis Sci.* 1995;36(Suppl):S972.
26. Schuman JS, Pedut-Kloizman T, Pieroth L, et al. Quantitation of nerve fiber layer thickness loss over time in the glaucomatous monkey model using optical coherence tomography. *Invest Ophthalmol Vis Sci.* 1996;37(Suppl):S1151.
27. Lloyd-Muhammad RA, Chung PY, Schuman JS, et al. Asymmetric cupping versus asymmetric discs in glaucoma suspects. *Invest Ophthalmol Vis Sci.* 1996;37(Suppl):S1093.
28. Roh S, Noecker RJ, Schuman JS, et al. Effect of optic disk drusen on nerve fiber layer thickness measured by optical coherence tomography (OCT). *Invest Ophthalmol Vis Sci.* 1996;37(Suppl):S1096.

# SECTION 3

# MEASURING OCULAR BLOOD FLOW

# Imaging of Blood Flow in Glaucoma

*Alon Harris, PhD, Louis Cantor, MD,
Larry Kagemann, MS*

## INTRODUCTION

At the June 1996 meeting of the European Glaucoma Society in Paris, several hundred ophthalmologists were asked if measurement of ocular blood flow was important in the management of their glaucoma patients. The ophthalmologists voted two to one "yes." While intraocular pressure (IOP) remains the primary focus in glaucoma treatment, assessment of ocular blood flow and the effects of IOP medications on blood flow are now important considerations in many clinics around the world. In this chapter we will review the hemodynamic assessment techniques of scanning laser ophthalmoscopy and color Doppler imaging (CDI). We will consider what may be learned about the glaucomatous eye with these two modalities. We will examine the etiologic and empirical studies that have moved the study of glaucoma into surprising new and promising directions: the study of ocular blood flow.

## WHY LOOK AT BLOOD FLOW IN GLAUCOMA?

### History

MacKenzie, in his 1833 book *Treatise on the Eye*, noted that the eyes of some glaucoma patients felt hard by palpation.[1a] This was the first association of glaucoma and ocular hypertension. In 1857, von Graefe first described glaucoma in the absence of ocular hypertension.[1b] von Graefe's theory met great resistance. Within the 24 years separating the two works, the role of hypertension in the pathogenesis of glaucoma had gained such wide acceptance in the scientific community that von Graefe, under the pressure of his peers, renounced his theory. It would be another 75 years until Elschnig,[1c] in 1928, would confirm von Graefe's observation of glaucoma in the absence of hypertension.

In 1892, Wagemann and Salzmann suggested the potential role of vascular factors in glaucoma.[2a] Convinced that ocular hypertension was not the sole contributing factor in glaucoma, Elschnig expanded on the vascular theory. After numerous exams, Elschnig observed that glaucomatous discs presented reduced capillary beds. He concluded that reduced nerve head perfusion resulted from the passage of vitreous into the cavernous disc due to IOP, whether high or normal. Belief that vascular defects resulted from IOP insult would continue for many years. Through the 1930s and 1940s, various authors demonstrated that increased IOP could reduce retinal vascular pressure and visual fields.[2b,2c]

In 1940, Duke and Elder excised a number of early stage glaucomatous eyes.[3a] They found evidence of sclerosis within the retrobulbar vessels. This vascular defect had produced ischemia resulting in softening of the optic nerve tissue. This finding demonstrated the potential presents of blood flow defects preceding and contributing to the type of neural damage observed in glaucoma. Loewenstein, in 1945, found that thrombotic occlusions of small ocular vessels were often implicated in disc cupping.[3b] Loewenstein's work was confirmed by Cristini 6 years later.[3c] Using anatomical methods, Cristini was able to determine that ischemia within the nerve head caused both optic disc cupping, and deformation within the laminar region. Cristini concluded that ischemia due to reduction in capillary networks within the optic nerve head (ONH), as observed by Elschnig nearly 25 years previously, was capable of producing lacunar degeneration.

The 1950s saw work that began to link visual function with blood flow parameters. Harrington, in 1959, studied the relationship between systemic blood pressure and visual field loss in primary open-angle glaucoma and normal tension glaucoma.[4a] This work was expanded by various other authors from the 1960s through the present.[4b-4e] The relationship between blood pressure and visual function remains an area of interest, though blood pressure measured in the arm is far removed from the pressures observed in the ophthalmic and other ocular arteries. More direct, yet circumstantial, evidence exists.

## Circumstantial Evidence

The Framingham Eye Study, The Beaver Dam Eye Study, and The Baltimore Eye Survey demonstrated that 40% to 60% of glaucoma patients have "normal" pressure, uncharacteristic of the high IOP traditionally identified as the cause of glaucomatous damage. This led both science and medicine to look more closely at the etiology of glaucoma, especially its vascular component. Utilizing fluorescein fundus angiography, Hayreh demonstrated that normal tension glaucoma patients exhibited reduced optic disk fluorescence.[5] From this, Hayreh concluded that reduced blood supply may be a permanent defect since the reduced fluorescence may be due to decreased vascularity.

Utilizing fluorescein angiography, Hitchings and Spaeth examined a group of low-tension glaucoma and chronic open-angle glaucoma patients.[6] They found that normal tension glaucoma patients exhibited localized hypoperfusion of the ONH, while the chronic open-angle group exhibited a combination of localized and diffuse areas of hypoperfusion. It was concluded that vascular changes may occur in glaucoma.

Corbett and Phelps believed that the possibility of a hemodynamic contribution to the damage which occurs in glaucoma merited some investigation. In 1985, they published a study in which they looked for clinical or radiographic evidence of cerebral atrophy in normal tension glaucoma patients. Since the blood supply to the eye is closely tied to the cerebral blood supply, and assuming some defect in ocular blood flow, they hypothesized that some evidence of cerebral disorder may be observed in normal tension glaucoma patients. Quite unexpectedly during their investigation, however, they discovered that an unusually large percentage of their patients reported a history of common or classic migraine.[7] This unexpected finding raised the possibility that since migraine is thought to be an ischemic disorder associated with vasospasm, normal tension patients may suffer an ischemic disorder which contributes to their glaucomatous condition as well as to their migraines. They followed up with a study that questioned normal tension, primary open-angle glaucoma, and ocular hypertensive patients about headaches. They discovered that normal tension glaucoma patients did indeed suffer from headaches more frequently than any other group. This was especially surprising considering the age of these patients. Headaches are less common among the elderly, yet this group of elderly patients suffered headaches more frequently than the younger, normal, healthy control subjects.[8]

Gasser and Flammer observed that many of their normal tension glaucoma patients reported (when asked, not necessarily voluntarily) that they suffered from cold hands. Intrigued, they performed a study in which patients with visual field loss but normal IOPs were subjected to cold water hand immersion immediately before a visual field examination.[9] The vasospasm-induced by this pretreatment with cold water caused a marked deterioration in their visual fields. The test was repeated after administration of 10 to 20 mg of nifedipine, a calcium channel blocker. Patients who demonstrated a vasospasm-induced field deterioration in the first test demonstrated an improvement of visual field performance with the nifedipine. Their work suggests a link between the level of blood flow and visual function, as well as the possibility of treatment for vasospasm in low or normal tension glaucoma.

## Empirical Evidence

In our lab at the Indiana University School of Medicine, we have used color Doppler ultrasound to document a difference in the ocular blood flow characteristics of normal tension glaucoma patients as compared to age-matched controls, and the ability to alleviate these differences using a vasodilatory agent.[10]

The ophthalmic artery systolic and diastolic blood velocity in a group of normal tension glaucoma patients was measured using pulsed color Doppler ultrasound imaging techniques (to be discussed in depth in the following sections). Similar measurements were obtained from a group of age-matched controls. The diastolic velocity of the glaucoma patients was significantly lower than that of the normals. From this information, we calculated the resistive index (also discussed in depth in the following sections) for both groups. The resistive index of the glaucoma patients was significantly higher, suggesting a greater resistance to flow or vasospasm in this group. Carbon dioxide, a potent vasodilator, was then added to the air of the groups until their end tidal $CO_2$ content reached a 15% increase.[11] Under the vasodilatory conditions, the differences in diastolic velocity and resistive index vanished. Based on our data, we were able to conclude that some normal tension glaucoma patients suffer from reversible ocular vasospasm.

## What About Primary Open-Angle Glaucoma?

Several large epidemiologic studies[12-14] have followed populations and patient groups in order to learn more about who develops glaucoma, and what, if any, risk factors may be used in trying to predict who merits close monitoring. As is well known, ocular hypertensives are at risk for developing field loss over time. In 1979, however, Hart et al followed the status of a group of 92 ocular hypertensives.[15] After 5 years, 64% of the ocular hypertensives exhibited no visual field defects, disc cupping, or disc pallor. Similarly, depending on the study used for

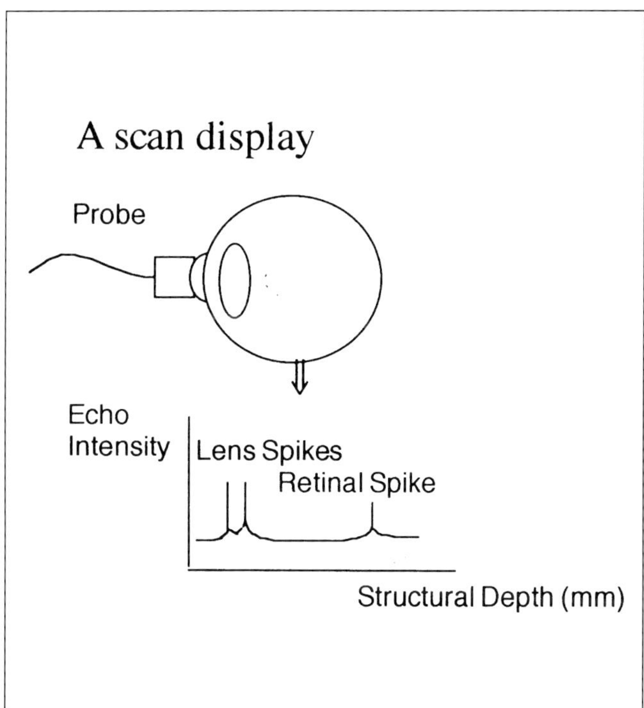



**Figure 8-1.** A-scan ultrasound uses echoes from internal structures to determine their depth.

data, 40% to 60% of the patients who do develop visual field loss never exhibit IOPs above the normal range. Until now, studies looking for evidence of vascular pathologies in glaucoma have primarily focused on normal tension glaucoma, as this disease lacks other documented explanations of a mechanism of damage. We have extended our work to include primary open-angle glaucoma patients, and have found evidence for ocular vasospasm in some percentage of patients.[16] Currently, it appears that the prevalence of ocular vasospasm in primary open-angle glaucoma patients is lower than in normal tension patients, but does exist and merits further investigation.

## THE BASIC PHYSICAL PRINCIPLES OF ULTRASOUND

### Introduction

Ultrasound is an imaging technology that uses echoes to locate structure. The first major attempt to use soundwave and echo technology was a failed attempt to locate the wreck of the Titanic in 1912. Similarly, early efforts in medical uses of ultrasound met the same fate. Like many technologies we enjoy today, we can thank the massive military research effort during World War II for ultrasound. The push for a practical and working SONAR (SOund Navigation And Ranging) system removed many technical barriers. Successful medical applications began soon after World War II in the late 1940s and early 1950s.[17]

## Mechanics of Ultrasound Scanning and Probes

Medical ultrasound is based on the movement of soundwaves through the body. The soundwave is projected into the body, and when it strikes an anatomic structure, some of the wave is reflected or echoed. The reflected soundwave is detected by the same probe which emitted the wave.

By definition, an A-scan, or axial scan, is a simple depth finding scan used to locate the distance to various structures on a line from the probe (Figure 8-1).

The echoes created by the various objects are represented by spikes in the display. A-scans are typically used in ophthalmology to accurately measure the axial length of the eye from the anterior surface of the cornea back to the anterior surface of the lens, and finally the anterior surface of the retina.

B-scans can be thought of as a group of adjacent A-scans, in which the height of the spike is displayed as a shade of gray (Figure 8-2).

If we picture the a scan probe sweeping over the eye from top to bottom, we would have a number of A-scan spikes as seen on the right. These spikes represent structure. We can display structure as white against a black background. The B-scan display below the spike graph was constructed from the map of A-scan spikes.

Functionally, a B-scan probe consists of many A-scan probes side by side in a row. Each scans in a line and receives echoes. The B-scan image we see clinically is a composite of the individual A-scan type of signals produced by each element of the linear array.

## Properties of Sound and Their Relationship to Probe Limitations

The movement of the soundwave through the body is governed by the relationship between velocity, frequency, and wavelength:

$$v = f \times \lambda$$

with v equal to velocity, f equal to frequency, and $\lambda$ equal to wavelength. As you can see by this relationship, the same frequency probe will produce different wavelengths within the body, depending on the velocity of sound through that type of tissue. The velocities of sound through a variety of materials are listed in Table 8-1.

Clinically, this is important because the best resolution that an ultrasound unit may have is a single wavelength.

Let's say you are considering a unit that features a 7.5 MHz linear probe. From Table 8-1, we see that the velocity of sound in water or soft tissue is 1540 m/s. The smallest structure that you would be able to resolve would be:

$$1540 \text{ m/s} = 7,500,000 \text{ Hz} \times \lambda$$
$$\lambda = 1540/7,500,000 = 0.000205 \text{ m, or } 0.2 \text{ mm}$$

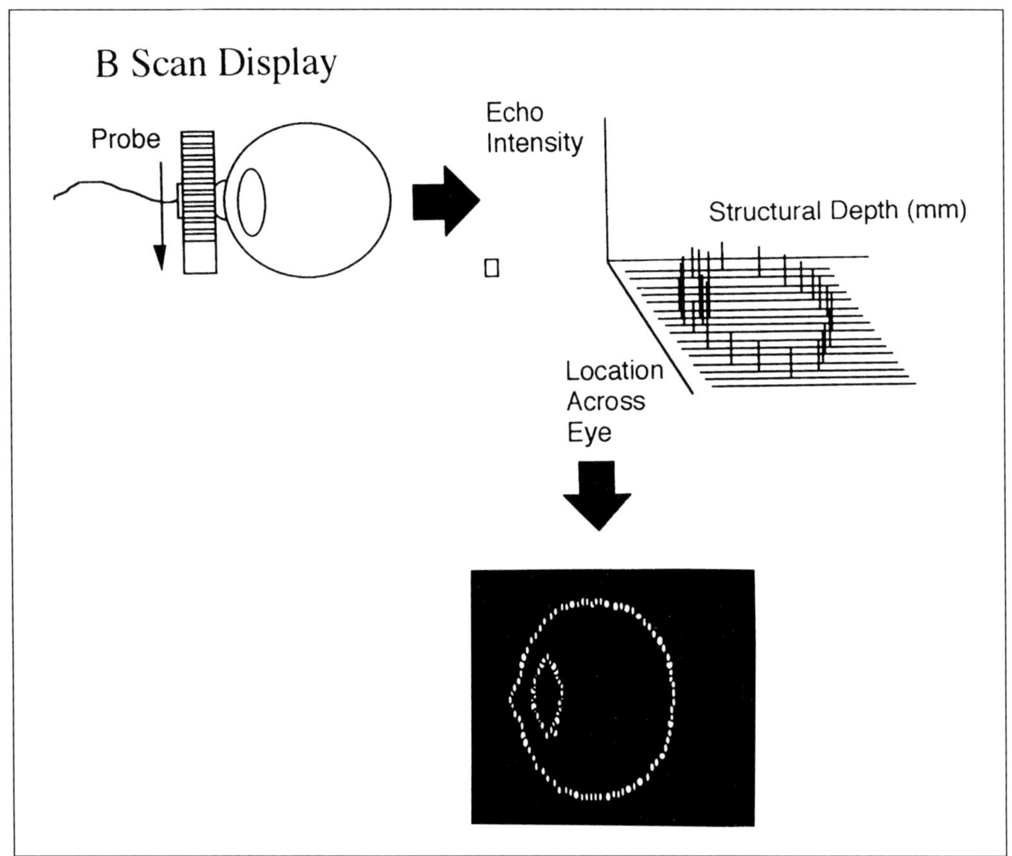



**Figure 8-2.** B-scans consist of a row of A-scans. Structural depths along each position on the probe are assembled to form a planar image.

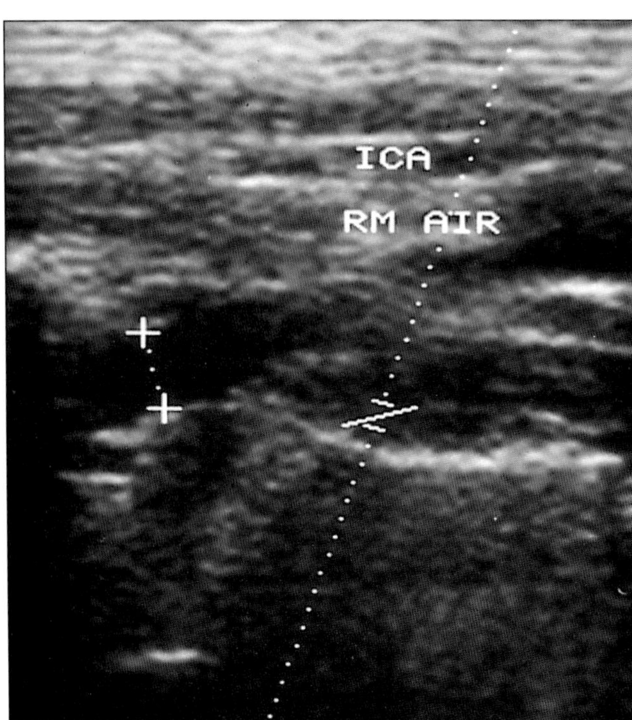



**Figure 8-3.** A B-scan image consists of pixels, each representing the echo intensity received from that location in the body.

Table 8-1

**Velocity of Sound in Various Biological Materials**

| Material | Velocity (m/s) |
| --- | --- |
| Air | 331 |
| Fat | 1450 |
| Castor oil | 1500 |
| Water (50°C) | 1540 |
| Human soft tissue | 1540 |
| Brain | 1541 |
| Liver | 1549 |
| Kidney | 1561 |
| Blood | 1570 |
| Muscle | 1585 |
| Ocular lens | 1620 |

Each pixel or dot on the display screen of this ultrasound would represent a piece of tissue 0.2 mm, or 200 microns, in diameter. The grainy composite image of a normal B-scan ultrasound image is composed of these pixels (Figure 8-3).

## Mechanics of Doppler Shifts

The Doppler effect is the change in perceived frequency of a wave emitted by a moving source. The effect was first described by Christian Doppler in 1843.[18] When a stationary

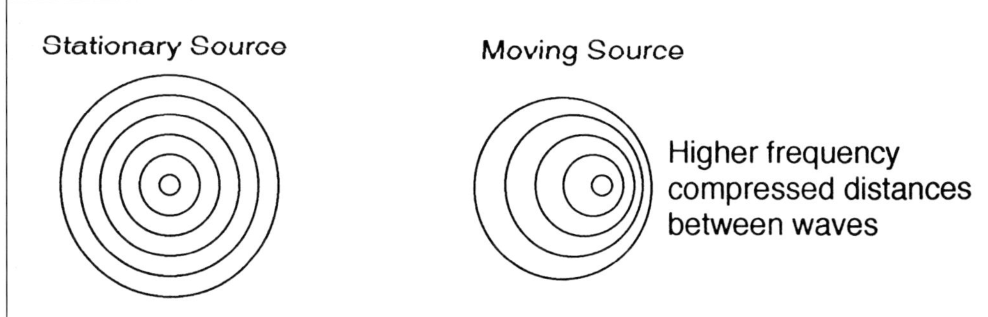


**Figure 8-4.** Soundwaves in front of a moving source are compressed. Soundwaves trailing a moving source are separated.

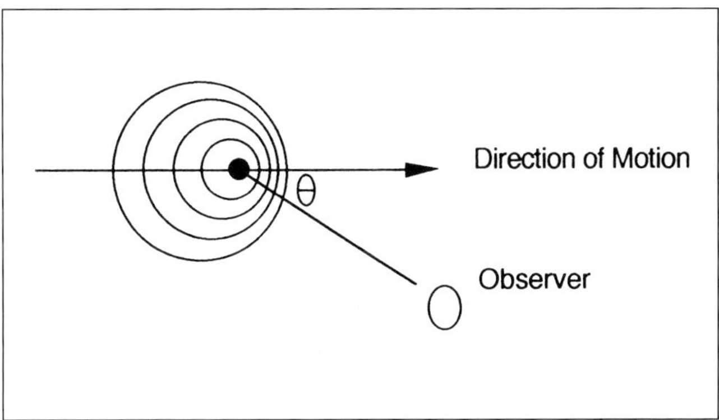


**Figure 8-5.** The frequency observed from a moving source depends on the relative location of the observer.

source creates a sound, the soundwaves propagate away from the source in all directions (Figure 8-4).

When a source is moving, the soundwaves in front of the source tend to be compressed. From the time that the source has emitted a soundwave to the time the next wave is emitted, the source will have moved slightly toward the existing wave. In this way, the motion of the sound source distorts the wave pattern as seen above. Conversely, by moving away from pre-existing waves which trail the source, that same source will cause the distance from wave to wave to grow. The magnitude of the perceived shift in frequency may be calculated as:

$$\Delta f = \frac{2fV_{source}}{V_{sound}} \cos\theta$$

with $\Delta f$ equal to the Doppler shift in Hertz, f equal to the frequency of the incident soundwave, $V_{source}$ equal to the velocity of the moving source of sound, and $V_{sound}$ equal to the velocity of sound in that medium (see Table 8-1). If we consider moving blood to be moving sources of sound (or in this case echo), an ultrasound unit with a little computing power can use the Doppler equation to deduce the velocity of the blood in the body. This requires the probe to be sensitive to the frequency as well as the magnitude of returning echoes. Note from the Doppler equation, that the frequency shift is also subject to the angle between the vector of motion and the location of the observer (Figure 8-5).

In the case of blood flow in the body, only flow directly toward the probe will yield the full Doppler shift. If the flow is at some angle to the probe, it is necessary to correct for that angle in order to accurately calculate blood velocity. While it is theoretically possible to correct for any angle up to 89°, the potential for error due to incorrect angle correction becomes large.

Let us consider the effect of an error of only 1° in angle correction in two different situations. An angle correction of 20° when 21° is called for will result in a 0.6% error, while angle correction of 78° when 79° was called for would result in a 9% error. As a matter of good clinical practice, it is advised that no angle correction of over 60° be attempted.

Most CDI ultrasound units display moving blood by overlaying the b mode image with areas of color. Usually, red will represent flow toward the probe, and blue is used to represent flow away from the probe (Figure 8-6). It is important to remember that the color observed in a Doppler image does not necessarily represent arterial or venous flow. An ultrasound unit has no way of distinguishing whether flow is venous or arterial. The color assignments are based purely on the direction of flow. It is up to the technician's or observer's knowledge of anatomy and expected flow characteristics to decide which type or vessel is being imaged. If a vessel is displayed as blue, but a strong pulsation is observed, it is likely that the vessel in question is an artery flowing away from the probe. Likewise, a vessel displayed as red, but lacking any evidence of pulsation, is probably a vein flowing toward the probe.

As mentioned, by utilizing the Doppler equation and observing the echoed frequencies, an ultrasound unit with a little computing power is capable of measuring the blood velocities. A sample volume window is placed on the vessel of interest. When properly positioned, the unit can be set to analyze the frequency spectra and calculate the velocities present in the vessel within this window. When this is accomplished in real time, a velocity waveform is obtained. A discussion of the different parts of the waveform, and the information which may be obtained from the waveform follows in the next section.

**Figure 8-6.** Movement toward the probe is color coded red, usually caused by arterial blood. Movement away from the probe is color coded blue, usually caused by venous flow.

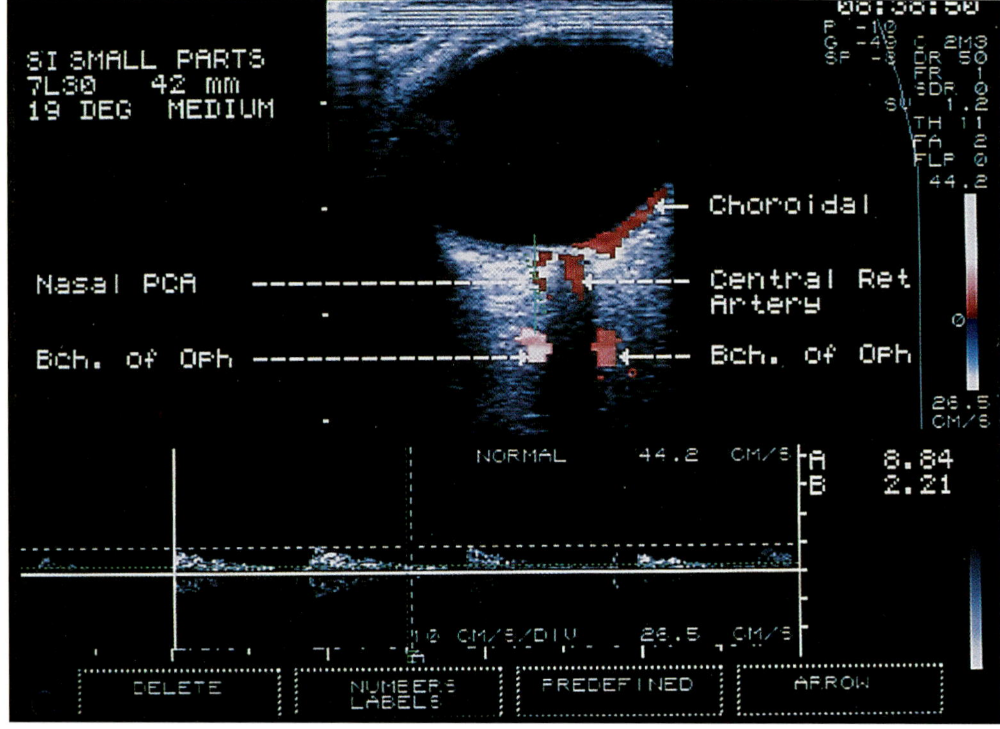


## Conclusions

Considering the size of ocular vessels, it is important to know the physical limitations of a particular probe frequency. When reading research publications, it is important to be aware of the limitations of resolution of various frequency probes. You will often find that one study conduced with a 2 MHz probe will reach different conclusions than one conducted with a higher frequency probe. You may also see that some systems will use a higher frequency for B-scan and CDI, while using a lower frequency for pulsed Doppler sampling of blood velocities. The spatial resolution of the B-scan of such a system is better than the spatial resolution of the sample window used to specify the location of pulsed Doppler sampling.

## WHAT DO WE IMAGE AND HOW DOES IT APPLY TO GLAUCOMA?

Glaucomatous damage occurs within the optic disc and the anterior optic nerve. In order to identify areas of ocular blood flow that are of particular interest in glaucoma, we will review nerve head anatomy and the vasculature which perfuses that area. With an understanding of the applicable vasculature, we can then examine the locations where measurement of blood velocity is possible using CDI.

The retina contains the ganglion cells from which the axons in the optic nerve originate. Ganglion cell bodies and the retinal portion of their axons are perfused by the central retinal artery. The relationship between ganglion cell metabolism and glaucomatous damage is not fully understood, but the health of ganglion cell bodies is thought to be pertinent to the progression of glaucoma. CDI may be used to quantify blood velocities of the central retinal artery immediately posterior to the globe.

The most anterior area of the ONH is the superficial nerve fiber layer (NFL). This is the area of nerve fibers visible by fundus examination as they converge at the disk and bend backward forming the optic nerve. This area, as with the ganglion cells discussed above, is perfused primarily by branches of the central retinal artery (Figure 8-7).

If a cilioretinal artery is present, it may also provide perfusion within the temporal quadrant of the ONH.

Immediately posterior to the superficial fiber layer, but anterior to the lamina cribrosa, lies the prelaminar region. This area consists primarily of nerve fibers collected into bundles and surrounded by glial cells (Figure 8-8).

As you can see in Figure 8-8, the prelaminar region is perfused by a capillary network which is independent of the capillaries in the adjacent choroid. Choroidal arterioles may reach across into the prelaminar region to provide some blood supply, but the choroidal capillaries do not extend over into the prelaminar region. There may also be contribution from arterioles reaching anterior and medially from the circle of Zinn-Haller. Both the circle and the surrounding choroid are fed by branches of the short posterior ciliary arteries (see Figure 8-8). Short posterior ciliary arteries approach the choroid, circle of Zinn-Haller, and optic nerve itself from temporal and nasal groupings of 10 to 15 arteries. Many of the short posterior ciliary arteries enter the globe posterior to the macula. It is important to remember that the thickness of the choriocapillaris is

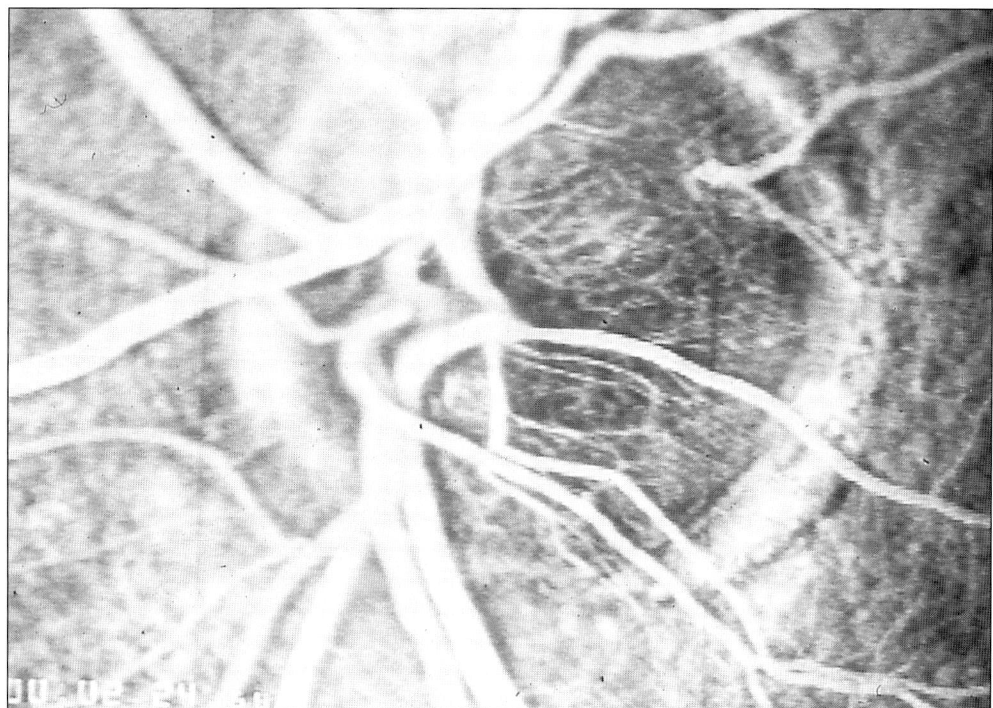

**Figure 8-7.** The superficial NFL is perfused by capillaries from the central retinal artery.

constant. The high density of choroidal arterioles behind the macula cause the choroid to be thickest here. The actual choriocapillaris is no thicker in this area than in the periphery.[19]

The lamina cribrosa region consists of tightly packed nerve fiber bundles as they pass though fenestrations in the collagen matrix. It is this collagen which supports the pressure gradient between the globe and optic nerve at the level of the lamina cribosa. This area of high mechanical stress is perfused by arterioles extending inward from the surrounding circle of Zinn-Haller. The circle itself is located around the lamina cribrosa within the body of the sclera. Once again, the circle is fed by branches of the short posterior ciliary arteries.

The retrolaminar region is the anteriormost section of the optic nerve. It consists of myelinated axons as they begin their trek to the lateral geniculate body. The retrolaminar region is perfused by the pial system, a dense meshwork of capillaries which lie around the outside of the core of nerve fibers. The pial system is fed directly by branches of the short posterior ciliary arteries, as well as posterior reaching arterioles of the circle of Zinn-Haller. The pial system also receives some branches from the central retinal artery as it courses through the center of the nerve (Figure 8-9).

Branches from the central retinal artery extend radially and anastomose with the capillary network of the pial system.

As you can see, the central retinal artery and short posterior ciliary arteries are the primary source of nutrients, oxygen, and waste removal in the area of glaucomatous optic neuropathy. The ability to quantify the blood velocities and resistive indices (discussed in the following sections) of these vessels has become invaluable in research, and is finding its way into the clinical environment.

The single source for these vital arteries is the ophthalmic artery. The only extracranial branch of the internal carotid artery, the ophthalmic artery is the source of the central retinal artery and the posterior ciliary arteries, as well as all other globe perfusing arteries. The posterior ciliary arteries branch into the various temporal and nasal posterior ciliary arteries. CDI is able to quantify blood velocity in the ophthalmic artery. Ophthalmic artery velocities can yield information concerning the resistance to flow in the vessels it feeds, those vessels being the immediate supply of blood to the tissue damaged in glaucoma.[9,20]

## PROCEDURES AND DATA INTERPRETATION

Data are obtained by direct ultrasound examination of the retrobulbar arteries discussed in the previous section. The patient reclines to 60° in a reclining dialysis chair. We chose these chairs because they are very comfortable for the patient, and allow easy and comfortable positioning of the patient for the technician. An ultrasonic coupling gel is applied to the probe, and the probe is gently placed on the closed eyelid. The mechanical pressure of the technician's hand due to the weight of his or her arm, probe, and cable is applied to the patient's forehead via the technician's palm, leaving the probe relatively weightless on the eye. This is well tolerated by the patient, and allows the technician to perform for extended periods without fatigue (Figure 8-10).

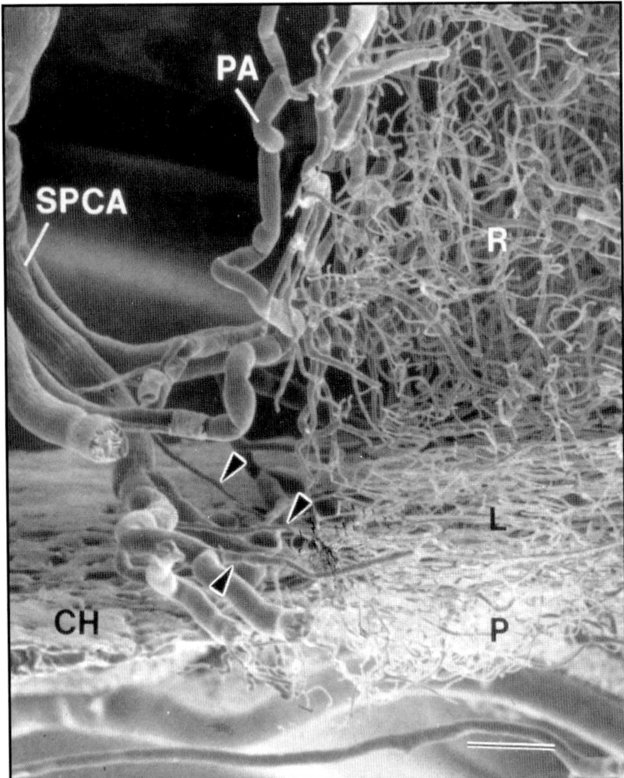



**Figure 8-8.** Capillaries of the prelaminar region are supplied both by choroidal arterioles as well as short posterior cilliary arteries.

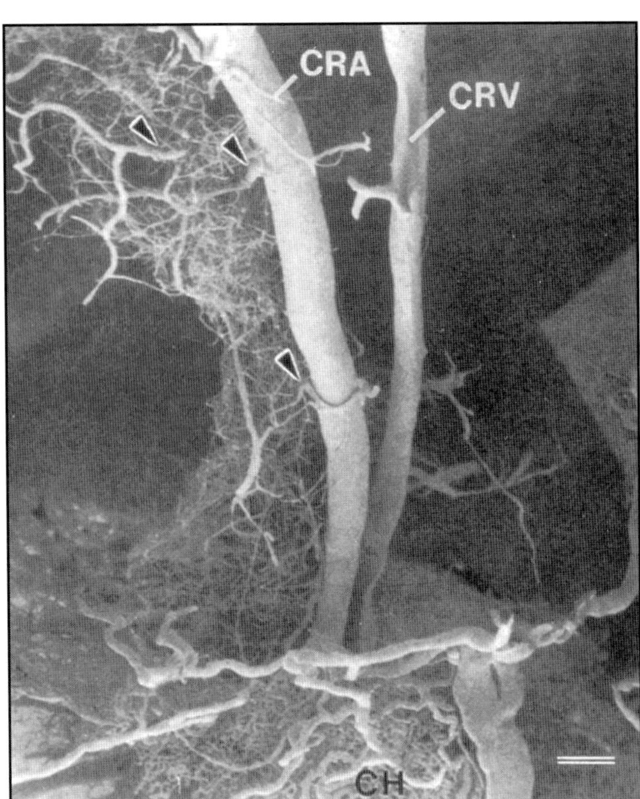



**Figure 8-9.** The pial system is primarily supplied by the circle of Zinn-Haller, though it also receives some supply from the intraneural central retinal artery.

Using the color Doppler ultrasound with at least a 5 MHz probe (7+ MHz preferred), we are able to obtain velocity readings from the ophthalmic artery, the central retinal artery, and the nasal and temporal posterior ciliary arteries as they enter the retrolaminar region of the optic nerve. In order to ensure reproducible data, we use various landmarks within the image when locating the area from which velocity samples are taken. The landmark used for the central retinal artery is based on an ultrasound artifact of the optic nerve. As the optic nerve approaches the globe, the nerve shadow visible in the B-scan portion of the ultrasound tapers down to form a small circle directly posterior to the globe. All CRA readings are taken by placing the Doppler sample window which operates using a pulsed repetition frequency within that circle. Similarly, readings are taken from the ophthalmic artery as it crosses the optic nerve, and on the nasal side of the nerve shadow. By using available anatomical landmarks within an image, we are able to obtain acceptable coefficients of reproducibility from an otherwise highly variable technique. The posterior ciliary arteries are sampled as they pierce the optic nerve to feed the pial system. When studying the changes in ocular blood flow of a patient over time, the baseline images are used to assure that velocity samples are taken in the same locations as the

Table 8-2

**Reproducibility of Color Doppler Imaging**

| | Coefficient of Variability (%) | | |
| --- | --- | --- | --- |
| Instrument | OA | CRA | PCA |
| Siemens Q2000 | | | |
| PSV | 12 | 25 | 19 |
| EDV | 6 | 11 | 25 |
| RI | 4 | 11 | 38 |
| | | | |
| Acuson 128 | | | |
| PSV | 6.5 | 5 | 37 |
| EDV | 11 | 12 | 39 |
| RI | 5 | 6 | 10 |

baseline readings. Using these techniques, we have published the reproducibility data seen in Table 8-2.[20,21]

When sampling the velocity profile of a vessel, most ultrasound units will produce an audio signal representative of the frequencies present in the blood velocities. Each artery has its own distinct characteristic waveform and sound.

The ophthalmic artery features the highest velocities of all arteries measured (Figure 8-11). Its waveform features a high systolic peak with a well-defined dichrotic notch. The

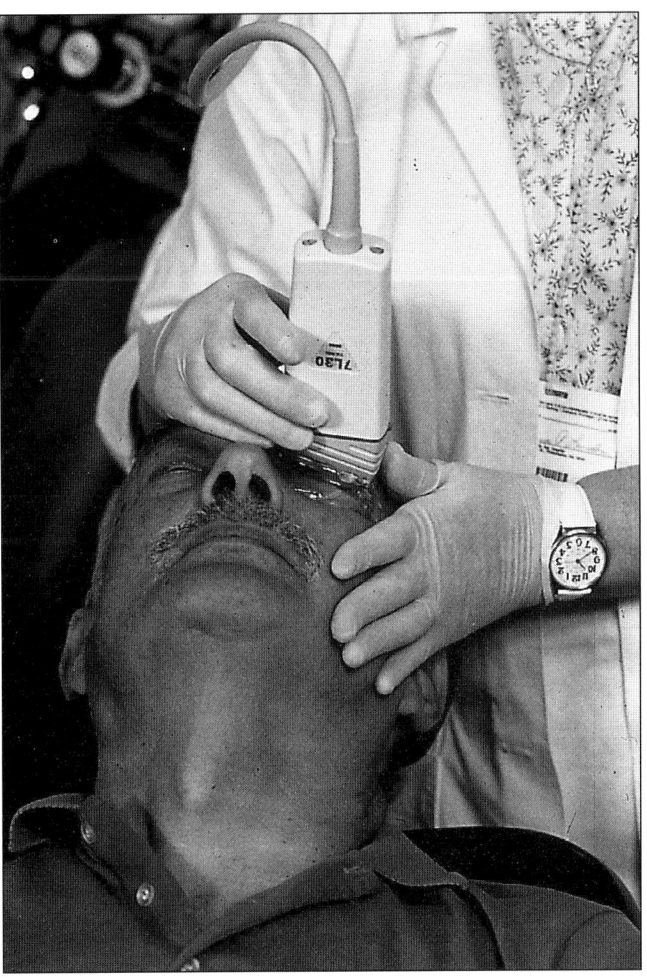

**Figure 8-10.** The probe is gently placed over the closed eyelid making contact through a coupling gel. The technician's palm rests on the forehead to avoid fatigue.

sound created for the ophthalmic artery, based on the frequencies created by the Doppler shifts, is a high raspy sound. The raspy quality is due to the wide range of velocities present in this vessel.

The central retinal artery waveform is similar to the ophthalmic artery waveform. The velocities present in the central retinal artery are only one third of those present in the ophthalmic artery. The dichrotic notch may or may not be present in the central retinal waveform. The sound produced for the central retinal artery is also raspy, but with a more muffled quality than that of the ophthalmic artery. The high frequencies of the ophthalmic artery are not present in the central retinal artery, but the central retinal artery does feature the same turbulent raspy quality.

The waveform of the short posterior ciliary arteries does not have a dichrotic notch. If one is seen, then the technician is sampling a direct branch of the ophthalmic artery, probably a posterior ciliary artery. You will also notice the lack of a distinct systolic peak. Most short posterior ciliary artery waveforms will appear to be simple bumps with some small trailing end diastolic velocity. The sound of the short posterior ciliary artery is a dull "wump wump" sound. The low velocities present have none of the raspy turbulent quality of the ophthalmic or central retinal arteries.

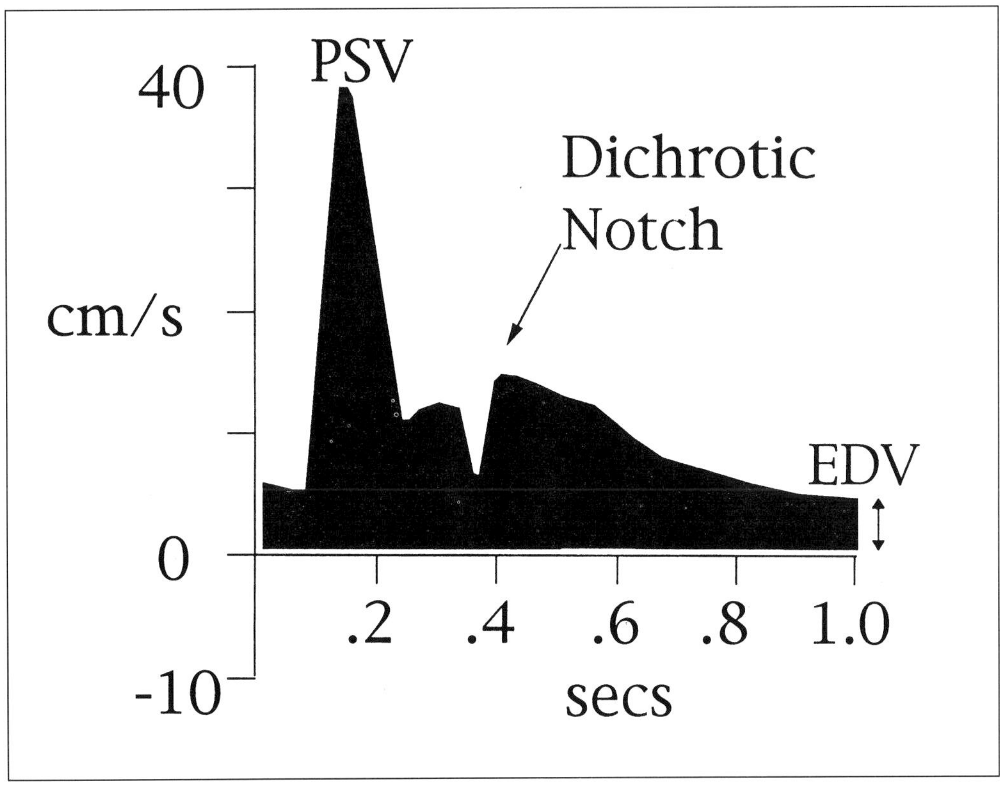


**Figure 8-11.** The ophthalmic artery produces a waveform including a distinct dichrotic notch.

The data taken from the CDI procedure are read from the waveforms (see the ophthalmic artery waveform in Figure 8-11). The highest point of the systolic peak is located by the technician as the peak systolic velocity (PSV). The lowest level of the diastolic plateau is located by the technician as the end diastolic velocity (EDV). From the two simple values obtained from this single measurement, a wealth of information may be obtained.

$$RI = \frac{PSV - EDV}{PSV}$$

$$PI = \frac{PSV - EDV}{MV}$$

Some authors have claimed that the Pulsatility Index (PI) should contain more information than the other indices since it is calculated using the mean velocity. This is because mean velocity calculation requires data across an entire cardiac cycle. It was assumed that an index containing data derived from the entire waveform would intrinsically contain more information than an index derived from two points. A study by Thompson et al[22] in 1988 found that this was not the case. They proposed that if the PI contained more information than a two-point index, then there would be a wide range of PI values for each of the simple index values. This was not the case. It turned out that the two-point indices correlated well with the more involved PI. The additional information involved in obtaining the PI resulted in no more information than was available from the simple two-point indices.

Pourcelot's resistive index (RI) is the percentage of the total velocity wave composed of pulsatile flow. If the RI was zero, the entire velocity would be non-pulsatile. If the RI was one, there would be only pulsatile flow. Resistive index is considered to be a measurement of resistance downstream or distal to the point of measurement.[23] Changes in a vascular bed's resistance to flow is reflected by changes in the RI.

As you can see, a talented and capable ultrasonographer will have a good knowledge of the anatomy of the globe, a steady hand, a good eye for waveforms, and a good ear for the sounds of the velocities. Each of these qualities is necessary for acceptable reproducibility with CDI.

If you recall, we have demonstrated the presence of reversible vasospasm in the ophthalmic artery in normal tension glaucoma patients. This increased resistance to flow and resulting decrease in flow values was not present in normals. When both groups were exposed to a vasodilator, the differences between the groups were eliminated. Using CDI technology, compromised flow in normal tension glaucoma patients was demonstrated. Some might claim that the reduced flow was the result of the disease, but if this were the case, why would a vasodilator cause the flow characteristics of normal tension glaucoma patients to match those of normals? In light of the absolute dependence of the optic disk on blood supplied from various branches of the ophthalmic artery, the importance of these CDI findings becomes evident. We look forward to increases in our understanding of the mechanism behind glaucoma being aided by CDI technology.

## SCANNING LASER OPHTHALMOSCOPY

Only 1 year after MacLean and Maumenee[24] performed a slit lamp fundus examination enhanced by an injection of 5% sodium fluorescein, Novotny and Alvis[25] first described photographic fluorescein angiography. Since that time, fluorescein angiography has been a vital tool in aiding our understanding of the normal physiology of perfusion of the retina and choroid and in understanding abnormalities of the same. However, photographic angiography suffers from low temporal resolution. Only one frame every several seconds may be obtained. The advent of the continuous imaging of video angiography increased the rate of image acquisition from one image every several seconds to approximately 20 to 30 images per second.[26] Standard video angiography is limited by low spatial resolution, as compared to the quality of photographic angiography. For years, there existed a void in angiography technology. The physician or scientist had an "either-or" choice of image quality or temporal resolution. The solution to this technology gap was first described by Webb et al[27] in 1980. Scanning laser ophthalmoscopy provides fast high quality images via a unique method of fundus illumination. Both photography and video techniques illuminate the entire fundus during the examination. The scanning laser ophthalmoscope (SLO) illuminates a single 10- by 10-micron point on the retina. The SLO measures the reflected light from each point, and assembles an image based on the pointwise reflection intensities. By only illuminating one point at a time, the illumination of the fundus is low relative to fundus photography and video angiography.[27] In addition, spatial resolution is increased through the use of confocal optics (Figures 8-12a and 8-12b).

By passing the reflected light through a confocal aperture, the point of illumination is only 300 microns thick. While this increases the amount of light needed for the examination, the total illumination required for the examination is still very low and easily tolerated by patients with a high degree of safety.

### Lasers

The Rodenstock SLO uses three lasers. They may be used in combination or alone to produce a variety of imaging modes. Each laser has its own strengths and weaknesses.

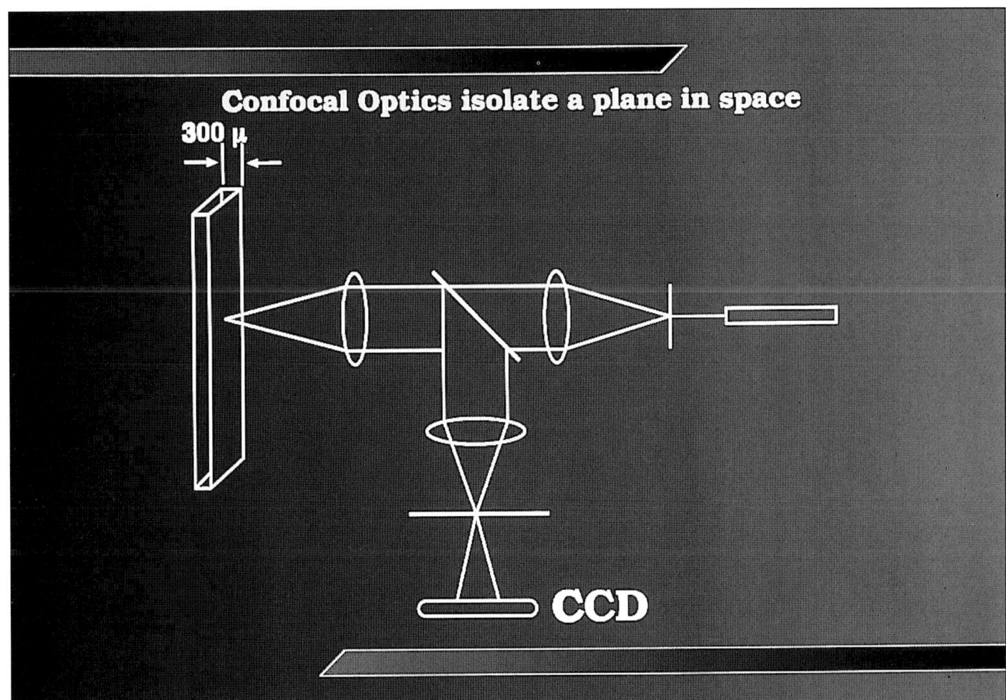


**Figure 8-12a.** Confocal optics isolate volumes of tissue within 300 micrometer focal plane.

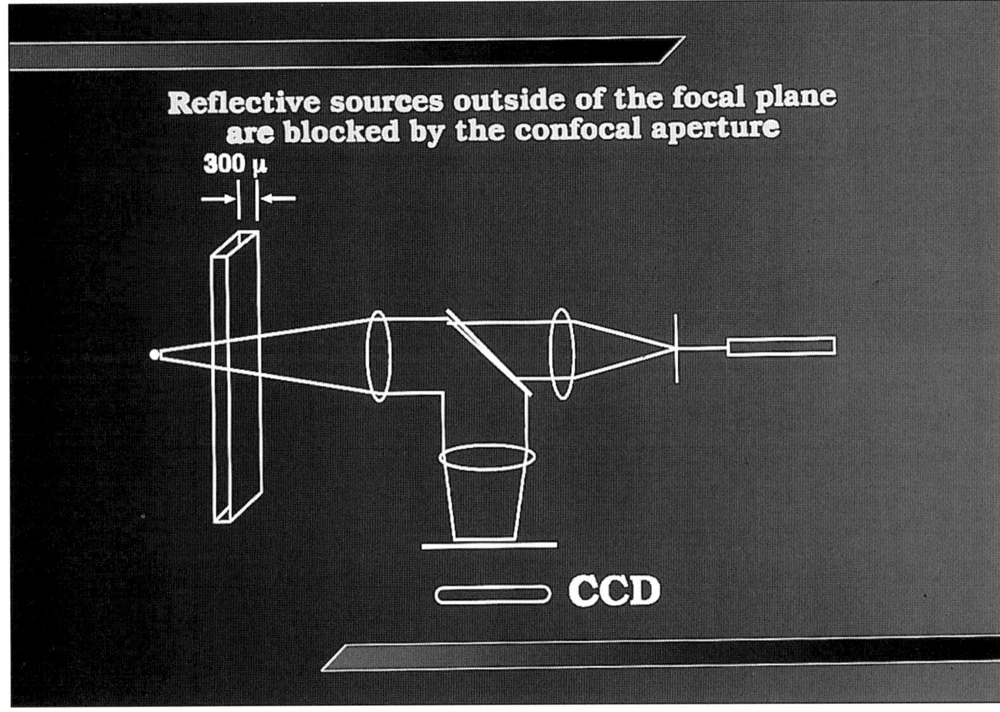


**Figure 8-12b.** Reflected light from other points on the xy focal plane is also blocked.

The 488-nm argon laser may be used for red-free imaging of the NFL, and is ideal for exciting fluorescein during angiography studies. The major problem with the argon laser is its lack of penetration power. If we look at an angiogram of the macular region (Figure 8-13), you will notice that the macular region is black. This lack of fluorescein is expected due the lack of retinal capillaries in this region, but why do we not observe a choroidal blush? The 488-nm light of the argon laser is unable to penetrate the retinal pigment layer. The fuscin pigment in the pigment layer and the xanthophyll pigment in the macula effectively block this wavelength of light. One might ask, if the pigment layer does block the argon light, why are we able to see choroidal flush in the periphery? The answer lies in the angle of penetration. Hayreh has observed

**Figure 8-13.** The avascular zone of the macular region does not present with choroidal blush due to the fuscin pigment in the macular pigment epithelium layer.

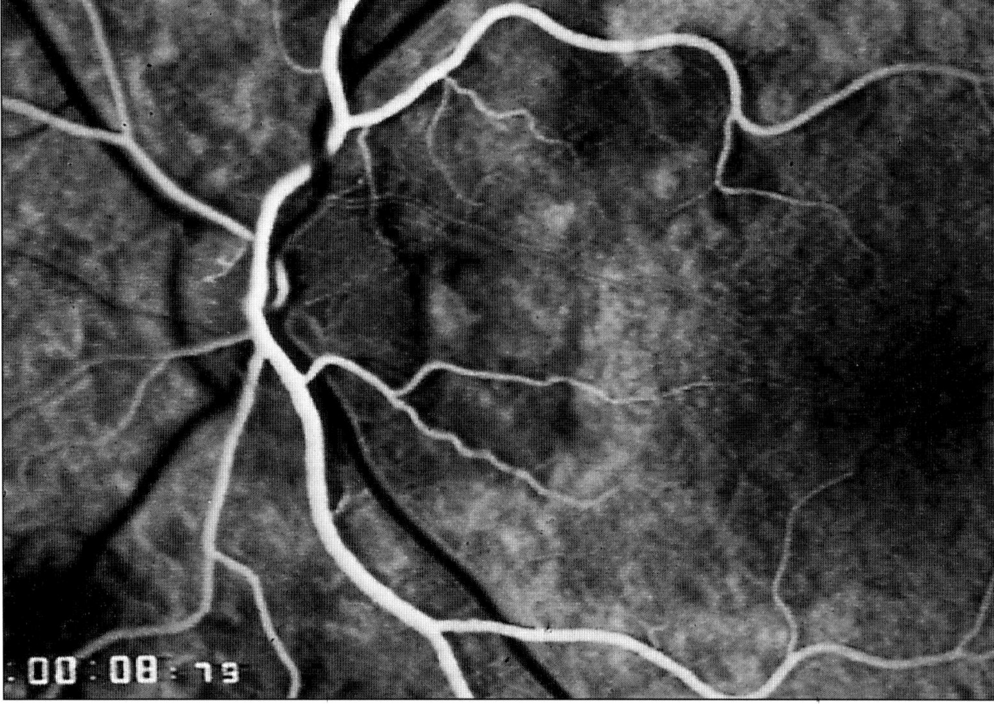


that light that approaches the retina at 90° to the surface is blocked by the retinal pigment layer. Light which approaches at some angle less than 90° seems better able to pass through the retinal pigment layer and therefore excite fluorescein in the choriocapillaris and produce choroidal blush.

The infrared laser produces a beam with a wavelength of 788 nm. Since absorption of light by the pigment layer begins to decrease at 660 nm, the infrared laser provides excellent penetration of the pigment layer. This allows study of choroidal circulation. Indocyanine green dye has a peak transmission frequency of 845 nm, and is adequately excited by the infrared laser, allowing angiographic studies of choroidal circulation.

The third laser in the SLO is a helium-neon laser. This laser produces a beam with a wavelength of 633 nm. While this beam is not normally used for imaging, it does provide an aiming beam for infrared studies, as the infrared beam is invisible to the operator, which makes aiming difficult. The helium-neon laser is also used to project static and video images onto the retina for perimetry, contrast, and other studies. Normal electroretinography, visual evoked potential, and perimetry tests illuminate a large section of retina. By using a stimulus generated by the SLO, the clinician may place a light stimulus onto any desired retinal location, and monitor that positioning via a real-time video monitor.

## Optics

Each of the three beams are aimed and detected through the same set of optics (Figure 8-14). A rotating polygon mir-

ror sweeps the beam horizontally across the retina. The beam is moved line by line vertically by a galvanometer-driven mirror. The movement required to cover a 40° field of view of the retina takes up only ~1 mm on the cornea. Reflected light passes through the scanning optics until it is separated from the incident light path by a partially reflecting mirror. The reflected light then passes through a confocal barrier, and finally is collected by a charge coupled device (CCD). The CCD is sensitive to wavelengths from 450 to 950 nm, and therefore sensitive to all of the laser wavelengths present in the SLO. The CCD's only job is to quantify the intensity of light being reflected from a single point. The CCD never "sees" the entire image at one time. It quantifies the light as some brightness level between black and white. A computer digitizes the signal from the CCD, assigning each point a number (black being zero and white being 255). This assignment of brightness point by point within a line, line by line within a frame goes on continuously as the SLO produces a stream of point brightness measurements. A video board within the SLO computer assembles the stream of brightnesses into the individual frames, and these frames are used to compose the video signal.

## Examination Procedure

Producing high quality SLO angiography examinations requires adherence to a strict protocol. In our clinic, we have, over time and experience, refined a method which we believe produces the highest quality examinations.

Before the examination begins, the unit is checked to

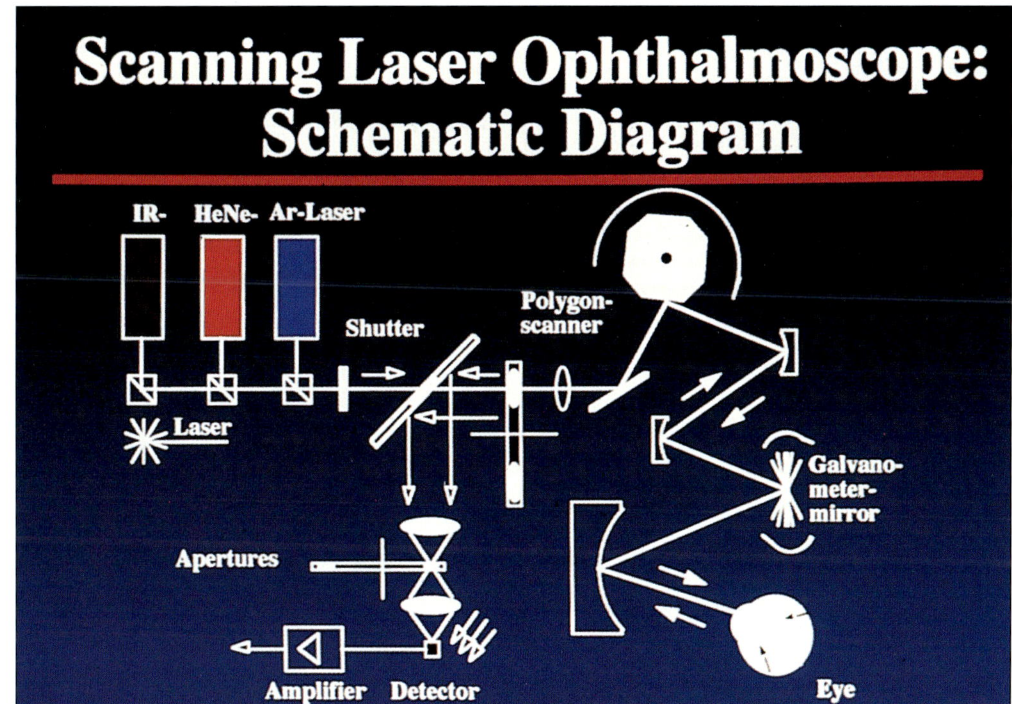


**Figure 8-14.** The lasers of the Rodenstock SLO travel a single optical path within the unit.

ensure that the optical path is dust free. The lasers of the unit are then set to zero. Two syringes are filled with Fluorescite and saline respectively. The syringes are connected so that the injection can easily be changed from fluorescein to saline and back.

We then are ready for the subject. We begin by talking with the subject in the room with the SLO running. The motor that turns the polygon mirror and the spinning mirror itself produce considerable noise. It is desirable that the subject be acclimated before the actual examination begins. This time is used to describe the procedure, explain what will be required of the subject, explain what type of discomfort may be caused by the injection of the fluorescein dye, what information we expect to gain from their examination, and most importantly, question the subject about allergies. Intravenous injection of the fluorescein may potentially cause a number of side effects including hives, itching, bronchospasm, and anaphylaxis. Even though the issue of potentially dangerous allergies is an exclusion criteria in SLO studies and was previously covered, the patient is questioned about allergies to iodine, shellfish, sulfa drugs, or dyes in general.

Once the procedure has been reviewed, the subject is positioned comfortably in the SLO unit, lateral canthus level with the positioning mark on the frame of the head rest. The subject is then prepared for dye injection. As the subject is prepared for injection, the laser power is adjusted for the examination. As the laser power is brought up, the beam is centered on the cornea of the dilated study eye. Focus is preset according to the refractive error of the subject, but fine tuning is often necessary to locate the surface of the NFL. The operator will, by voice command, direct the subject's gaze left or right, up or down, in order to center the ONH within the video frame. A S-VHS VCR is now started to record the examination. Several seconds of 40° and 20° red-free images are recorded (Figures 8-15a and 8-15b).

The red-free images are used for vessel measurements. Data analysis will be discussed in the following section. After completion of the red-free imaging, the patient is injected with the dye. As the injection is made, a video timer is started. This timer encodes the video signal with a clock signal with a temporal resolution of 1/100th of a second. A high concentration bolus is desired, so injection velocity is maximized. From the time of injection, several seconds will pass before dye appears in the eye. During this time, it is probable that the retinal vessels will be unseen. It is imperative that, during this time, the SLO operator keeps the beam on the center of the eye. With the increased intensity of the beam, a subject is prone to move, causing the ONH to become off center, or out of the frame entirely. If there is any doubt, the barrier filter should be removed momentarily to ensure proper positioning.

On appearance of the dye, the subject is calmly and reassuringly instructed to relax and try to maintain gaze without blinking. Inexperienced operators who exclaim "hold still now and keep your eye open" on seeing the dye may exacerbate blinking and eye motion. The initial angiogram is recorded until the retinal arteries have become dark again and choroidal blush has peaked. After the 40° angiogram is completed, a 20° angiogram of the perimacular area is obtained. In this image, dye appears as dots of hyperfluorescence surrounded by areas of hypofluorescence. These dots are

**Figure 8-15a.**
Red-free images are
obtained to measure
vessel diameter
using video
densitometry.

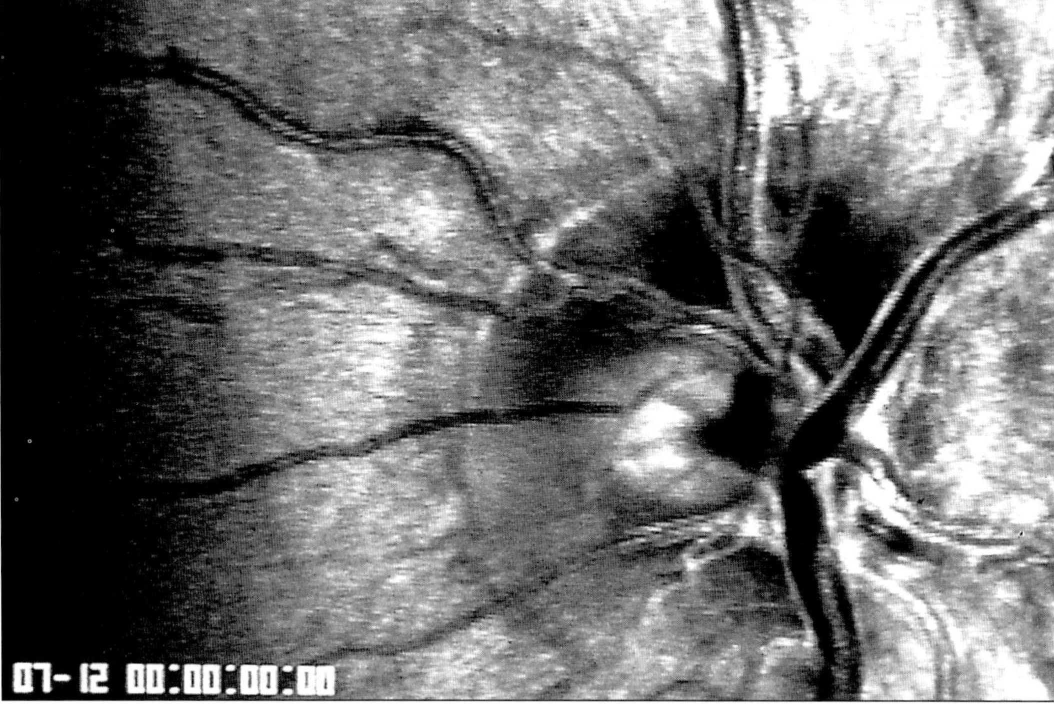


**Figure 8-15b.** Red-free
images are obtained to
measure vessel diameter
using video densitometry.

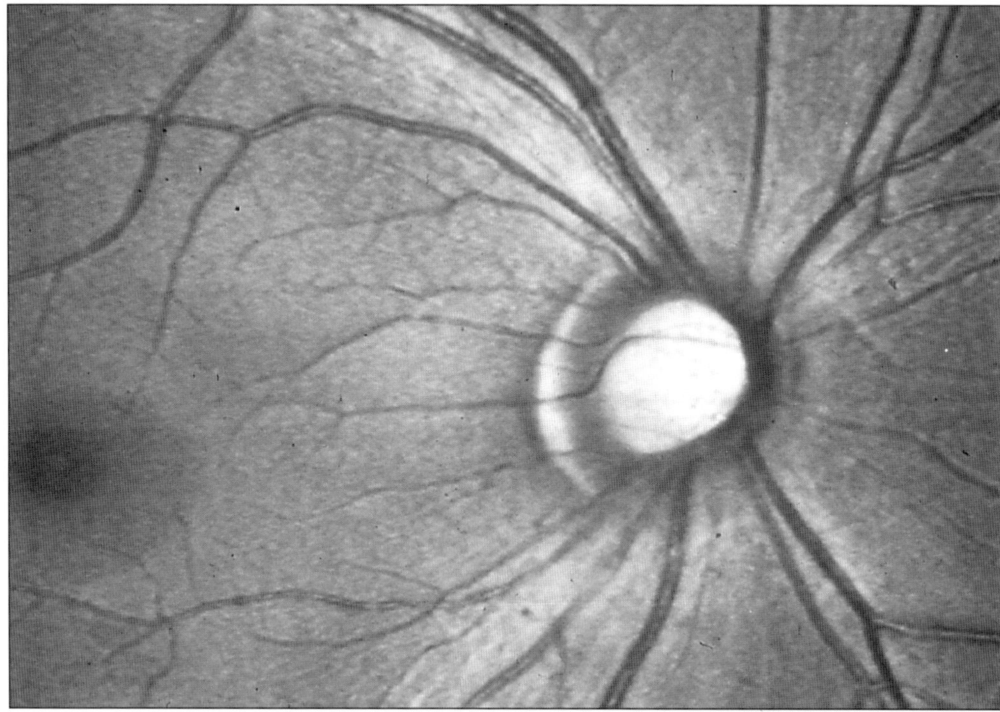

thought to be microdroplets of dye trapped between rouleaux formations passing through capillaries.[28] After several seconds of perifoveal recording, while the retina is still bright, gaze is returned to the starting nasal direction in order to image the capillary beds of the ONH. Capillary flow in the nerve head is recorded for 15 to 25 seconds. After this, the subject is told to sit back and the laser is turned off.

The subject is immediately questioned about any dizziness or nausea during the examination. If any sign of symptom is reported or observed, the subject is asked to sit for a few minutes. The SLO is turned off so the room can quiet down and the subject can have a chance to regain his or her strength. If dizziness is reported, blood pressure is taken. When the subject feels that any reactions to the dye (or needle stick) have passed, he or she is helped to his or her feet. As a matter of safety, the procedure is posted in the examination room.

## Examination Analysis

The videotaped SLO angiography examinations are analyzed by an HRX video image analysis system running customized software. A PC-driven unit, the HRX contains enough memory to hold 12.8 seconds of digitized video with a frame-grabbing speed of 20 frames per second. It also contains a wide variety of image processing and enhancement features. Our laboratory has developed a software package with a number of special features designed to facilitate SLO video analysis. These include frame alignment algorithms, user-defined line measurement, and area of interest pixel value averaging throughout a video segment.

## Pre-Analysis Calculations

Analysis begins by computing the 40° and 20° pixel size based on measurements of the subject's axial eye length and corneal curvature. These values are entered into the Littman formula[29]:

$$\text{Correction factor} = 0.01 \times (aA^2 - bA + c)$$

where a, b, and c are tabular values based on corneal curvature, and A is ametropia measured in diopters. This correction factor is used to correct for magnification effects that occur when characteristics of the subject's eye vary from the assumed norm. With no correction and normal length and curvature, the SLO has pixel sizes of approximately 9 by 7 microns and 12 by 13 microns depending on field of view setting. With the actual pixel sizes known, the red-free portion of the examination is digitized. From these images, retinal vessel diameters are measured by densitometry.

## Densitometric Measurement of Vessel Diameter

The analyst begins by entering the actual pixel size into the analysis software. This allows true distance measurements to be performed directly from the images by the computer. Lines are drawn across vessels. The analyst estimates the path of a line which lies at 90° to the vessel wall. The computer will then read the pixel values of the pixels which make up the line across the vessel (Figure 8-16).

Under red-free conditions, vessel walls will appear darker at the edges and lighter in the middle (Figure 8-17).

It is standard to use the half height of the densitometry curve to represent the inner wall of the vessel. The distance between the two half heights is measured to obtain the vessel diameter. From this, cross-sectional area is computed. This can be used to calculate estimates of blood flow based on measured velocity. This is also used simply to monitor changes in vessel diameter which may represent changes in the tone of the muscle of the vessel, in turn representing changes in the autoregulatory state of the vessel.

## Arm Retina Time and Dye Dilution Curves

The next segment of the examination digitized is a 10 to 12 second segment of the 40° field of view angiogram beginning immediately prior to the arrival of dye in the eye. These digitized data are enhanced to increase contrast so that the very first appearance of dye in the eye is easily visualized. In the frame where dye first appears, the clock reading is noted directly from the image. As you recall, a clock is started on injection of the dye. In order to get a rough indicator of circulatory health on the systemic level, the time that it takes for the dye to travel from the arm to the retina, the Arm to Retina Time, is recorded.

It is probable that the individual frames will not be in proper alignment with each other due to eye movements. In order to correct for this, the 240 individual digitized images must be aligned so that vessels appear to remain stationary throughout the digitized segment. To do this, the images are roughly placed into alignment by the analyst, and then the analysis software goes through the stack of digital images for fine alignment. With the images aligned, the analyst will choose a 3 by 3 pixel area on a proximal point of a retinal artery, on some distal point on that same artery, and on the vein that collects blood from that artery (Figure 8-18).

With these three areas defined, the analysis software goes through each image in the series and computes the average pixel intensity in each area. These intensities are graphed over time to produce dye dilution curves. The dye dilution curve contains a variety of information on the hemodynamics of the retina. The slope of the curve can be used to indicate the flow of the dye passing through the vessel; higher flow causes a vessel to brighten more quickly. The heel of the curve may be used to indicate the time of dye arrival at the specified point. By comparing the arrival times at two points on an artery, the analyst knows how long it took for the dye to travel between the two points. Using the known pixel size, the analysis software is capable of measuring the distance between the two points within one pixel distance. Knowing time and distance, the analyst is able to compute the velocity of the blood through the artery. Combining this velocity information with the cross-sectional area calculated from the diameter previously, the analyst can calculate blood flow.

Using the point on the vein, arrival time of dye in the vein and proximal point on the artery are compared to provide the Arteriovenous Passage time. This time is a measure of the general condition of retinal circulation: the lower the time, the more rapid the passage of blood through the retinal circulation.

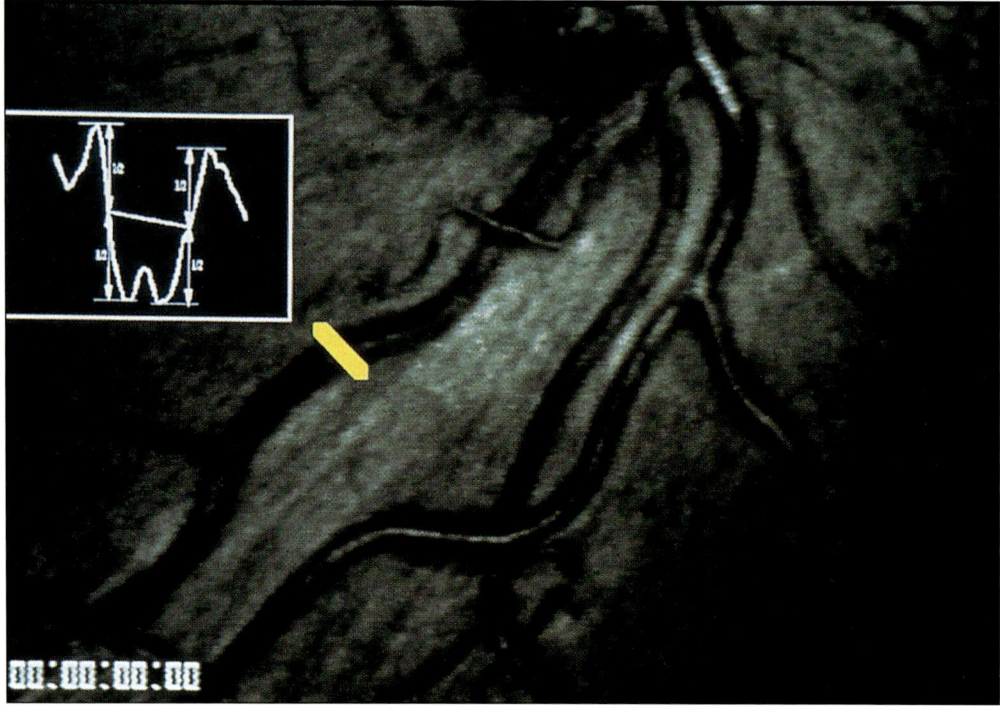

**Figure 8-16.** When making densitometry measurements, a line is placed across a vessel. The brightness of each point on the line is measured.

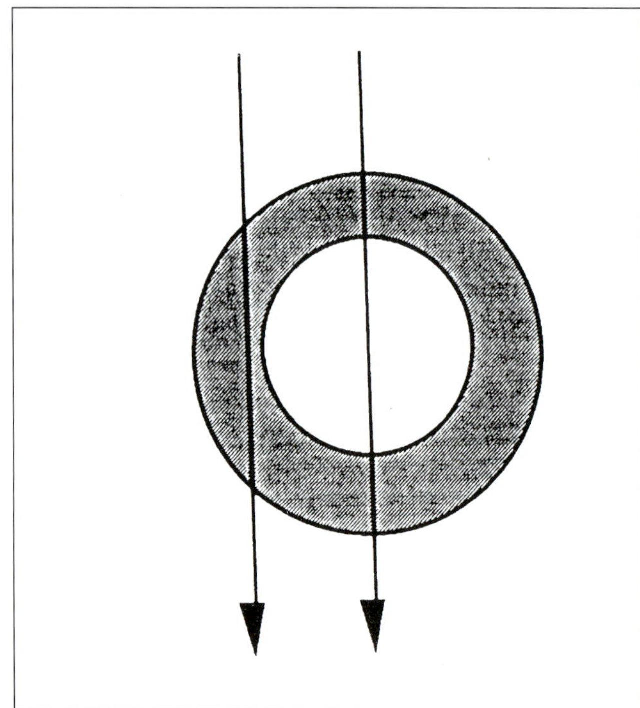

**Figure 8-17.** Densitometry assumes that the half height location of vessel brightness identifies the inner wall of the vessel.

### Capillary Transit Velocities

For this final phase of SLO analysis, we obtain the actual velocity of red blood cells as they pass through the capillaries of the perifoveal network and the surface NFL of the ONH. To do this, a segment of 20° video which contains vis-

ible hyperfluorescent particles is digitized. The calculated pixel size for the 20° view of the patient is entered, and the length of a capillary of interest is measured. Using the time code contained within the image, the analyst pages through sequential frames of the video to find a time when a particle enters and leaves the capillary of interest. In Figure 8-19, you see two sequential frames in which a hyperfluorescent particle is visible moving from the center of a capillary to the end of the capillary.

This is repeated for the passage of 10 to 15 particles, and the passage times are averaged. This process is repeated for 10 to 15 capillaries. Using capillary length measurements, the capillary transit velocities are calculated. All velocities are averaged, and the final average is reported as the capillary transit velocity. This procedure may be repeated on a video segment of the ONH surface in order to calculate the ONH capillary transit velocity. In a recent study,[30] capillary velocities of the ONH were found to be nearly twice as fast as the capillary velocities of the perifoveal capillaries. Values for all SLO parameters in normal subjects are listed in Table 8-3.

## OTHER CONFOCAL SCANNING LASER OPHTHALMOSCOPES

Rodenstock is not the only manufacturer of SLOs. The Rodenstock unit provides excellent image qualities and great flexibility in the number of possible uses for the unit: perimetry, red-free imaging, etc., but is weak in other areas. Its biggest weakness is the lack of numerical data available directly from the unit. Analysis of image data from the

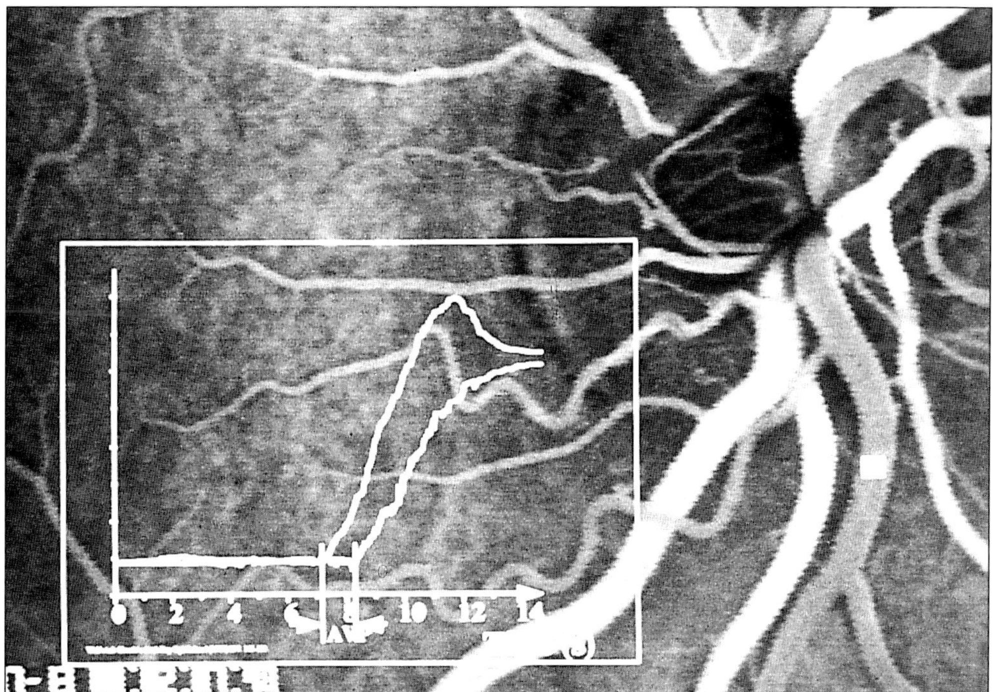

**Figure 8-18.** Dye dilution curves identify the initial appearance of dye within a vessel. Arteriovenous Passage time is the amount of time between first appearance of dye in a retinal artery and its collecting vein.

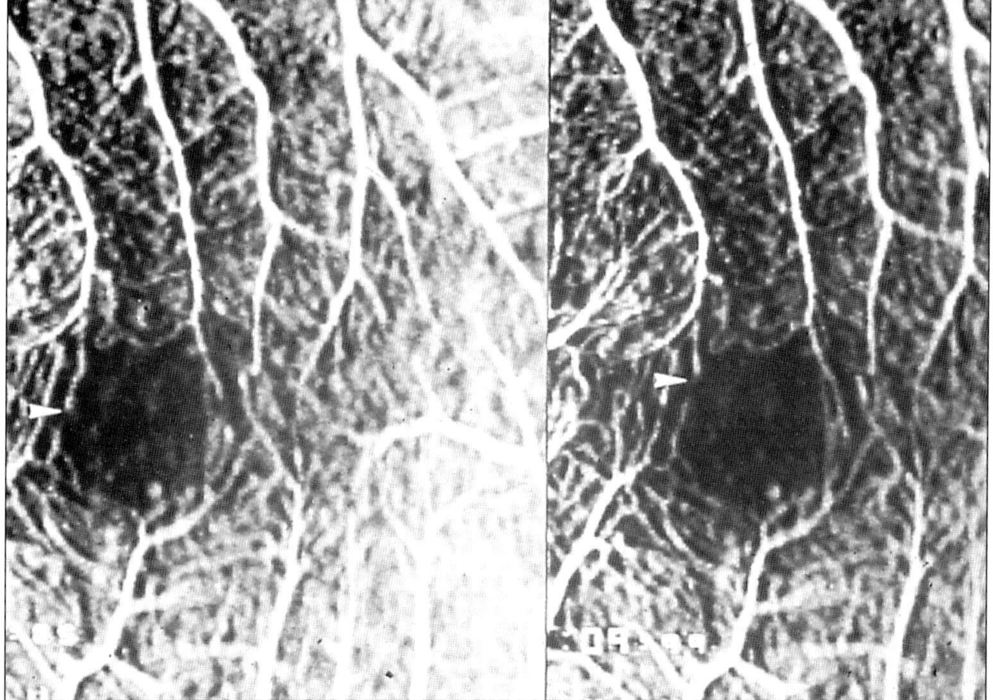

**Figure 8-19.** The arrows show the movement of a hypofluorescent area of capillary blood in two sequential video frames.

Rodenstock SLO requires an investment of time and money rivaling the cost of the SLO itself. Other SLO units on the market have been designed to be much more useful in the manner in which data are presented.

Heidelberg Engineering, GmbH produces a number of SLO devices, each designed to provide data immediately after the examination is complete. The newest Heidelberg device, the Heidelberg Retinal Angiography unit, will be dis-cussed later in the text and is beyond the scope of this chapter. We will briefly review the Heidelberg Retinal Tomograph (HRT) and Heidelberg Retinal Flowmeter (HRF) units.

## Heidelberg Retinal Tomograph

The HRT device utilizes confocal optics by using a moving focal plane to detect the surface of the ONH. This is discussed in greater detail in Chapter 4. Briefly, beginning with

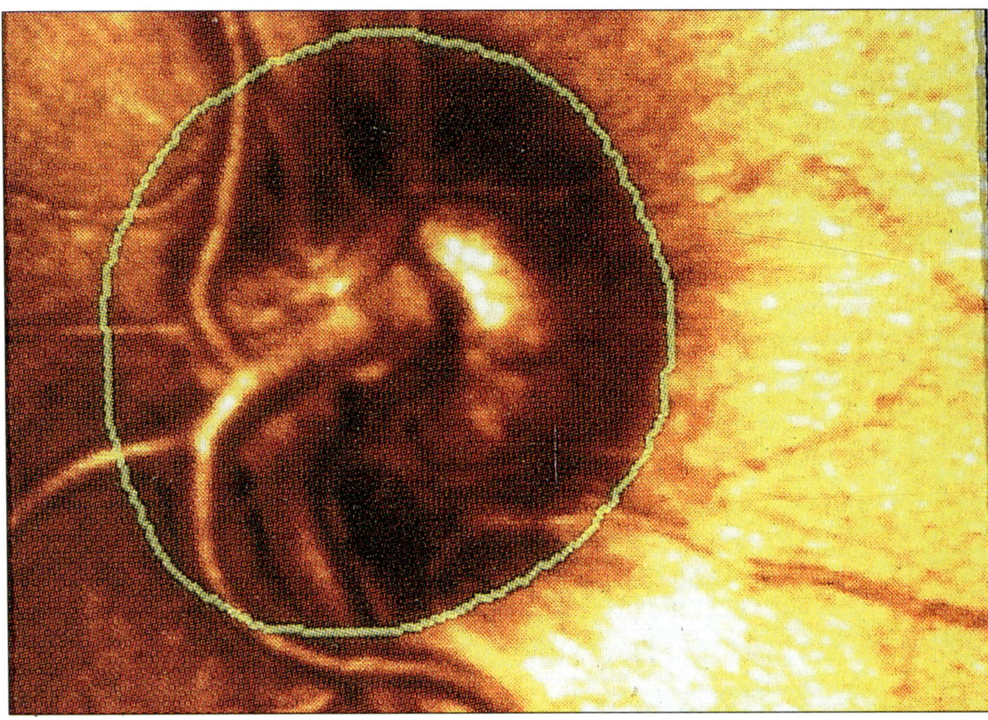

**Figure 8-20.** The Heidelberg Retinal Tomograph (HRT) creates a topographic map of the ONH.

```
Area:                        2.391 mm²
Effective area:              1.242 mm²
Mean radius:                 0.868 mm
Mean height of contour:      0.956 mm
Height variation contour:    0.288 mm
Volume below contour:        0.221 cmm
Volume below surface:        0.193 cmm
Volume above surface:        0.088 cmm
Mean depth ins. contour:     0.081 mm
Effective mean depth:        0.156 mm
Maximum depth in contour:    0.534 mm
Third moment ins contour:   -0.271 mm
```

**Figure 8-21.** The HRT produces a report containing a number of disk measurements and calculated indices.

### Table 8-3
### Normal Values of SLO Exam Parameters

| Parameter | Value |
| --- | --- |
| Arm Retina Time | 12.4±1.56 seconds |
| Mean Dye Velocity | 6.1±1.56 mm/s |
| Arteriovenous Passage Time | 1.64±0.3 seconds |
| Perifoveal Capillary Transit Velocity | 2.6±0.4 mm/s |
| Peripapillary Capillary Transit Velocity | 4.7±1.0 mm/s |

a focal plane anterior to the surface of the retina at the ONH, the HRT moves the focal plane posteriorly in 75-micron increments through the surface of the retina at the optic disc. After acquiring 32 optical slices, each image is divided into a 256 by 256 pixel square grid. Each retinal grid point is examined in each of the 32 images. The depth at which the brightest reflection was returned is assumed to be the surface of the retina at that grid point. By mapping out the surface depth at each grid point, the HRT creates a topographic map of the optic disc (Figure 8-20).

The brighter the color, the deeper the structure. The circle seen in Figure 8-20 of the image from the HRT is drawn by the user in order to locate the rim of the disk for the analysis software. With the rim defined, the software will provide a report containing a number of useful parameters (Figure 8-21).

As you can see, data analysis on the HRT does not require extensive processing time or an external processing system as does the Rodenstock SLO.

## Heidelberg Retinal Flowmeter

The HRF is a confocal scanning laser device which utilizes the Doppler effect. When light strikes moving blood cells, the reflected light is Doppler shifted as described in the third equation. With a bandwidth of 2000 Hz, the HRF is capable of detecting flow velocities of up to 0.78 mm/sec.

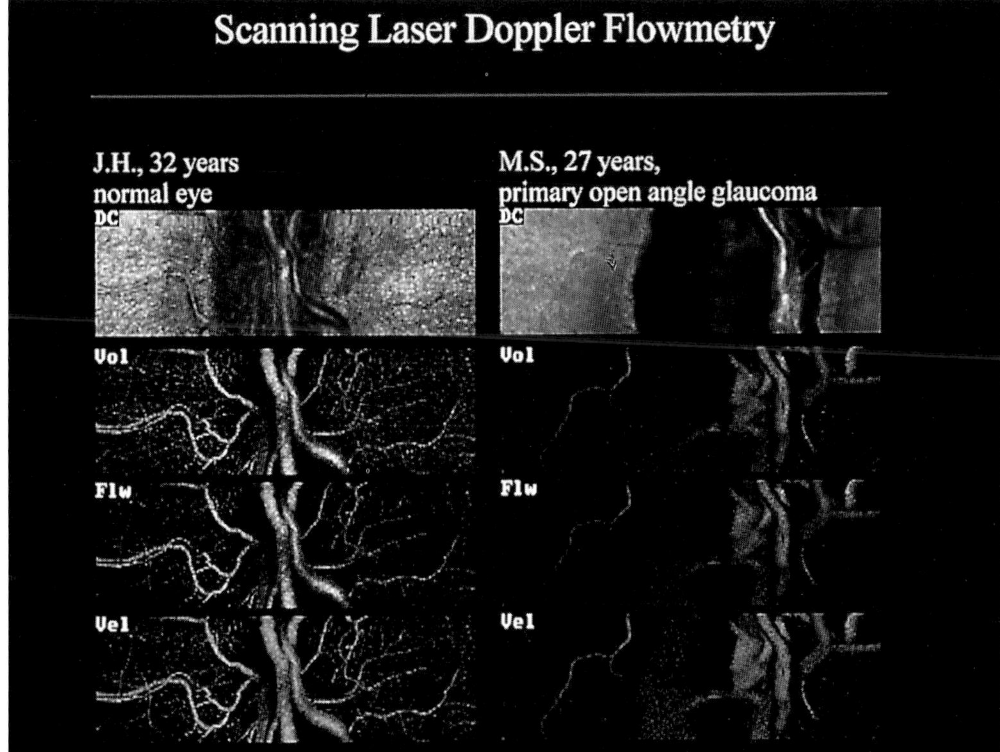


**Figure 8-22.** The Heidelberg Retinal Flowmeter (HRF) measures blood flow within 400 by 2560 by 640 micrometer volumes of retinal tissue. The user may probe individual 100 by 100 by 400 micrometer volumes of tissue for area measurements.

This range of measurement limits the validity of HRF measurements to capillary beds. As shown in Table 8-3, capillary velocities in retinal arteries as measured by the SLO were above the cut-off frequency of the HRF. This discrepancy between the two technologies merits further study.

By analyzing the frequencies contained in the retinal reflection, the HRF is able to calculate the amount of blood moving at various velocities, and compute blood flow within a 400-micron tissue slice. Unlike other laser flowmeters, which measure flow at a single point, the HRF produces a flow map. This map is an image of a 2560 by 640 micron section of retinal tissue. The user may place a digital "probe" or sample window at any point on the map to have the flow in that area displayed. A sample may also be obtained from a group of points to have the average flow within the box displayed. A sample HRF output using the default 100 by 100 micron window is shown in Figure 8-22.

## REFERENCES

1a. MacKenzie W. *Treatise on the Eye*. Boston, Mass: Carter, Hendee & Co; 1833.

1b. von Graefe. Die Iridectomie Bei Amaurose Mit Sehnervenexcavation. *Arch fur Ophthalmologie*. 1857;311-546.

1c. Elschnig. *Hendbuch der speziellen pathologiseher Anatomie und Histologie*. Berlin: Julius Springs; 1928;1.

2a. Wagemann A, Salzmann P. Anatomische Untersuchugen uber einseitige Retinitis Haemorrhagica mit Secundar-Glaucom nebst Mittheilungen uber dabei beobachtete Hypooyon-Keratitis. *Arch fur Ophthalmologie*. 1892;38:213.

2b. Lauber H. Treatment of atrophy of the optic nerve. *Arch Ophthalmol*. 1936;16:555-568.

2c. Reese AB, McGavic JS. Relation of field contraction to blood pressure in chronic primary glaucoma. *Arch Ophthalmol*. 1942;27:845-850.

3a. Duke, Elder S. Primary glaucoma as a vascular disease. *Ulster Med J*. 1953;221:1.

3b. Loewenstein A. Cavernous degeneration, necrosis, and other regressive processes in optic nerve with vascular disease of eye. *Arch Ophthalmol*. 1934;34:220-225.

3c. Cristini G. Common pathological basis of the nervous ocular symptoms in chronic glaucoma. *Br J Ophthalmol*. 1951;35:11-16.

4a. Harrington DO. The pathogenesis of the glaucoma field. *Am J Ophthalmol*. 1959;47:177-184.

4b. Sachsenweger R. *Klin Mbl Augenheilk*. 1963;142:625.

4c. Ebner R. Verhandlungen osterreichischen. *Ophthalmol Ges*. 1965:133.

4d. Leighton DA, Phillips CI. Systemic blood pressure in open angle glaucoma, low tension glaucoma, and the normal eye. *Br J Ophthalmol*. 1972;56:447-453.

4e. Tielsch JM, Katz J, Sommer A, Quigley HA, Javitt JC. Hypertension, perfusion pressure, and primary open angle glaucoma. *Arch Ophthalmol*. 1995;113:216-221.

5. Hayreh SS, Walker W. Fluorescent fundus photography in glaucoma. *Am J Ophthalmol*. 1967;63:982-989.

6. Hitchings RA, Spaeth GL. Fluorescein angiography in chronic simple and normal tension glaucoma. *Br J Ophthalmol*. 1977;62(20):126-132.

7. Corbett JJ, Phelps CD, Eslinger P, Montague PR. The neurologic evaluation of patients with low-tension glaucoma. *Invest Ophthalmol Vis Sci*. 1985;26:1101-1104.

8. Phelps CD, Corbett JJ. Migraine and low-tension glaucoma. A case

control study. *Invest Ophthalmol Vis Sci.* 1985;26:1105-1108.

9. Gasser P, Flammer J. Influence of vasospasm on visual function. *Documenta Ophthalmologica.* 1987;66:3-18.

10. Harris A, Sergott R, Spaeth GL, et al. Color Doppler analysis of ocular vessel blood velocity in normal tension glaucoma. *Am J Ophthalmol.* 1994;118:642-649.

11. Kety SS, Schmidt CF. The effects of altered arterial tensions of carbon dioxide and oxygen and cerebral blood flow and cerebral oxygen consumption of normal young men. *J Clin Invest.* 1948;27:484.

12. Kahn HA, Leibowitz HM, Ganley JP, et al. The Framingham Eye Study. I. Outline and major prevalence findings. *Am J Epidemiol.* 1977;106:17-32.

13. Tielsch JM, Katz J, Singh K, et al. A population based evaluation of glaucoma screening: the Baltimore eye survey. *Am J Epidemiol.* 1991;134:1102-1110.

14. Klein B. Klein R, Sponsel W, et al. Prevalence of glaucoma: the Beaver Dam eye study. *Ophthalmology.* 1992;99:1499-1504.

15. Hart WM, Yablonski M, Kass MA, Becker B. A multivariate analysis of the risk of glaucomatous visual field loss. *Arch Ophthalmol.* 1979;97:1455-1458.

16. Harris A, Evans DW, Kagemann L. Vasospasm in primary open angle glaucoma. Submitted for 1996 American Academy of Ophthalmology abstract.

17. Curry TS, Dowdey J, Murry R. *Christensen's Introduction to the Physics of Diagnostic Radiology.* 4th ed. Malvern, Pa: Lea & Febiger; 1990.

18. Marion J, Hornyak W. *Physics for Science and Engineering, Part 1.* Philadelphia, Pa: CBS College Publishing.

19. Hayreh SS. Anterior ischaemic optic neuropathy II. Fundus on ophthalmoscopy and fluorescein angiography. *Br J Ophthalmol.* 1974;58:964-980.

20. Harris A, Williamson T, Martin B, et al. Test/retest reproducibility of color Doppler imaging assessment of blood flow velocity in orbital vessels. *J Glaucoma.* 1995;4:281-286.

21. Williamson T, Harris A. Major review: color Doppler ultrasound imaging of the eye and orbit. *Surv Ophthalmol.* 1996;40:255-267.

22. Thompson R, Trudinger B, Cook C. Doppler ultrasound waveform indices, A/B ratio, pulsatility index, and Pourcelot ratio. *Br J Ophthalmol.* 1988;95:581-588.

23. Pourcelot L. Applications cliniques de l'examinen Doppler transcutane. *Inserm.* 1974;34:213-240.

24. MacLean A, Maumenee A. *Am J Ophthalmol.* 1960;50:3.

25. Novotny H, Alvis D. A method for photographing fluorescein in circulating blood of the human eye. *USAF Sch Aviat Med.* 1960;60:1-4.

26. Heuven W, Schaffer C. Advances in televised fluorescein angiography. *Fluorescein Ang ISFA.* Tokyo, Japan: Igaku-Shoin; 1973:10-14.

27. Webb R, Hughes G, Delori F. Flying spot TV ophthalmoscope. *Appl Opt.* 1980;19:2991-2997.

28. Nasemann J, Burk R. *Scanning Laser Ophthalmoscopy and Tomography.* München, Germany: Quintessenz Verlags GmbH; 1990.

29. Littman H. Determination of the true size of an object on the fundus of the living eye. *Klin Mbl Augenheilk.* 1988;192:66-67.

30. Arend O, Harris A, Remky A, Martin B. Scanning laser ophthalmoscopy based evaluation of epipapillary velocities: a novel approach. Submitted for publication.

# Confocal Tomographic Angiography of the Optic Nerve Head in Glaucoma

*Shlomo Melamed, MD, Sara Krupsky, MD,
Giora Treister, MD*


## INTRODUCTION

The exact mechanism of injury of nerve fibers of the optic nerve in glaucoma is still unclear. The mechanical theory suggests that stretching of the lamina cribrosa causes blockage of axoplasmic flow in the nerve fibers. The vascular theory proposes that impaired blood supply to the optic nerve head (ONH) causes death of nerve fibers. The important role of the ONH perfusion has been discussed in low-[1] as well as high-tension glaucoma.[2,3] The concurrence of splinter hemorrhages, peripapillary choroidal atrophy, and sectoral damage pattern of the disc in certain glaucoma patients may serve as supportive evidence for the role of localized vascular impairment in glaucoma.[4,5]

The blood supply of the ONH is complex. Retinal vessels supply the most superficial layer of the ONH. The prelaminar region is supplied especially by the peripapillary choroid and the short posterior ciliary arteries, while the laminar region is supplied by the short posterior ciliary arteries.[3,6] By using fluorescein angiography, several investigators have already reported on filling defects at the superficial and peripapillary retinal vessels in glaucoma,[7,8] and these defects could be correlated with visual field defects.[9] However, the limitations of conventional fluorescein angiography do not allow an accurate evaluation of the blood supply of the deeper regions of the nerve, such as the lamina cribrosa, due to the poor penetration of this dye through the ONH and the pigment epithelium. The use of the dye indocyanine green (ICG) has proven to be superior to fluorescein for visualization of the choroidal vasculature due to its emission at the infrared wavelength and better penetration through the pigment epithelium.[10] Recent developments in scanning laser ophthalmoscopy allow low light level illumination and excellent resolution through the application of digitized imaging techniques. The technology of the confocal tomography system enables us to acquire a three-dimensional map of the ONH.[11,12] The combination of these new developments in image analysis and the advent of ICG angiography should offer the advantage of visualizing the vascular pattern of the deeper portions of the ONH, including the lamina cribrosa.[13,14] Such integration of these technologies was made possible in the new Heidelberg Retinal Angiograph instrument (HRA). This chapter describes our experience with confocal tomographic angiography (CTA) in various conditions of glaucoma patients.

## MATERIALS AND METHODS

### Confocal Tomographic Angiography

The confocal laser scanning system (Heidelberg Retina Tomograph [HRT], Heidelberg Engineering, Heidelberg, Germany) uses a 795-nm laser source to excite the ICG. A barrier filter with cut-off at 810 nm blocks reflected light and permits detection of ICG fluorescence. A second laser source (830 nm) is used to align the system prior to injection. The laser beam is focused to the retina, manually adjusting for spherical aberrations between -12 and +12 D in steps of 0.25 D. The area of interest can be scanned in 10°, 20°, or 30° field of view.

Images appear continuously on the computer monitor and only selected images are acquired and saved to the hard disk. Images can be acquired in a manual single image acquisition mode, using an operating panel button or a foot switch. Images can also be acquired in a tomographic automatic mode: once the scan depth is determined by the operator (1 to 7 mm), the system creates 32 equally spaced tomographic images. A special program enables the enhancement of the differences in ICG fluorescence at the extremes. This is achieved by cut-off of 2.5% of the fluorescence at each edge with adjustment of the fluorescence curve. Consequently, areas with no fluorescence are displayed in red color, while areas of maximal fluorescence (usually the large retinal vessels) appear in green color.

## Indocyanine Green Angiography

ICG (Cardio-Green, Becton-Dickinson, Md) 25 to 50 mg was diluted according to manufacturer recommendations and injected to the antecubital vein, followed by 5 cc saline flush.

## Patient Population

All patients had a complete ophthalmological examination, including best corrected visual acuity, applanation tonometry, slit lamp examination, ophthalmoscopy, and CTA. In addition, all patients with glaucoma underwent visual field tests (either the Goldmann or the Humphrey 24-2 program), ONH photography, and confocal laser scanning tomography (using the HRT). Patients with known allergy to iodine, liver disease, or pregnancy were excluded from the study. All patients signed a detailed informed consent prior to the injection of ICG.

## Normal Optic Nerve Head

CTA was performed in 30 patients with normal-looking optic nerves, in whom ICG had already been indicated for macular pathology; another group of 10 patients with unilateral glaucoma and a normal optic disc were also evaluated.

## Glaucomatous Optic Nerve Head

Patients with glaucoma with either sectoral notching of the ONH or severe glaucomatous cupping underwent CTA. A correlation between the specific glaucomatous visual field loss and the ONH pathology was made, using HRT, CTA, and the Humphrey visual field analyzer (programs 24-2 or 10-2).

### Sectorial Damage of the Disc

Eighteen patients with sectorial notching to the rim were studied. Patient 1 representing this group was a 72-year-old male who had primary open-angle glaucoma in both eyes. Visual acuity was 20/40 in both eyes and intraocular pressure (IOP) was 16 and 18 mmHg in the right and left eyes, respectively, on timolol 0.5% B.I.D. Ophthalmoscopy revealed an inferior notching reaching the rim of the disc in both eyes. Superior visual field loss was present in both eyes, correlating well with the location of disc damage. Patient 2, with inferior visual field loss in the right eye, was also chosen for demonstration.

### Very Advanced Optic Nerve Damage

Twelve patients with very advanced cupping of the ONH were studied, and the results of the CTA were correlated with the confocal laser scanning tomography and the visual fields.

Patient 3, one of these patients, had end-stage chronic angle closure glaucoma in both eyes. Visual acuity was limited to light perception in the right eye and 20/30 vision in the left eye. His IOP was 59 mmHg in the right eye and 51 mmHg in the left eye despite therapy with timolol 0.5% B.I.D. and acetazolamide 500 mg B.I.D. po. The cornea and lens were clear in both eyes. Ophthalmoscopy revealed absolute glaucomatous cupping (C/D=1.0) in the right eye and pretotal cupping (C/D=0.95) in the left eye. Gonioscopy disclosed a totally closed angle around 360° in both eyes. Visual field in the left eye was limited to a central island of 5°.

## Effect of Trabeculectomy

Seven patients with uncontrolled IOP were studied before and within 1 week after a successful trabeculectomy. Patient 4, a 75-year-old female with pseudoexfoliation glaucoma (PXF), presented with IOP of 36 mmHg in the right eye despite maximally tolerated medical therapy and argon laser trabeculoplasty 2 years prior to her current admission. As her optic disc was found to be severely damaged (C/D of 0.9) and her visual field disclosed only a small central island of 10°, she underwent trabeculectomy in her right eye. Seven days after surgery her IOP was 4 mmHg, with a clear cornea, deep anterior chamber with no bleb leak. Both laser confocal scanning tomography (with HRT) and CTA were performed using the same parameters 1 day before and 7 days after the trabeculectomy.

## Various Types of Visual Field Defects

Several patients with advanced glaucomatous optic nerve damage presented with different patterns of visual field loss. In most of the cases, a good correlation could be made between the visual field pattern and the vascular impairment to the optic disc.

### Cecocentral Scotoma

A 65-year-old female with a history of low-tension glaucoma, affecting mainly the left eye (Patient 5). Her IOP was 18 mmHg in both eyes, with C/D=0.8 in the left eye and C/D=0.6 in the right eye. The visual field was normal in the right eye and displayed a cecocentral scotoma in the left eye.

### Tunnel Vision

A 78-year-old female with end-stage glaucoma in the left eye (Patient 6). IOP was 28 mmHg despite maximal medical therapy, with pretotal cupping of the disc and tunnel vision.

### Bilateral Arcuate Scotomata

A 73-year-old male with advanced glaucoma in the left eye, with controlled IOP at 17 mmHg using timolol 0.5% B.I.D. His visual field disclosed superior and inferior arcuate scotomata (Patient 7).

## Wide Cups with Normal Visual Field

Four patients with very wide cups and narrow rims but with normal visual fields were also tested.

## RESULTS

CTA of the ONH was very well tolerated by all patients examined, with no allergic reactions or nausea experienced by any patient.

In all patients we were able to differentiate between superficial blood vessels at the level of the optic nerve rim from those lying in a deeper level, in the cup, by using the confocal tomography system. However, we were not able to define the origin of these vessels, either from the peripapillary choroidal system or the short posterior ciliary arteries, as their filling time was rather quick. Also, although solitary blood vessels could be delineated with good resolution, much of the deep blood supply of the optic nerve was visualized as a fine network of arborizing miniature vessels resulting in diffuse fluorescence, representing the microvascular pattern of the optic nerve. About 30 minutes after the injection of ICG, dye was no longer detected in the blood vessels.

## Normal Looking Optic Discs in Non-Glaucomatous Patients

CTA of the normal discs disclosed a high resolution display of the superficial blood vessels. Confocal tomography using 1.0 to 3.5 D of divergence allowed penetration into the deeper layers of the nerve, delineating the distribution of the deeper microvasculature (Figures 9-1a through 9-1c). Figure 9-1d displays another example of a normal disc. It could be argued that a diffuse microvascular filling pattern of the rim and its slopes was the common denominator in the normal discs.

## Localized Notching of the Optic Nerve Head

In Patient 1, the inferior notching in both optic discs correlated with the absence of ICG fluorescence in these locations, as well as the superior visual field defects. The dark sectoral area at the inferior part of the disc persisted throughout the depth of the disc, indicating no blood flow to this region in both eyes. Figures 9-2a and 9-2b illustrate both optic nerves while Figures 9-2c and 9-2d demonstrate the CTA of these discs. Figure 9-2e demonstrates the superior visual field loss in the left eye. Figures 9-3a and 9-3b illustrate the CTA of Patient 2, which shows a superior filling defect which correlates well with the inferior field loss.

## Severe Glaucomatous Cupping of the Optic Nerves

In some patients, despite a very similar ophthalmoscopic view of the large and deep cupping of the optic discs, substantial differences in the pattern and intensity of CTA could

be demonstrated. Also, in some eyes, although ophthalmoscopy could not reveal any vascular pattern at the level of the lamina cribrosa, CTA disclosed perfused vessels at this plane. As an example, Patient 3 had very severe glaucoma with total cupping (cup-to-disc ratio of 1.00) and light perception only in the right eye with cup-to-disc ratio of 0.95, visual acuity of 20/30, and tunnel vision limited to 5° in the left eye. CTA demonstrated trunks of vessels across the plane of the lamina cribrosa in both eyes, but no microvascular pattern could be detected (Figures 9-4a and 9-4b).

## Effect of Trabeculectomy

In Patient 4, pretrabeculectomy CTA performed at an IOP of 36 mmHg, disclosed very poor filling of blood vessels throughout the ONH area. This pattern was evident in all planes tested, indicating poor perfusion of superficial and deep vessels. Five days after trabeculectomy, at an IOP of 4 mmHg with no bleb leak, CTA revealed a newly perfused group of deep vessels at the inferotemporal region of the disc. In addition, some congestion of superficial blood vessels with no extravascular leakage could be detected. Confocal laser tomography of the ONH disclosed a reduction in mean cup depth from 0.428 to 0.125 mm as well as a reduction in cup area from 1.505 to 0.724 mm² after trabeculectomy.

Consequently, focusing on the blood vessels at the laminar plane required less dioptric power in the post-trabeculectomy examination (-1.0 D compared to -2.25 D prior to surgery) (Figures 9-5a through 9-5f).

## Various Types of Visual Field Defects

In Patient 5, presenting with severe optic disc damage and a cecocentral scotoma, CTA disclosed absolute loss of the microvascular pattern in the horizontal region of the affected disc (Figures 9-6a through 9-6c).

CTA performed in Patient 5, who presented with pretotal cupping of the optic nerve and tunnel vision, disclosed a complete loss of blood supply in the superior and inferior regions of the disc, leaving an arborizing vessel supplying only the midtemporal region. The existence of this remnant blood supply might explain the maintenance of tunnel vision in this patient, with a relatively intact maculopapillary bundle (Figures 9-7a through 9-7c).

In Patient 7, who had superior and inferior arcuate scotomata, the CTA demonstrated loss of vascular supply superiorly and inferiorly in an "hourglass" appearance (Figures 9-8a through 9-8c).

In three patients with normal visual fields and wide cups, CTA disclosed a normal pattern of vascularity with no filling defects at the optic nerve (Figure 9-9).

**Figures 9-1a-c.** CTA of a normal, non-glaucomatous ONH. a) The most superficial layer of retinal vessels (0.0 D). b) A mid-depth plane showing the microvascular pattern of the rim and its slopes (1.25 D). c) A deep plane demonstrating laminar vessels, previously undetected when focusing on the superficial plane (3.25 D).

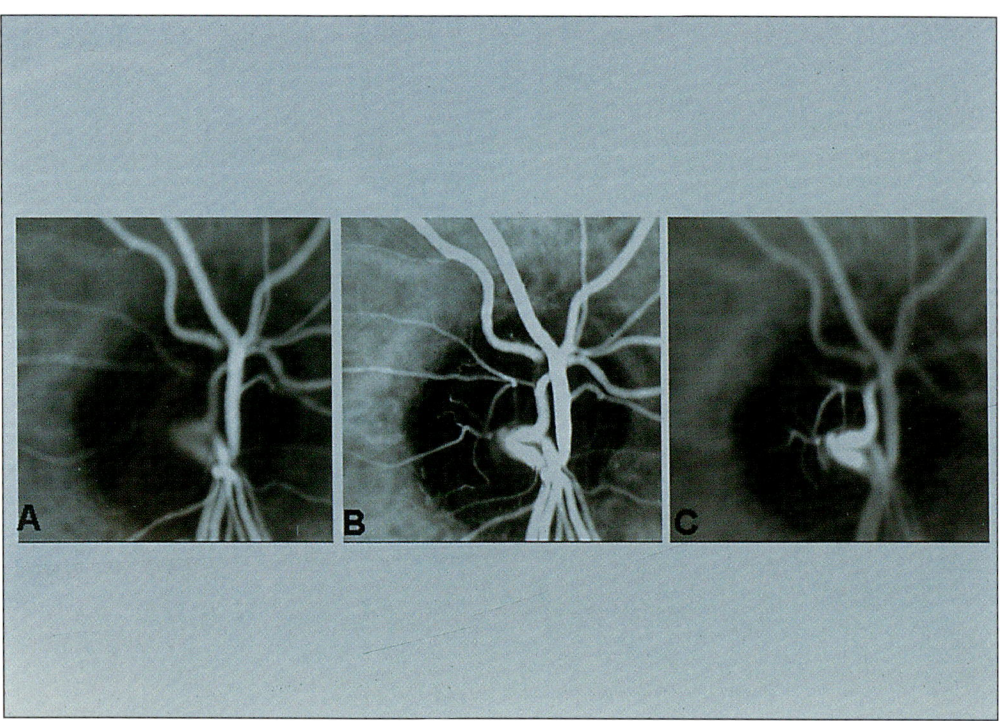


**Figure 9-1d.** Another example of normal microvascular distribution.

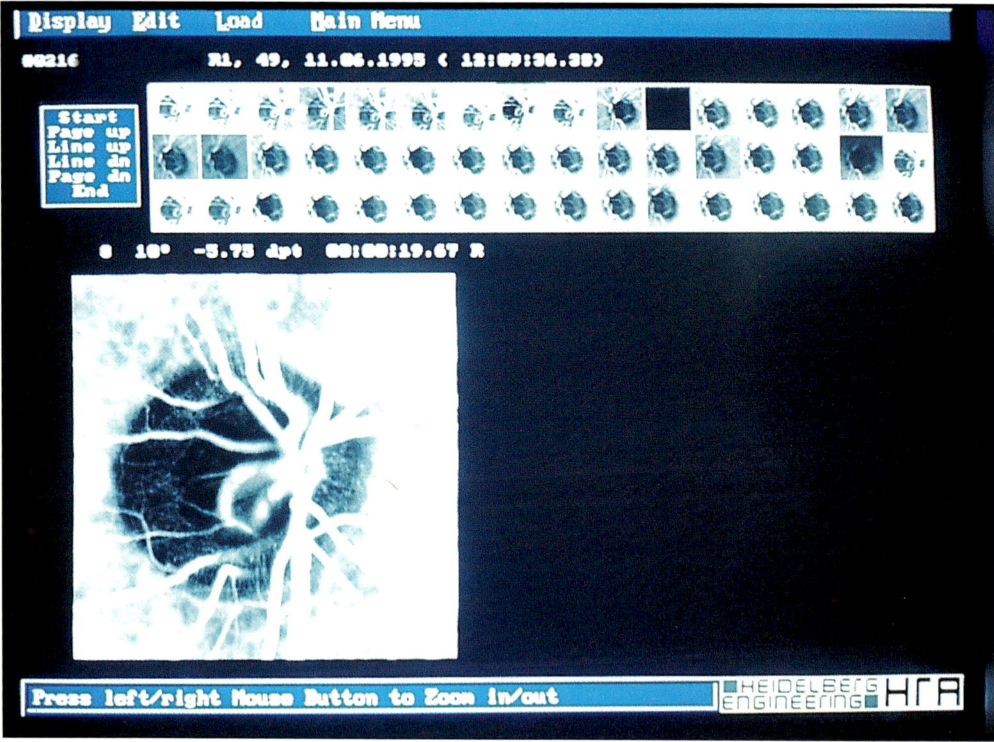

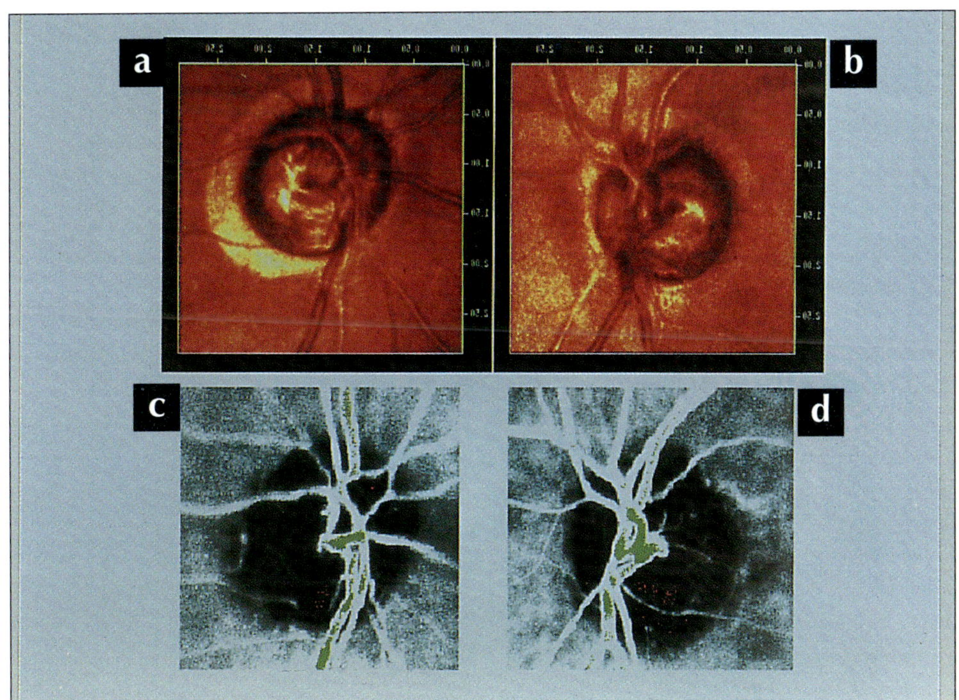

**Figures 9-2a-d.** CTA of the optic nerve with inferior sectoral notching. Patient 1: Both optic nerves had inferior notching to the rim associated with superior visual field defects. Figures a and b describe the optic nerves in the right and left eyes respectively (HRT). Figures c and d illustrate their corresponding CTAs, which demonstrate an absolute inferior filling defect, better enhanced by cutting 2.5% of fluorescence from each edge of the grayscale. Red represents no fluorescence while green represents maximal fluorescence.

**Figure 9-2e.** The superior visual field loss in left eye.

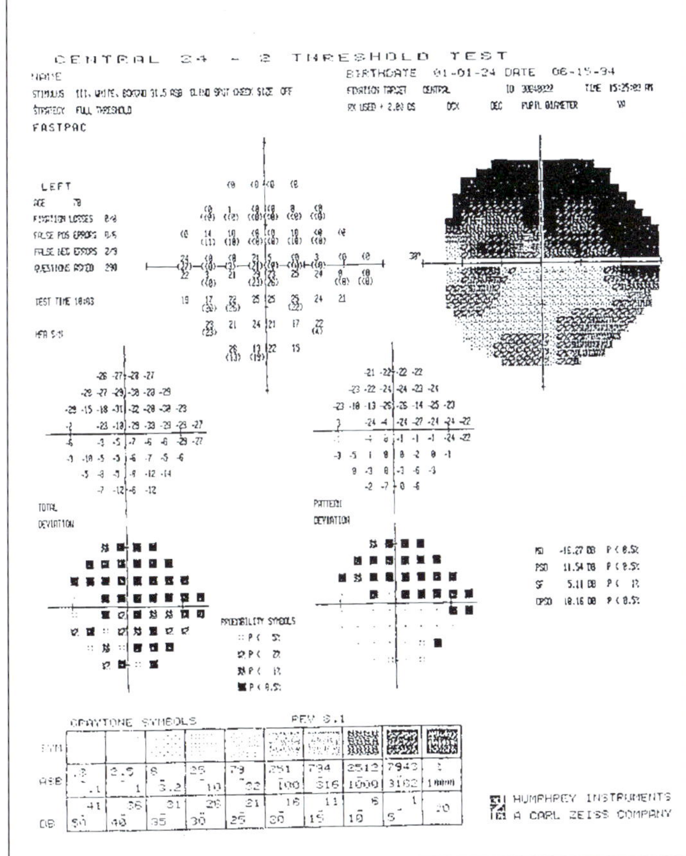

**Figure 9-3a.** CTA of the optic nerve with superior sectoral damage. Patient 2 with inferior visual field loss in the right eye. This figure shows the absolute superior filling defect.

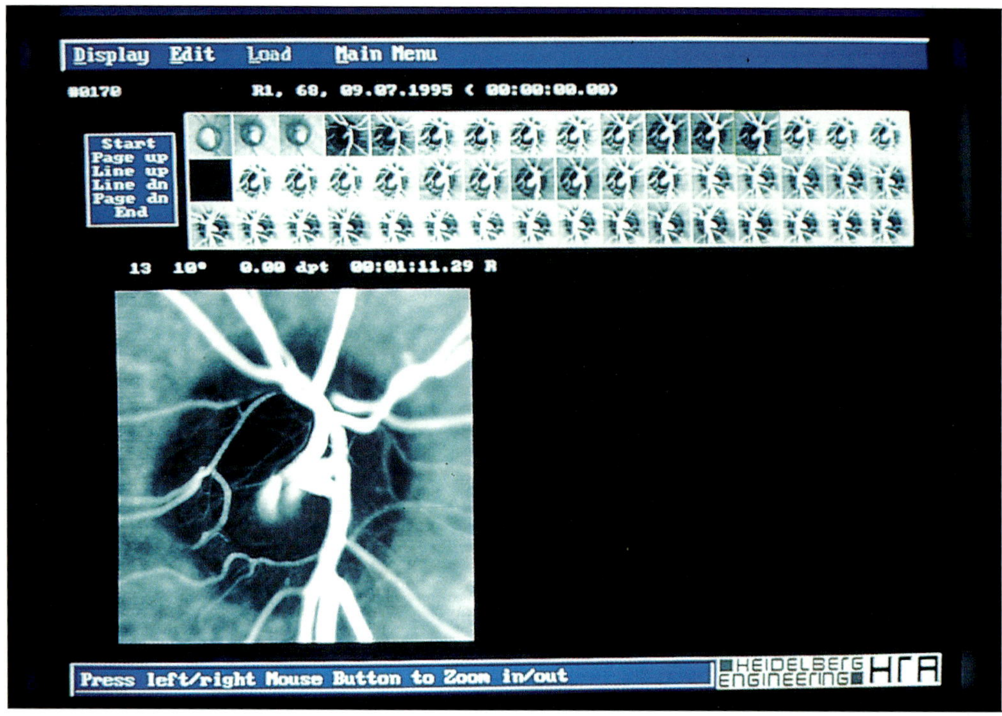


**Figure 9-3b.** The 5% fluorescence cut-off program further enhances the absolute superior filling defect.

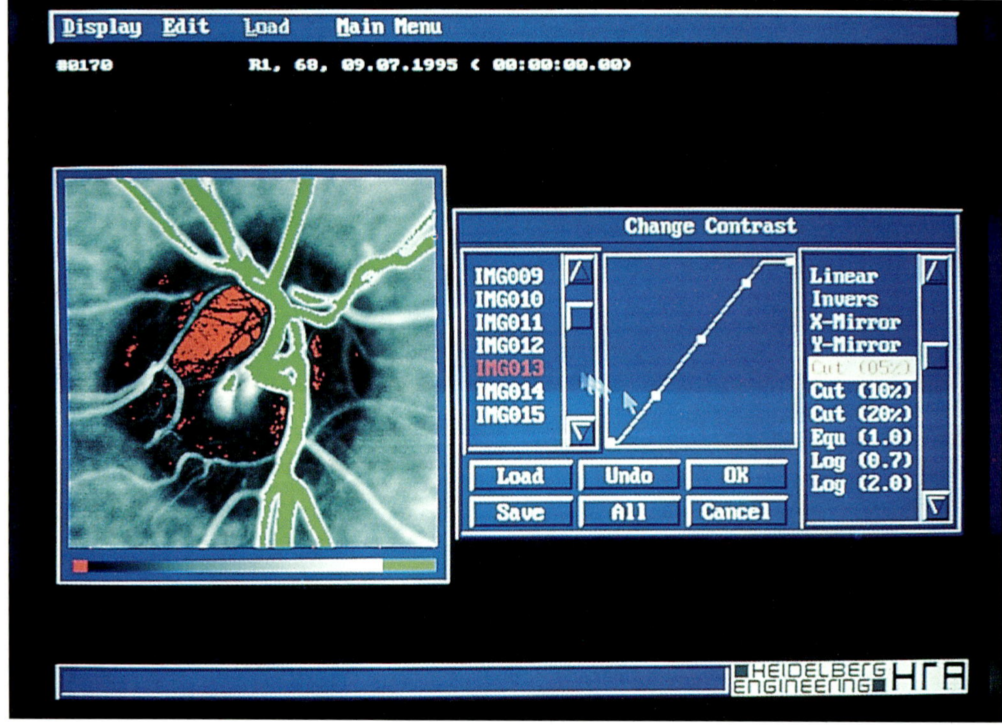

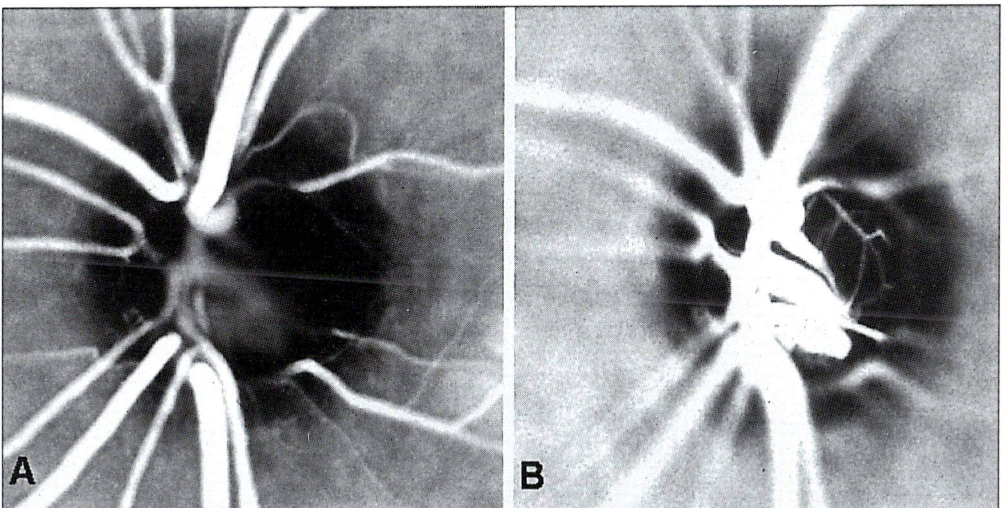

**Figures 9-4a-b.** CTA in severe glaucomatous cupping of the ONH. a) Patient 3 with end-stage chronic angle closure glaucoma. The superficial layer of the left disc (-1.0). b) The existence of "trunks" of blood vessels without microvascular pattern in the deeper plane (-4.0 D).

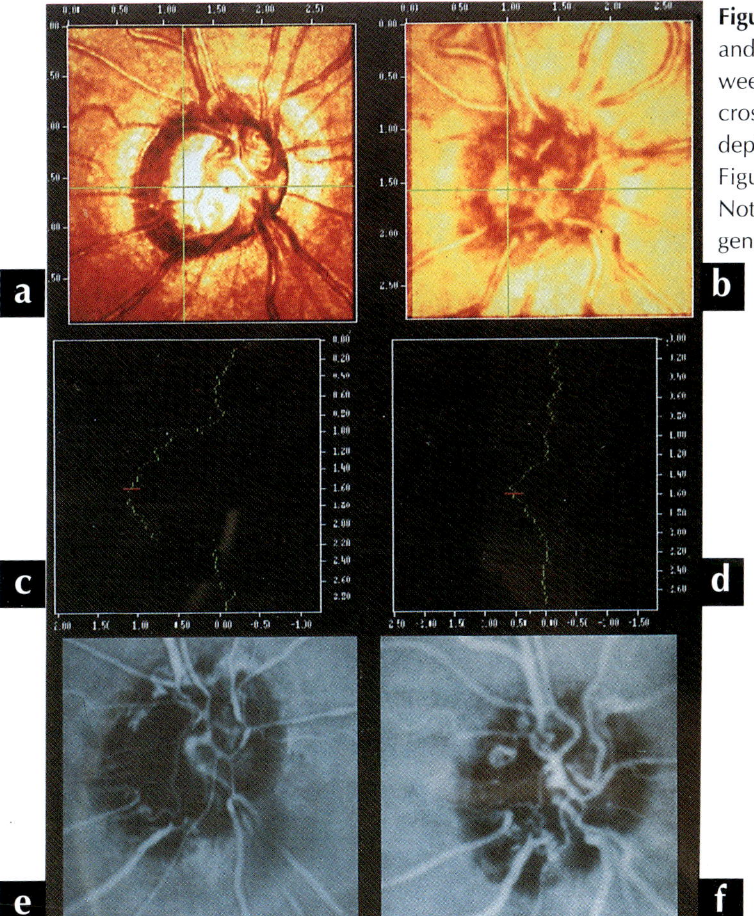

**Figures 9-5a-f.** CTA before and after trabeculectomy. Figures a and b describe confocal tomography performed before and 1 week after trabeculectomy. Figures c and d depict the vertical cross-section of the cup before and after trabeculectomy. Cup depth of 0.428 mm before and 0.125 mm after surgery. Figures e and f show the CTA before and after trabeculectomy. Note perfusion of deep inferotemporal vessels (arrow) and generalized congestion of all vessels (-1.0 D).

**Figure 9-6a.** Cecocentral scotoma. Patient 5: CTA of the left eye demonstrates absolute loss of the microvascular pattern in the mid-temporal sector of the disc (Figures 9-6a and 9-6b) with the corresponding cecocentral scotoma (Figure 9-6c).

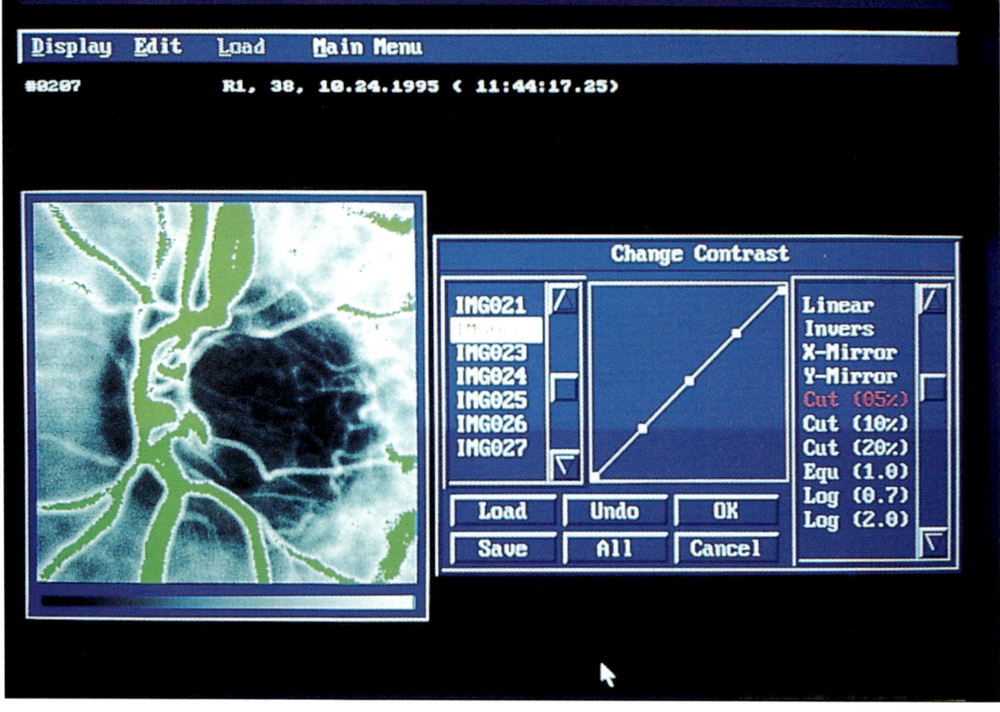


**Figure 9-6b.** Mid-temoral sector of disc.

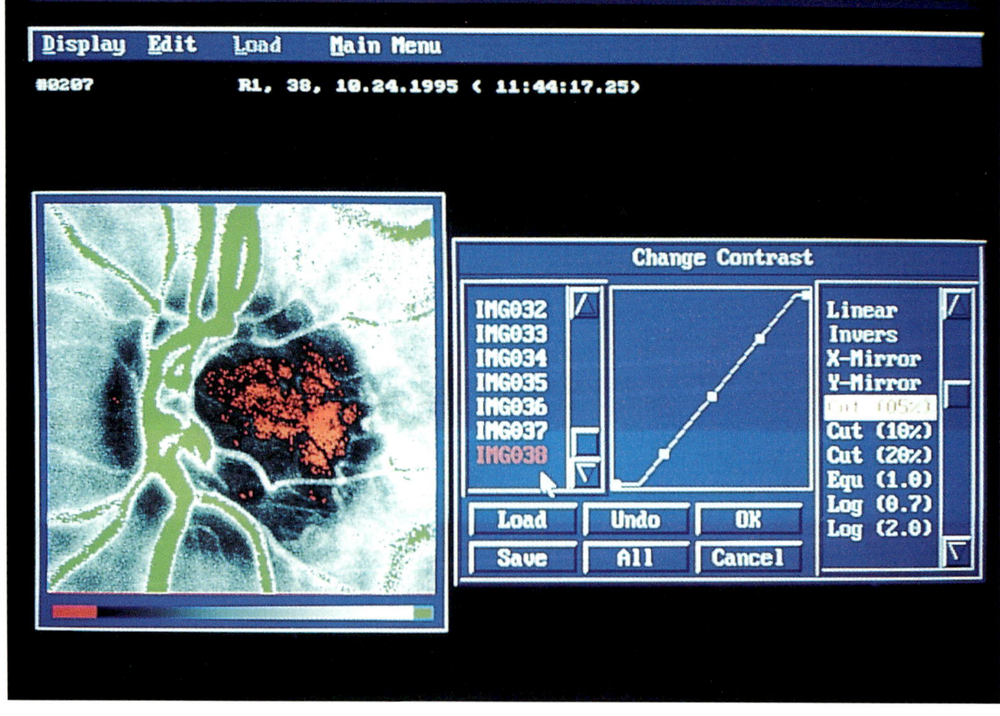

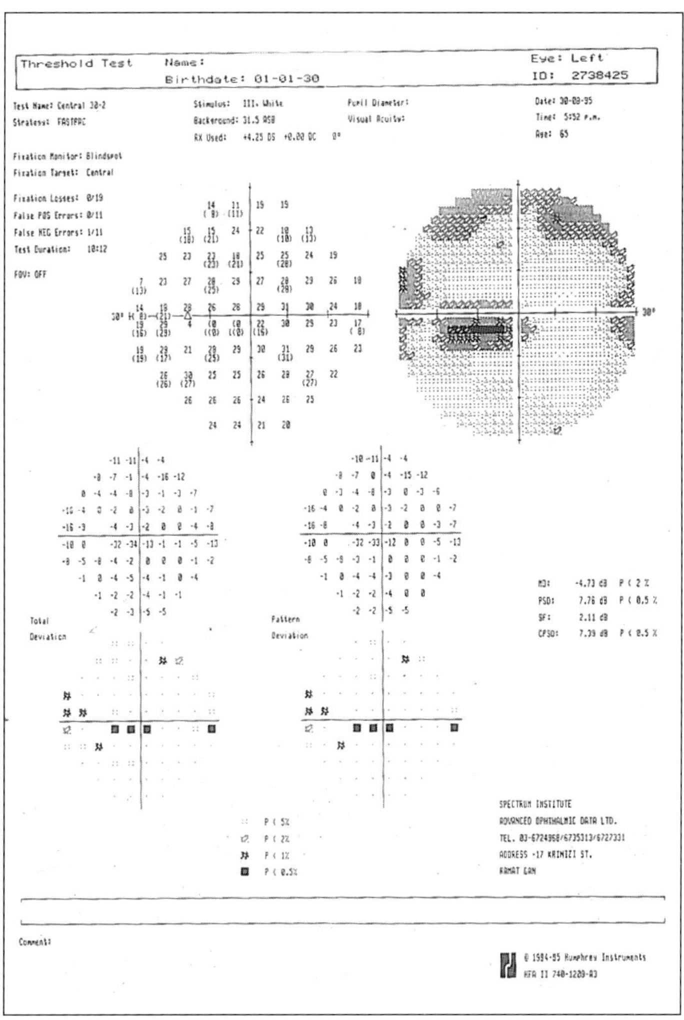

**Figure 9-6c.** Corresponding cecocentral scotoma.

**Figure 9-7a.** Tunnel vision. Patient 6 with pretotal cupping of the optic nerve. CTA disclosed an almost complete loss of blood supply, leaving a single arborizing vessel supplying only the mid-temporal region.

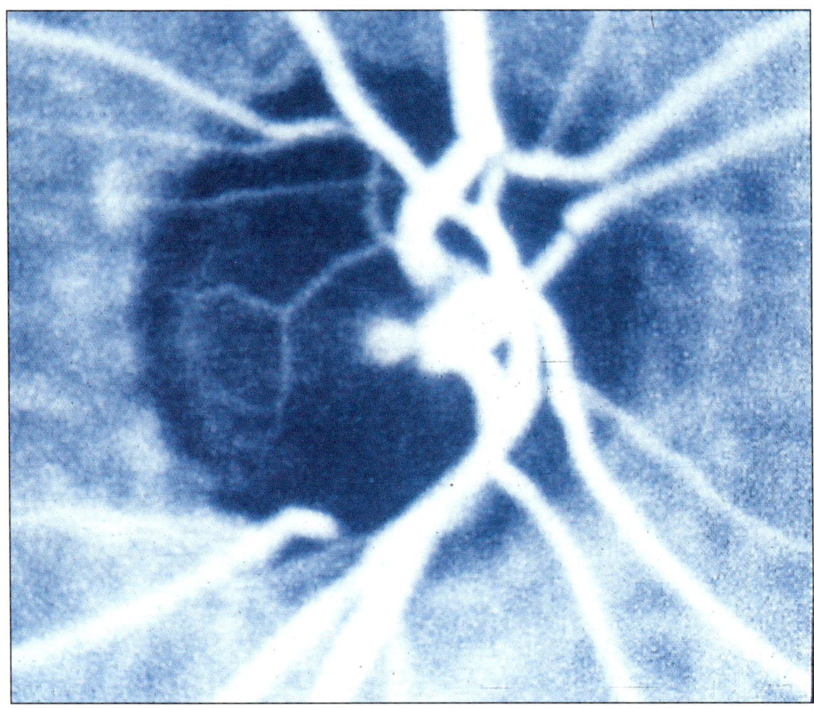

**Figure 9-7b.** Tunnel vision. Patient 6 with pretotal cupping of the optic nerve. CTA disclosed an almost complete loss of blood supply, leaving a single arborizing vessel supplying only the mid-temporal region.

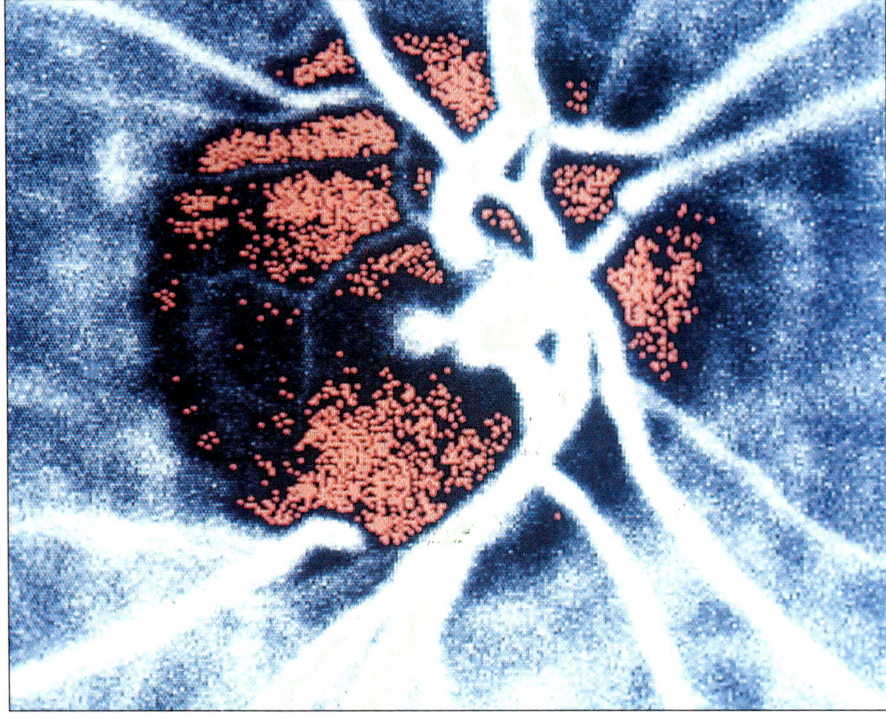

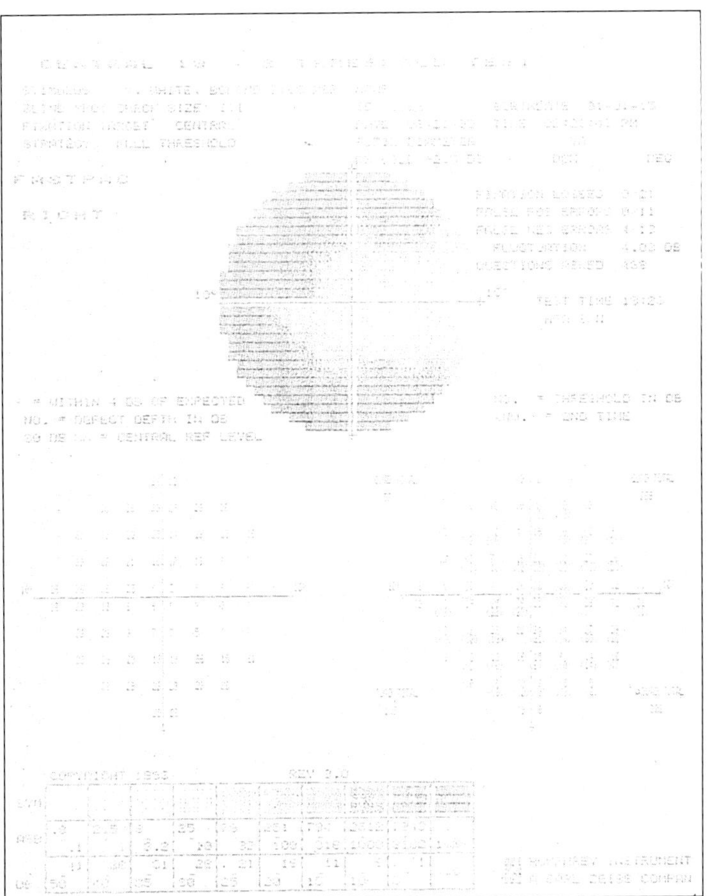

**Figure 9-7c.** This remnant blood supply may explain the maintenance of tunnel vision, with relatively intact maculopapillary bundle.

**Figure 9-8a.** Superior and inferior arcuate scotomata in Patient 7 who had both superior and inferior arcuate field defects.

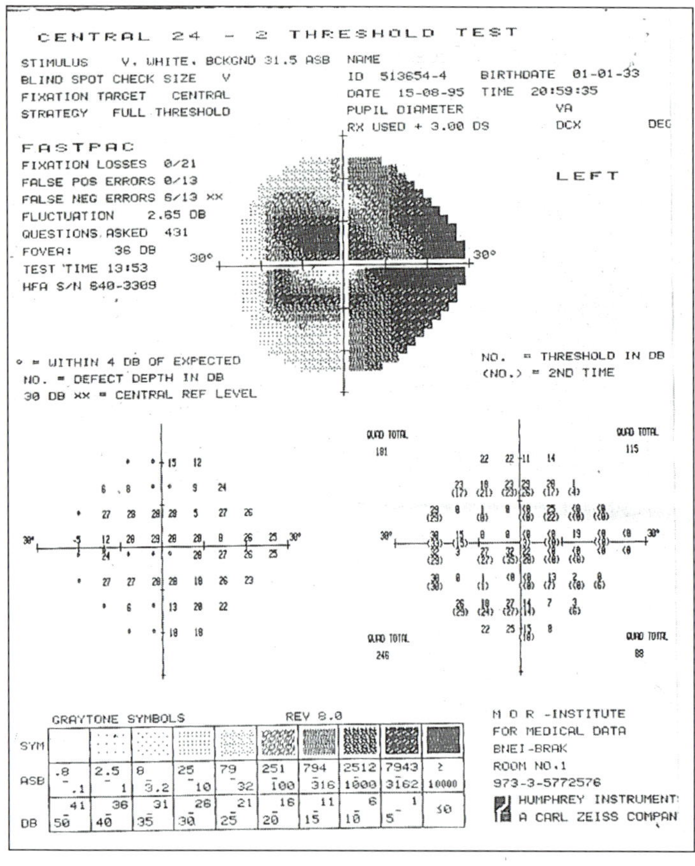

**Figure 9-8b.** CTA showed loss of perfusion superiorly and inferiorly in an "hour-glass" shape.

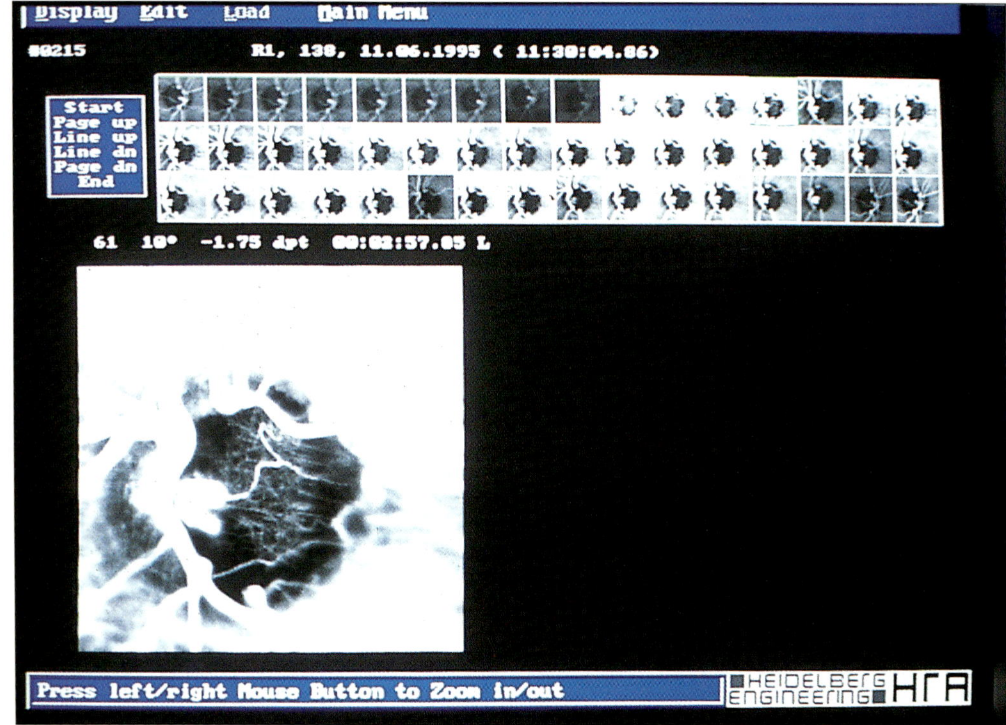

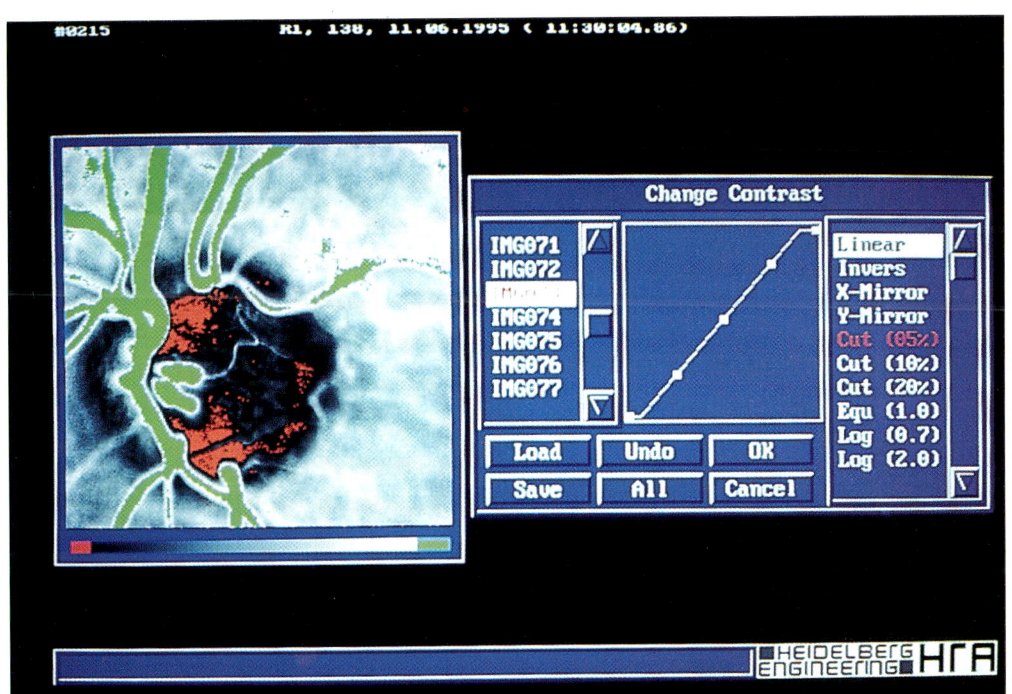

**Figure 9-8c.** CTA showed loss of perfusion superiorly and inferiorly in an "hourglass" shape.

## DISCUSSION

Impairment of blood supply to the ONH in glaucoma has already been accepted by many as a major mechanism contributing to glaucomatous damage.[1,2] Because of its variable arterial origins, small vessel caliber and multilaminate architecture, the microvascular circulation of the ONH is very complex and hard to evaluate with our current technology.[6] Traditional fluorescein angiography has demonstrated various alterations in the vascular pattern of the ONH in glaucoma, such as increased incidence of ONH filling defects,[7] their typical location near the superior and inferior poles of the disc,[8] their specificity for glaucoma when located in the cup wall,[15] and the correlation of their size with the severity of the visual field defect.[9] In addition, linkage between axon loss and vascular damage could also be supported by correlating nerve fiber layer defects with fluorescein filling defects.[16]

However, due to the poor penetration of fluorescein through the optic nerve tissue, only the superficial vessels of the optic nerve and peripapillary region can be visualized. As glaucomatous damage, mechanical or vascular, is believed to occur at the level of the lamina cribrosa, fluorescein angiography is inherently insufficient to disclose vascular alterations confined to that level. Further technological development allowed digital image analysis of video fluorescein angiography to be obtained with a scanning laser ophthalmoscope. Using this technology, videotaped sequences were digitized and capillary blood velocity was calculated.[17] ICG angiography has the advantage of better visualization of the choroidal vasculature as well as better tolerance by the patient.[10] Confocal imaging with scanning laser tomography can generate optical sectioning of the ONH and the peripapillary region.[11,12] Thus, only the application of ICG angiography combined with the advent of confocal tomography made it possible to analyze the vascular pattern from deeper focal planes of the optic nerve.

Our clinical experience with CTA was very encouraging. One of the main challenges is to establish a normal range for the vascular pattern of the ONH. Hayreh[3] has already described the marked interindividual variation in the blood supply of the optic nerve. He found variations in the number of short posterior ciliary arteries supplying the eye and the area of supply to the ONH by each artery.[18]

Although we were able to differentiate deep from superficial blood vessels, we encountered variations in pattern and intensity of fluorescence in the normal discs. Diffuse microvascular filling of the slopes of the rim wall and the rim itself with no detectable filling defects was the common finding in the normal ONHs. This pattern of microvascularization throughout the optic nerve area was demonstrated in all normal eyes and it may indicate good perfusion to the ONH. Further development of imaging programs which will enable the detection of relative differences in ICG fluorescence is needed for more accurate evaluation of this microvascular system.

In this study, we tested a relatively small number of glaucoma patients, so obviously, no conclusion can be made as to the typical alterations of the vascular system in this disease. However, with this limitation in mind, it was very encourag-

**Figure 9-9.** Normal visual field with wide optic nerve cup. CTA discloses normal distribution of optic nerve blood vessels with no filling defects.

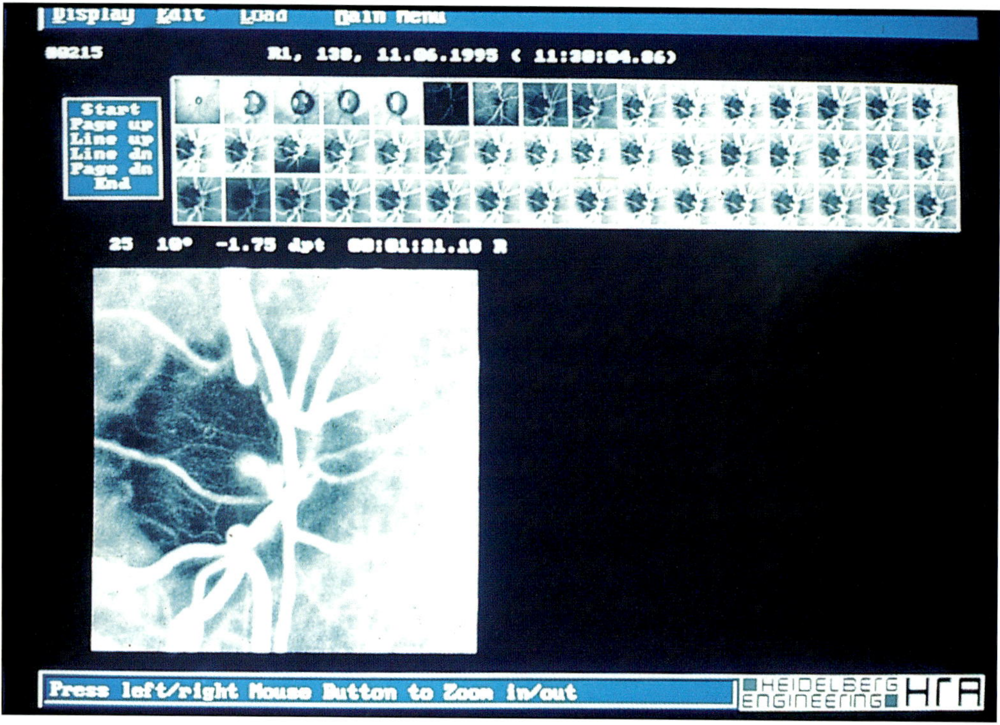

ing to learn that CTA provides valuable information about the optic nerve vascular pattern of various conditions in glaucomatous eyes. Especially interesting and encouraging was our growing experience with correlation to various types of visual field defects and compromised perfusion of respective regions of the optic nerve.

It was most intriguing to learn that in eyes with absolute damage to the optic nerve from very advanced glaucoma, despite their identical ophthalmoscopic presentation, CTA disclosed clearly detectable variations in the deep vascular pattern. In some patients with end-stage glaucoma, the ONH was devoid of ICG fluorescence throughout its cup, while in a disc with a similar ophthalmoscopic view, a vascular pattern was clearly evident at the same level. Interestingly, there were only trunks of vessels demonstrated at the laminar level of these damaged discs, without arborization into a microvascular pattern. This finding may indicate that there is an important role for the capillary system in the pathogenesis of glaucomatous damage. Further studies into the clinical importance of this finding and the correlation with visual field abnormalities are needed.

As evaluation of vascular pattern differences on the basis of comparing relative variations in ICG fluorescence is still under development, at the current stage we can use CTA to detect regions of localized ischemia to the ONH. In patients with sectoral disc changes, we could correlate lack of ICG fluorescence in the affected region (indicating compromised blood supply) with the associated visual field defects. It was interesting that several patients who had inferior or superior notching with respective superior and inferior visual field defects, there was absolutely no ICG fluorescence in the superficial as well as the deep layers of the disc. It remains to be seen whether the demonstration of blood vessels in a damaged zone of the ONH may be associated with no or less visual field loss. If so, CTA might have a very important prognostic value in the future.

Other patients representing a variety of visual field loss patterns demonstrated compromised perfusion to sectors directly related to the visual field loss. For example, in eyes with tunnel vision, CTA demonstrated remnant perfusion of the mid-temporal region (from MPB), possibly explaining the maintenance of central vision in these severely damaged discs. Also, an eye with a cecocentral scotoma disclosed no perfusion in this mid-temporal region, while eyes with bilateral arcuate scotomas had an hourglass appearance of no perfusion as shown by CTA. The correlation between vascular supply and functional capacity of the nerve fibers gets further support by showing "normal" appearance of microvascular pattern without filling defects in subjects with wide cups and normal visual fields.

Another interesting finding was the demonstration of "newly perfused" deep blood vessels at the inferotemporal region of the disc after trabeculectomy. It is conceivable that in this patient with uncontrolled PXF glaucoma the elevated IOP of 36 mmHg caused posterior displacement and stretching of the lamina cribrosa with collapse of some of the remaining blood vessels. After trabeculectomy, with the sharp reduction of IOP to 4 mmHg, the lamina cribrosa

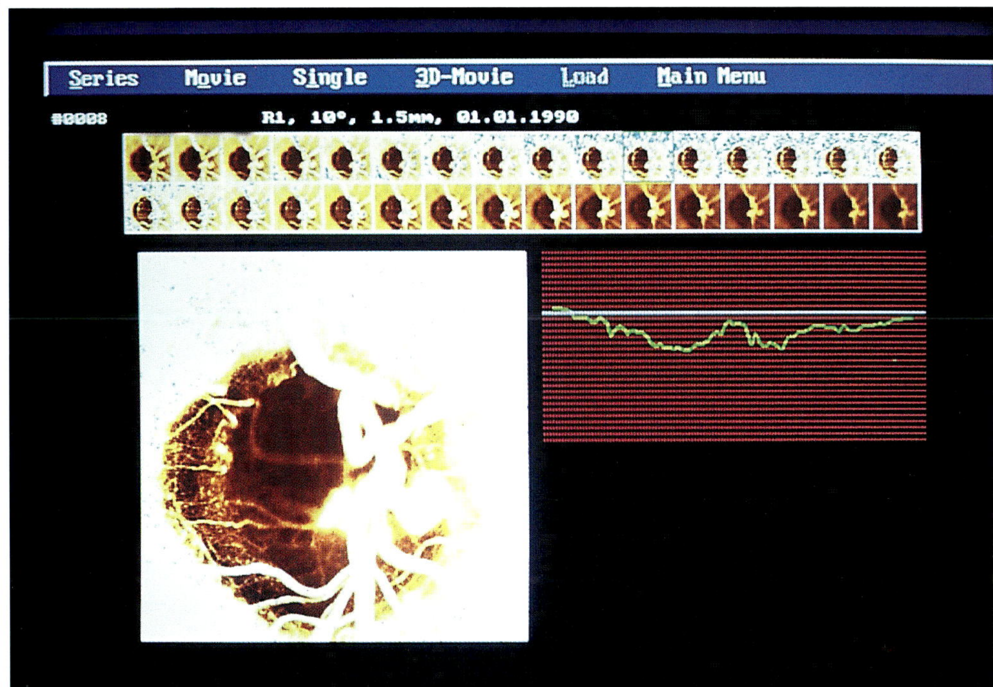

**Figure 9-10a.**
Determination of optic nerve layers in relation to tested plane by CTA. A case with superior relative filling defect in the right eye. Note indicator of plane depth in Figure 9-10a points to superficial layer while in Figure 9-10b it correlates with the bottom of the cup (laminar region). Such a program allows more accurate correlation of tested planes with nerve layers.

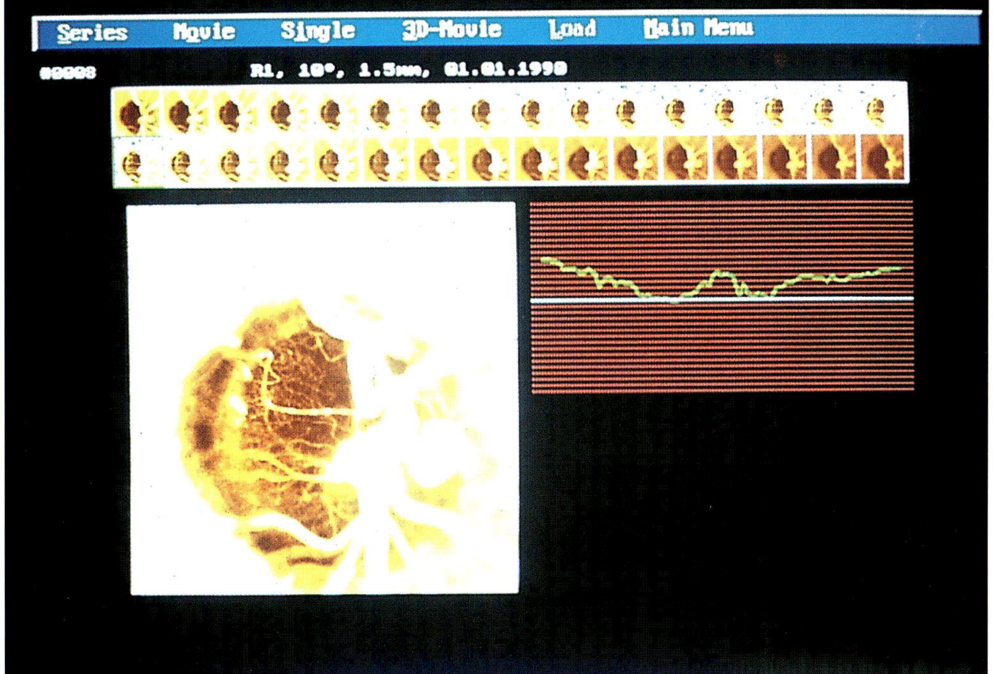

**Figure 9-10b.**
Determination of optic nerve layers in relation to tested plane by CTA. A case with superior relative filling defect in the right eye. Note indicator of plane depth in Figure 9-10a points to superficial layer while in Figure 9-10b it correlates with the bottom of the cup (laminar region). Such a program allows more accurate correlation of tested planes with nerve layers.

recoiled forward, with subsequent relief of pressure from adjacent vessels. Consequently, in this patient, the infero-temporal vessels were reperfused. Further support for this is given by the measurements of cup depth before and after surgery performed by the confocal laser scanning ophthalmoscope. In this patient, cup depth was reduced from 0.428 mm before to 0.125 mm after trabeculectomy, clearly indicating movement forward of the lamina cribrosa in this case.

It still remains to be seen whether the reperfusion of the optic nerve is long-standing and whether it carries with it some improvement of visual functions as described before.[19] Also, our preliminary experience with such patients shows that many of them show no change in perfusion after trabeculectomy. So, apparently, reperfusion after IOP reduction depends also on the extent and chronicity of the optic nerve damage.

Despite our success in delineating deep blood vessels of the ONH and demonstration of some interesting features in the glaucomatous discs, we have to emphasize that CTA is a new technology which will require modifications and improvements. One of the main problems is to accurately correlate each plane with the laminar or prelaminar regions. Premeasurement of cup depth by confocal laser scanning ophthalmoscopy is of value in the assessment and determination of the position of the lamina cribrosa and its related vascular pattern. Such a program enabling parallel viewing of plane depth and optic cup contour may be helpful in better definition of the actual tissue tested. Such a program is now available, and a representative case is shown in Figures 9-10a and 9-10b.

At the current state-of-the-art, the HRA does not have the ability to convert the confocal tomographic pattern into a three-dimensional display of fluorescence. Thus, analysis of location and fluorescence intensity of disc vessels may encounter some difficulty in certain eyes. In summary, our preliminary results with the application of CTA confirm that evaluation of the deep and superficial vessels of the ONH is feasible using this technique. CTA may become a powerful tool in evaluating the blood supply of the glaucomatous optic nerve.

## REFERENCES


1. Carter CJ, Brooks DE, Doyle DL, et al. Investigations into a vascular etiology for low-tension glaucoma. *Ophthalmology.* 1990;97:49.
2. James B. Blood flow in the pathogenesis of glaucoma. *Curr Opin Ophthalmol.* 1993;4:65-72.
3. Hayreh SS. Blood supply of the optic nerve in health and disease. In: Lambrou GN, Greve EL, eds. *Ocular Blood Flow in Glaucoma.* Amsterdam: Kugler & Ghedini; 1989:3-48.
4. Diehl DL, Quigley HA, Miller NR, et al. Prevalence and significance of optic disc hemorrhage in a longitudinal study of glaucoma. *Arch Ophthalmol.* 1990;108:545.
5. Jonas JB, Nguyen XN, Gusek GC, et al. Peripapillary retinal vessel diameter in normal and glaucoma eyes. *Invest Ophthalmol Vis Sci.* 1989;30(Suppl):429.
6. Sugiyama K, Cioffi GA, Bacon DR, et al. Optic nerve and peripapillary choroidal microvasculature in the primate. *J Glaucoma.* 1994;3(Suppl 1):S45-S54.
7. Spaeth GL. *The Pathogenesis of Nerve Damage in Glaucoma: Contributions of Fluorescein Angiography.* New York: Grune & Stratton; 1977.
8. Fishbein SL, Schwartz B. Optic disc in glaucoma. *Arch Ophthalmol.* 1977;95:1975.
9. Nanba K, Schwartz B. Fluorescein angiographic defects of the optic disc in glaucomatous visual field loss. In: Greve EL, Heijl A, eds. Fifth International Visual Field Symposium. Boston, Mass: Junk; 1983:67-73.
10. Flower RW, Hochheimer BF. A clinical apparatus for simultaneous angiography of the separate retinal and choroidal circulation. *Invest Ophthalmol Vis Sci.* 1973;12:248-261.
11. Webb RH, Hughes GW, Delori FC. Confocal scanning laser ophthalmoscope. *Appl Opt.* 1987;26:1492-1499.
12. Weinreb RN, Dreher DW, Bille JF. Reproducibility of topographic measurements of the normal and glaucomatous ONH with the laser tomographic scanner. *Int Ophthalmol.* 1989;13:25-29.
13. Sheider A, Schrodel C. High resolution indocyanine green angiography with the scanning laser ophthalmoscope. *Am J Ophthalmol.* 1989;108:58-459.
14. Weinreb RN, Bartch DU, Freeman RW. Angiography of the glaucomatous optic nerve head. *J Glaucoma.* 1994;3(Suppl):S55-S60.
15. Adam G, Schwartz B. Increased fluorescein filling defects in the wall of the optic disc cup in glaucoma. *Arch Ophthalmol.* 1980;98:1590.
16. Nanba K, Schwartz B. Nerve fiber layer and optic disc fluorescein defects in glaucoma and ocular hypertension. *Ophthalmology.* 1988;95:1227.
17. Cantor LB, Harris A, Wolf S et al. Measurement of superficial ONH capillary blood velocities by scanning laser fluorescein angiography. *J Glaucoma.* 1994;3(Suppl):S61-S63.
18. Hayreh SS, Baines JAB. Occlusion of the posterior ciliary artery: 3. Effects on the ONH. *Br J Ophthalmol.* 1972;56:754-764.
19. Epstein DL. *Chandler and Grant's Glaucoma.* 3rd ed. Philadelphia, Pa: Lea & Febiger; 1986: 88-97.

# SECTION 4

# ANTERIOR SEGMENT IMAGING

# Practical Uses of Ultrasound Biomicroscopy in Glaucoma

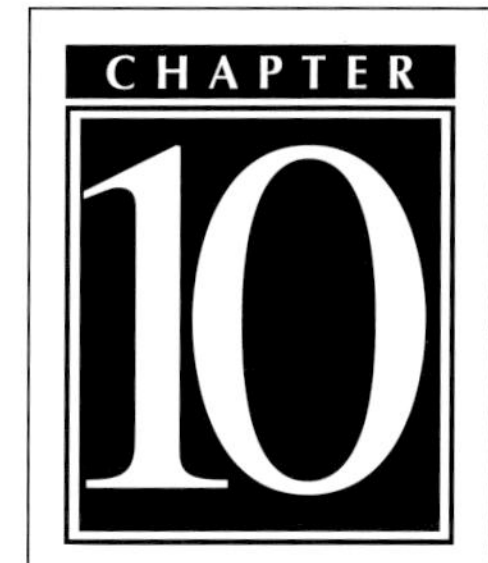


*Robert Ritch, MD, Jeffrey Liebmann, MD,
Raymond Iezzi, MD, Celso Tello, MD*

The ultrasound biomicroscope (UBM, Humphrey Instruments, Inc, San Leandro, Calif) provides high resolution, two-dimensional imaging of the anterior segment.[1,2] It has been useful in elucidating the anatomic correlates of a wide variety of disorders, including anterior segment tumors,[3,4] angle-closure glaucoma,[5-10] malignant glaucoma,[11,12] pigment dispersion syndrome (PDS),[13,14] trauma,[15] and inflammatory disease.[16-18] Ultrasound biomicroscopy has also been useful in the evaluation of surgical procedures and their complications, including filtration bleb structure,[19] intraocular lens haptic position,[20] keratorefractive surgery,[21] surgical complications,[22,23] and intraocular foreign bodies.[24,25]

## THREE-DIMENSIONAL IMAGING

We have described a method for three-dimensional reconstruction of UBM images.[26] Our particular unit incorporates a 50 MHz transducer, giving a resolution of approximately 50 microns, a field of view of 5 mm, and a scan penetration of 4 to 5 mm. All scanning is performed with the patient supine under standardized room lighting conditions. Eye cup immersion scanning is performed with a real-time image update rate of eight frames per second.

Multiple, sequential, parallel, aligned images are acquired using a motorized scanning control arm incorporating a motor that moves the attached ultrasound probe along the z-axis at a precise constant velocity to complement the x- and y-axis sweep of the transducer (Figure 10-1). The controlled scanner movement along the z-axis produces a real-time ultrasound panoscopic view of the eye with a slice thickness of 50 microns. These slices are obtained by digitizing the real-time videotape output of the UBM with a digital

video frame-grabber, using 640 by 480 pixels at eight frames per second. A standard Macintosh IIfx personal computer, equipped with 32 megabytes of RAM and a SuperMac Digital Film VideoCapture Board are used for video processing and three-dimensional image reconstruction.

Multiple, parallel, aligned ultrasound images are stored as Macintosh-based digital Quicktime movies. Using this data compression storage format, Quicktime movies are filed on a floppy disc. Digitized video images are then assembled to generate three-dimensional images using commercially available voxel-processing software (VoxBlast, Vay Tech, Inc, Fairfield, Iowa and Voxel View Mac, Vital Images, Inc, Fairfield, Iowa).

Figures 10-2a and 10-2b show a three-dimensional reconstruction of a cyst located at the iridociliary junction, indenting the peripheral iris and narrowing the anterior chamber angle in a woman who presented with a small iris elevation at 9 o'clock. The multiloculated nature of the cyst cannot be appreciated in a two-dimensional image.

Figures 10-3a through 10-3d show a posterior chamber intraocular lens, one of the haptics of which is displaced posteriorly to the ciliary sulcus, migrating outward along the pars plana in a 70-year-old woman who presented with blurred vision. The intraocular lens is a complex structure that cannot be imaged in any single two-dimensional plane. Figures 10-4a and 10-4b show a functioning, elevated, ischemic bleb. Three-dimensional reconstruction can delineate internal bleb anatomy, including the scleral flap, fistula, internal ostium, and conjunctiva-tenon's-episcleral interface. The entire drainage track from the anterior chamber to the subconjunctival space can be imaged three-dimensionally.

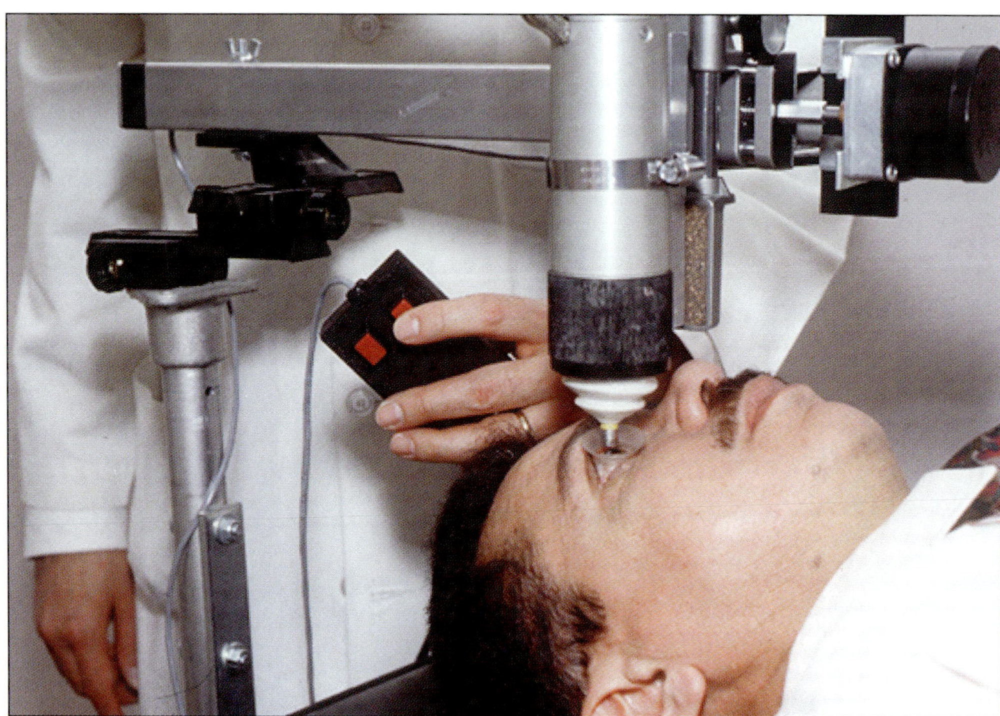

**Figure 10-1.** Motorized scan control arm, providing controlled scanner movement along the Z-axis. Reprinted with permission from Iezzi R, Rosen RB, Tello C, et al. Personal computer-based three-dimensional ultrasound biomicroscopy of the anterior segment. *Arch Ophthalmol.* 1996;114:520-524. Copyright 1996, American Medical Association.

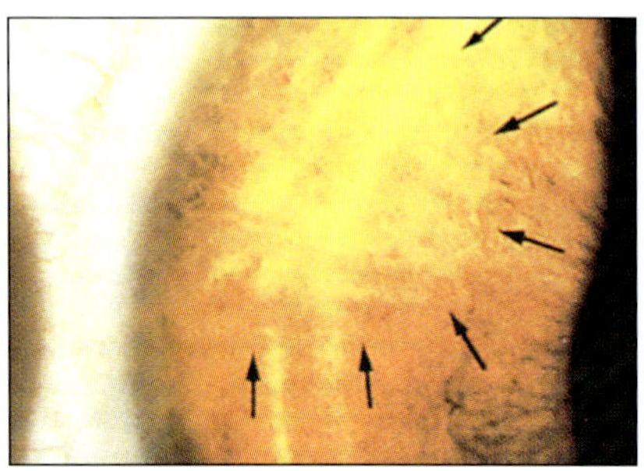

**Figure 10-2a.** Small iris elevation at 9 o'clock (small arrows). Reprinted with permission from Iezzi R, Rosen RB, Tello C, et al. Personal computer-based three-dimensional ultrasound biomicroscopy of the anterior segment. *Arch Ophthalmol.* 1996;114:520-524. Copyright 1996, American Medical Association.

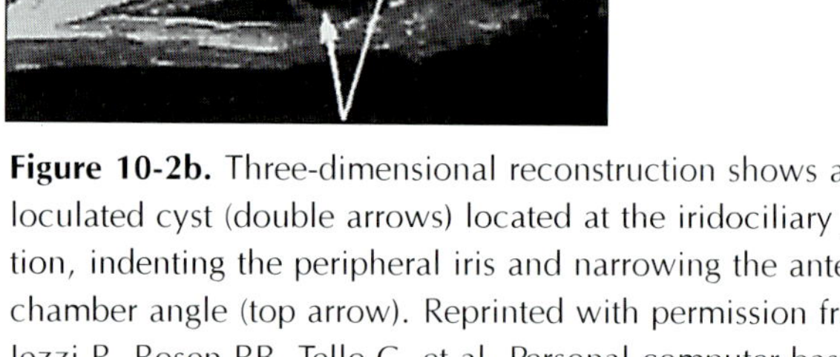

**Figure 10-2b.** Three-dimensional reconstruction shows a multi-loculated cyst (double arrows) located at the iridociliary junction, indenting the peripheral iris and narrowing the anterior chamber angle (top arrow). Reprinted with permission from Iezzi R, Rosen RB, Tello C, et al. Personal computer-based three-dimensional ultrasound biomicroscopy of the anterior segment. *Arch Ophthalmol.* 1996;114:520-524. Copyright 1996, American Medical Association.

## PIGMENT DISPERSION SYNDROME

Ultrasound biomicroscopy has been extremely important in helping us to elucidate the underlying pathophysiology of PDS and pigmentary glaucoma (PG) and also to correlate pathophysiology with approaches to treatment.

PDS and PG are characterized by loss of the pigment granules from the iris pigment epithelium (IPE) and their deposition throughout the anterior segment. The classic diagnostic triad consists of corneal pigmentation (Krukenberg spindle); slit-like, radial, mid-peripheral iris transillumination defects; and dense trabecular pigmentation. The iris insertion is typically posterior and the peripheral iris tends to have a concave configuration.

PDS was originally described in 1949 by Sugar and Barbour,[27] who described two young men with Krukenberg spindles and hyperpigmentation of the trabecular meshwork, and considered it a specific but rare disease. In 1966, Sugar[28] summarized 147 cases in the world literature, mentioning several additional features, including bilaterality, frequent association with myopia, greater incidence in men than in women, and a relatively young age of onset. In 1979, Campbell[29] proposed the pathogenesis to involve mechanical damage to the IPE during rubbing of the posterior iris against the anterior zonular bundles during physiologic pupillary movement.

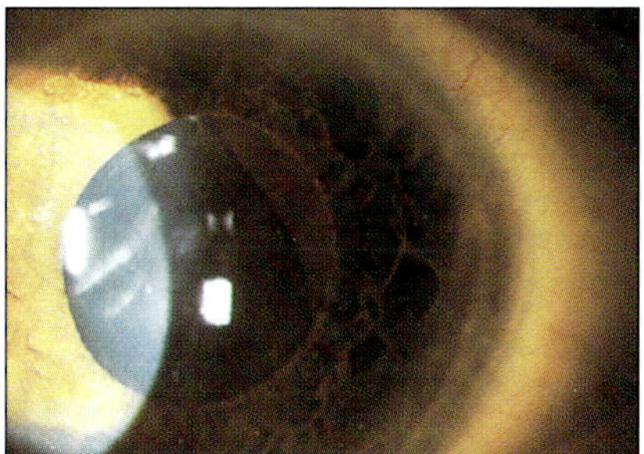

**Figure 10-3a.** Nasally shifted posterior chamber intraocular lens. Reprinted with permission from Iezzi R, Rosen RB, Tello C, et al. Personal computer-based three-dimensional ultrasound biomicroscopy of the anterior segment. *Arch Ophthalmol.* 1996;114:520-524. Copyright 1996, American Medical Association.

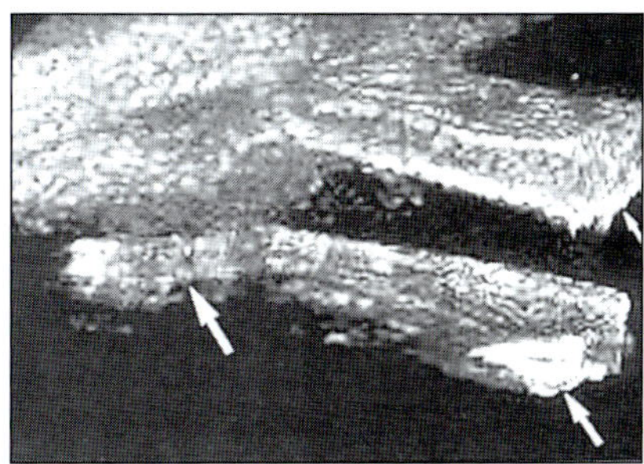

**Figure 10-3b.** Three-dimensional reconstruction showing haptic (left arrow), optic (lower arrow), and iris. Reprinted with permission from Iezzi R, Rosen RB, Tello C, et al. Personal computer-based three-dimensional ultrasound biomicroscopy of the anterior segment. *Arch Ophthalmol.* 1996;114:520-524. Copyright 1996, American Medical Association.

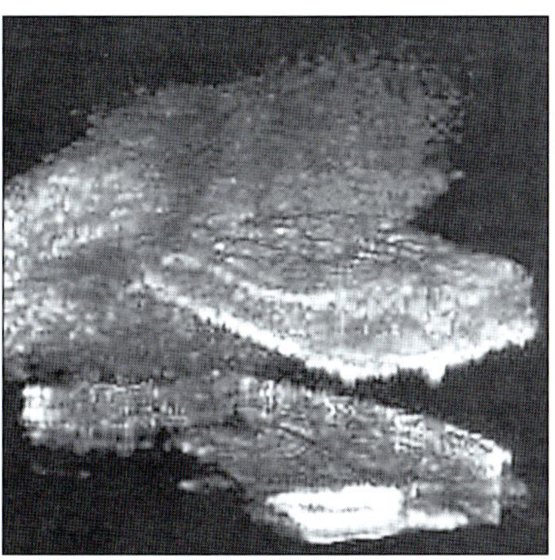

**Figure 10-3c.** Rotated view. Reprinted with permission from Iezzi R, Rosen RB, Tello C, et al. Personal computer-based three-dimensional ultrasound biomicroscopy of the anterior segment. *Arch Ophthalmol.* 1996;114:520-524. Copyright 1996, American Medical Association.

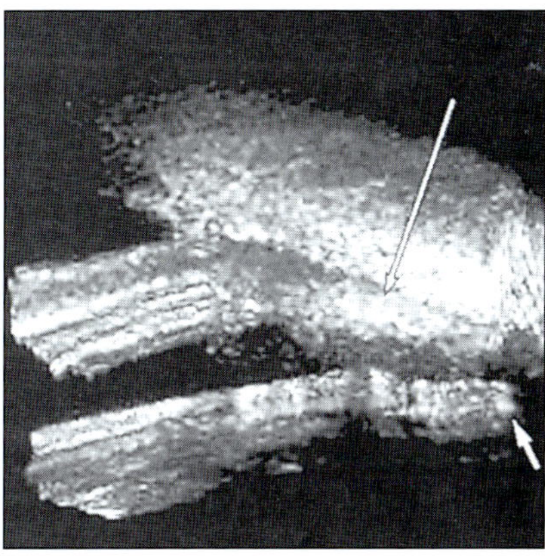

**Figure 10-3d.** Displacement of one haptic (right arrow) posteriorly to the ciliary sulcus migrating outward along the pars plana. Ciliary body (top arrow). Reprinted with permission from Iezzi R, Rosen RB, Tello C, et al. Personal computer-based three-dimensional ultrasound biomicroscopy of the anterior segment. *Arch Ophthalmol.* 1996;114:520-524. Copyright 1996, American Medical Association.

## Clinical Findings

Loss of iris pigment appears clinically as a midperipheral, radial, slit-like pattern of transillumination defects seen most commonly inferonasally and more easily in blue eyes than in brown eyes. Although the defects can sometimes be seen by retroillumination, they are more easily detected by a dark adapted examiner using a fiberoptic transilluminator in a darkened room. Corneal endothelial pigment generally appears as a central, vertical, brown band (Krukenberg spindle). The anterior chamber is deeper both centrally and peripherally than can be accounted for by sex, age, and refractive error.[30]

The angle is characteristically wide open, with a homogeneous, dense hyperpigmented band on the trabecular meshwork. The iris insertion is posterior and the peripheral iris approach is often concave. The iris is most concave in the midperiphery. Pigment is also deposited on Schwalbe's line, on the iris surface, on the zonules,[31-33] and on the posterior capsule of the lens (Zentmayer ring).

PDS is associated with a high incidence (6% to 8%) of retinal detachment.[34-36] The incidence is independent of miotic treatment.[35] The incidence of lattice degeneration appears to be higher for all degrees of myopia in patients with PDS[37] than in the general population.[38]

## Natural History

The mean age of onset of PDS remains unknown, but is probably in the early 20s for most patients, although some present in the teens, and women tend to have a higher age at the time of diagnosis and onset of glaucoma. The phenotypic expression of this autosomal dominant disorder varies widely. Referral practices tend to have patients with more

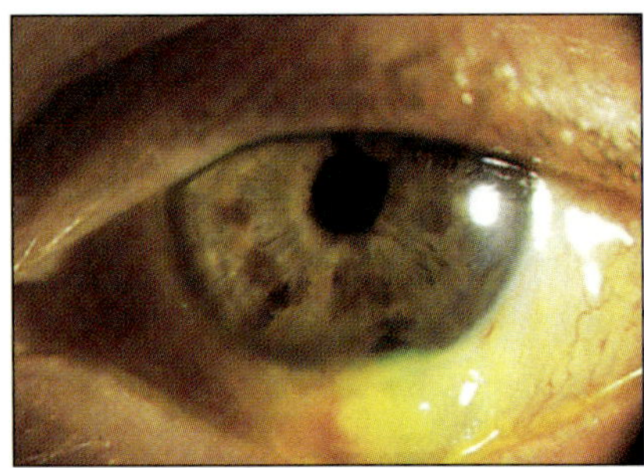

**Figure 10-4a.** Functioning, elevated, ischemic bleb. Reprinted with permission from Iezzi R, Rosen RB, Tello C, et al. Personal computer-based three-dimensional ultrasound biomicroscopy of the anterior segment. *Arch Ophthalmol.* 1996;114:520-524. Copyright 1996, American Medical Association.

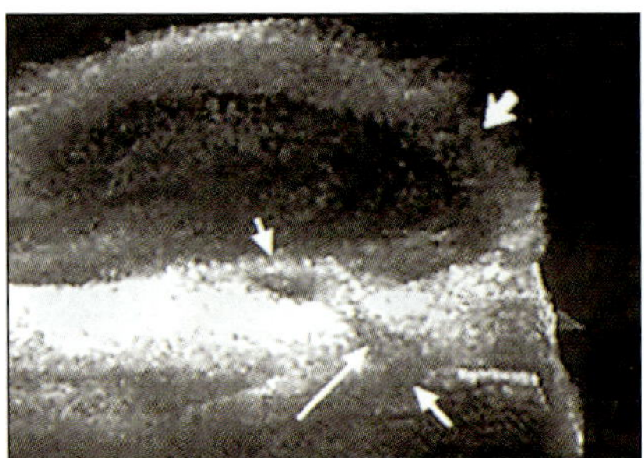

**Figure 10-4b.** Three-dimensional rotational animation with volumetric resampling. Scleral flap, patency of the transscleral fistula, internal ostium, and bleb are visible (arrows left to right, respectively). Reprinted with permission from Iezzi R, Rosen RB, Tello C, et al. Personal computer-based three-dimensional ultrasound biomicroscopy of the anterior segment. *Arch Ophthalmol.* 1996;114:520-524. Copyright 1996, American Medical Association.

extensive involvement, although even in these patients, the diagnosis is often missed. More subtle manifestations may never be detected because of a lack of suspicion on the part of the examiner, unawareness of the examiner of pathognomonic signs in patients with mild phenotypic involvement, failure to perform slit-lamp examination in patients presenting for refraction, and simply lack of an eye examination.

The severity of both PDS and PG decreases in middle age when pigment liberation ceases, at least in the majority of patients. Lichter and Shaffer[39] observed decreased pigment in the trabecular meshwork in 10% of 102 cases, concluding that pigment could pass out of the meshwork with age. Transillumination defects may disappear,[29,40] most likely by migration of pigment epithelial cells adjacent to the defects. The intraocular pressure (IOP) may return toward normal.[40-42] Some patients treated with long-term miotic therapy have been able to reduce or discontinue treatment for glaucoma.[41,43] Older patients presenting with glaucoma may have only very subtle manifestations, if any, of PDS, and may be misdiagnosed as primary open-angle glaucoma or low-tension glaucoma.[44] Remission of PG has also been reported following glaucoma surgery[35] and following lens subluxation.[45]

Trabecular pigmentation is initially dense and homogeneous for 360°. With age and clearance of pigment from the angle, it becomes lighter and more localized to the filtering portion of the meshwork, while it disappears from Schwalbe's line and the scleral spur. When the trabecular meshwork begins to recover, the normal pigment pattern reverses and the pigment band becomes darker superiorly than inferiorly. We have termed this the "pigment reversal sign" and, in older patients, it may be the only finding suggestive of previous PDS (Figures 10-5a and 10-5b).

## Ultrasound Biomicroscope Findings

The UBM has enabled us to further elucidate the pathophysiology of PDS.[13,14,46-52] The iris appears to be too large relative to the size of the anterior segment (Figures 10-6a and 10-6b). This may predispose to iridozonular contact, which also appears to be facilitated by a congenitally more posterior iris insertion in patients with PDS when compared to age-, sex-, and refraction-matched controls.[51]

Lid blinking may be important in the physiology of aqueous humor flow. When blinking is prevented in patients with PDS, aqueous builds up in the posterior chamber and the iris assumes a planar or even a convex configuration.[14,53] As the iris gradually flattens, iridolenticular contact diminishes (Figure 10-7). Blinking acts mechanically to alter anterior segment anatomy. Campbell[53] proposed that a blink initially deforms the cornea, transiently increasing IOP and pushing the iris posteriorly against the lens. After a blink, the concave iris configuration returns in all eyes.[14] During blinking of the nictitating membrane in the chick eye, the cornea indents in a wave from the periphery to the center and anterior chamber depth decreases (Figures 10-8a and 10-8b).[54] We have hypothesized that blinking acts as a mechanical pump to push aliquots of aqueous humor from the posterior to the anterior chamber.[55] A pressure wave begins at the iris periphery and moves centrally, pushing the iris posteriorly toward the zonules and pushing aqueous before it into the anterior chamber. Abnormally extensive iridolenticular contact in eyes with PDS prevents equilibration of aqueous between the two chambers (reverse pupillary block).[53,56] At the same time, the iris reassumes its concave configuration. The now increased volume of aqueous in the anterior chamber helps to maintain the midperipheral iris concavity.

Iridolenticular contact also increases with increasing myopia, independent of the presence of PDS.[14] This may

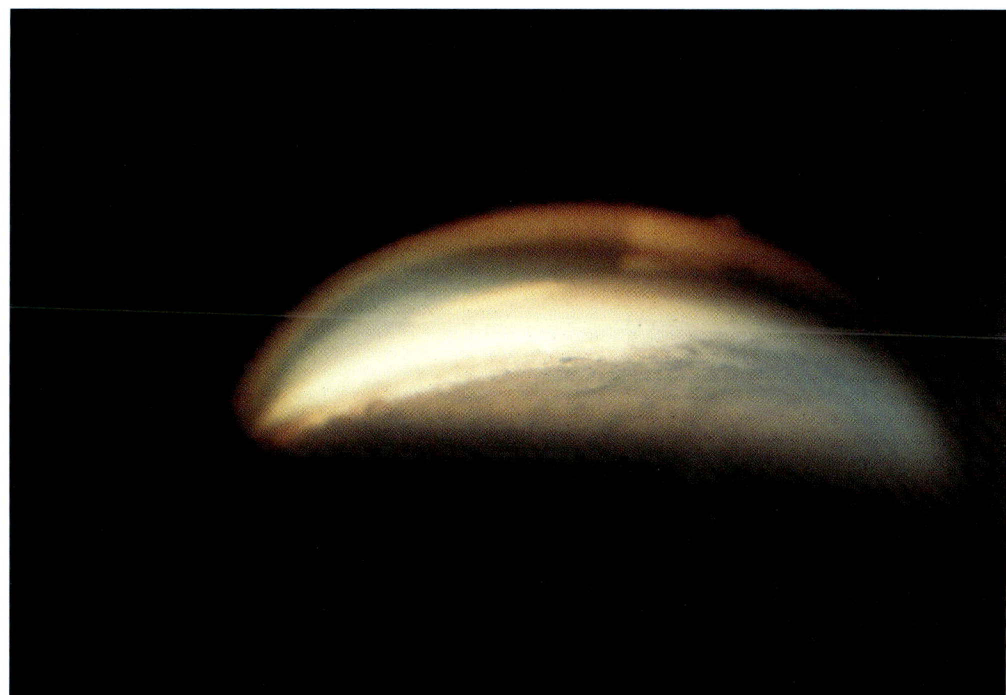

**Figure 10-5a.** Pigment reversal sign in a 48-year-old man. Inferior angle. Reprinted with permission from Ritch R. A unification hypothesis of pigment dispersion syndrome. *Trans Am Ophthalmol Soc.* In press.

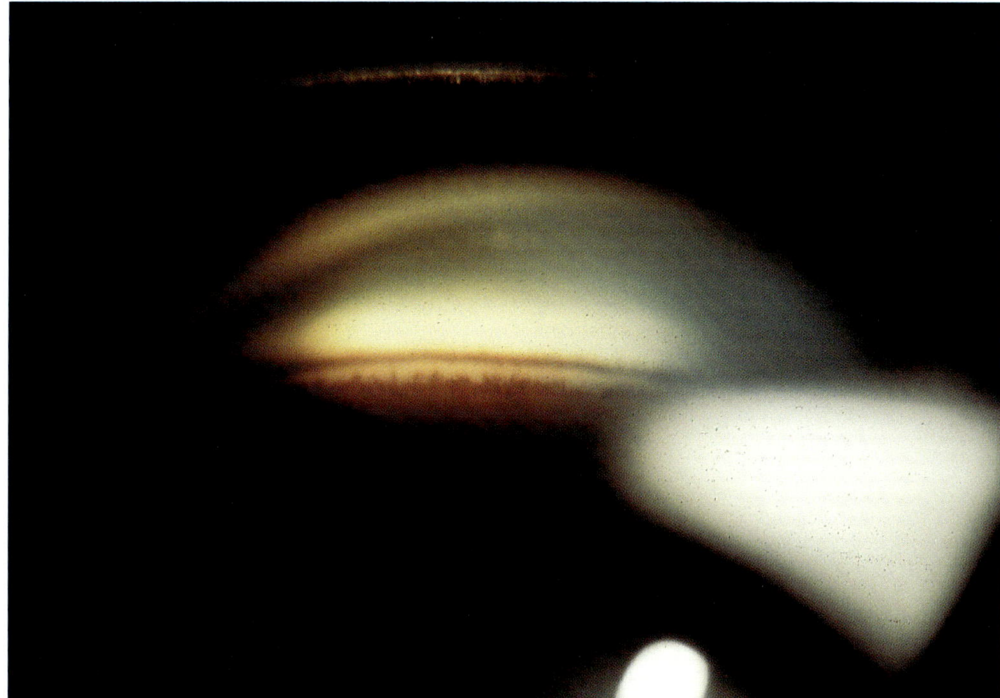

**Figure 10-5b.** Superior angle. The pigment is denser in the superior angle. Note that the pigment band has sharp anterior and posterior margins and appears smooth, indicating that this pigment was deposited in the past and is now localized to the region of the filtering portion of the trabecular meshwork. The iris is inserted posteriorly. Reprinted with permission from Ritch R. A unification hypothesis of pigment dispersion syndrome. *Trans Am Ophthalmol Soc.* In press.

explain why myopia enhances the phenotypic expression of the genetic abnormality underlying PDS.

Accommodation may also affect iris contour (Figures 10-9a and 10-9b).[14,57] In normal eyes, it causes an iris concavity indistinguishable from that in PDS. Aqueous in the anterior chamber is forced into the angle recess and the peripheral iris becomes more concave. As accommodation is relaxed, the iris resumes its initial configuration. UBM during accommodation in eyes with PDS shows iridozonular contact at the lens margin, consistent with the usual position of iris transillumination defects.[58]

Pilocarpine eliminates the iris concavity and iridozonular contact, producing a convex rather than a planar configuration, identical to the configuration produced by inhibition of blinking. Laser iridectomy relieves reverse pupillary block by allowing aqueous to flow from the anterior to the posterior

**Figure 10-6a.** Ultrasound biomicrograph of a normal eye.

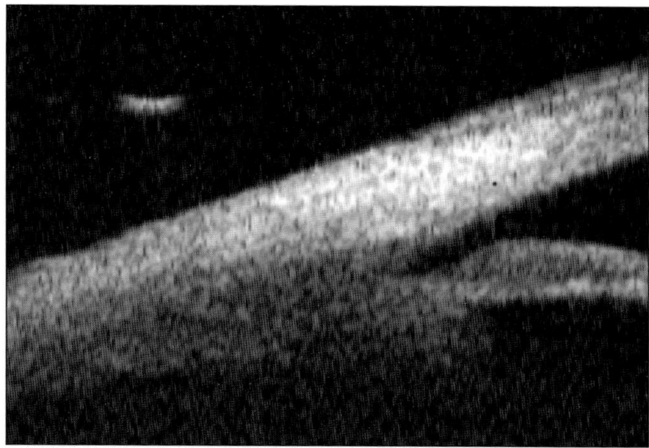

**Figure 10-6b.** Ultrasound biomicrograph of an eye with PDS. The iris is large relative to the size of the anterior segment and the midperipheral concavity is prominent. There is extensive iridolenticular contact. Reprinted with permission from Ritch R. A unification hypothesis of pigment dispersion syndrome. *Trans Am Ophthalmol Soc.* In press.

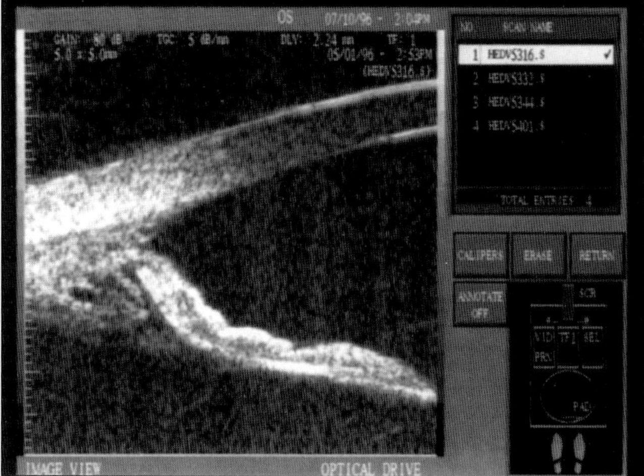

**Figure 10-7.** Inhibition of blinking for several minutes results in expansion of the posterior chamber, a convex iris configuration, and loss of iridolenticular contact in this eye of a patient with PDS. Despite lack of iridolenticular contact, aqueous pressure in the posterior chamber is sufficient to maintain the iris in a convex position. Reprinted with permission from Ritch R. A unification hypothesis of pigment dispersion syndrome. *Trans Am Ophthalmol Soc.* In press.

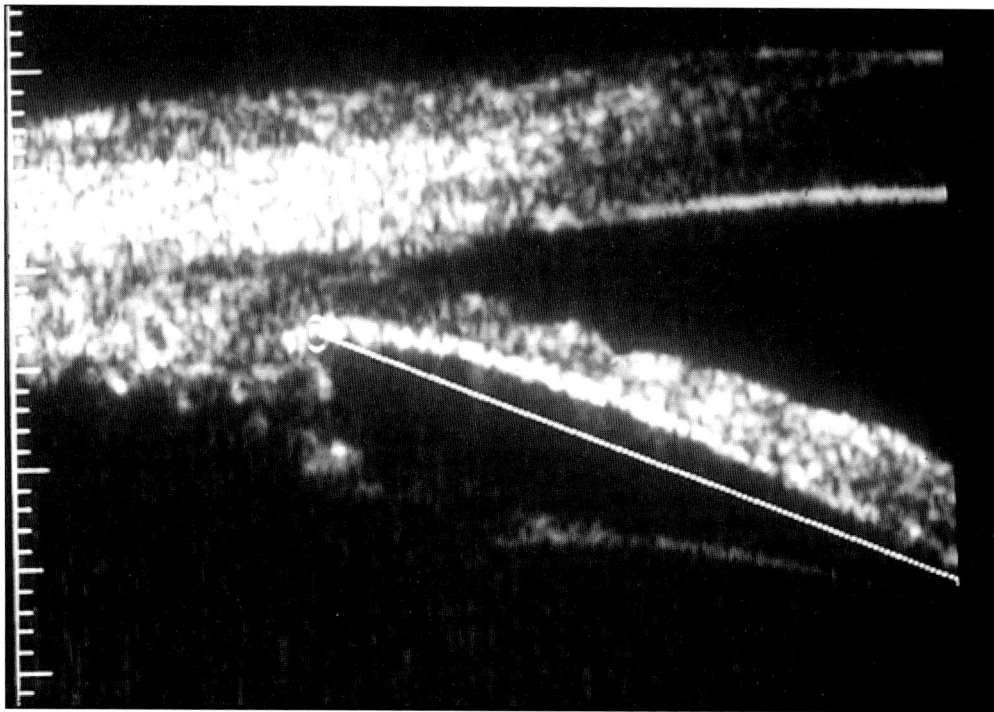

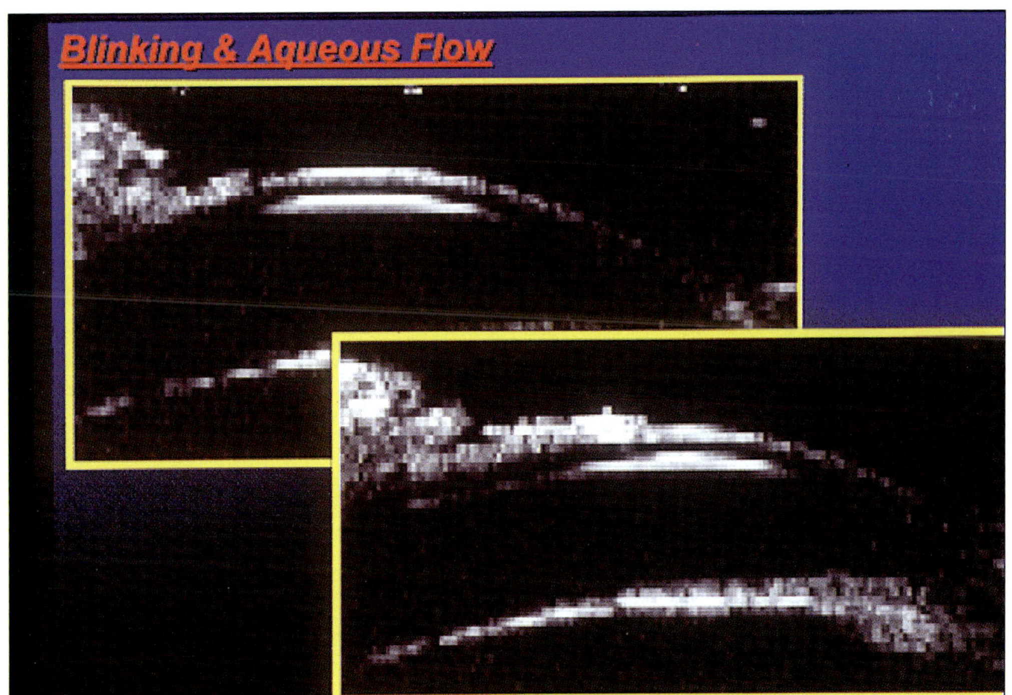



**Figure 10-8a.** Chick cornea prior to blinking of the nictitating membrane. Reprinted with permission from Ritch R. A unification hypothesis of pigment dispersion syndrome. *Trans Am Ophthalmol Soc.* In press.

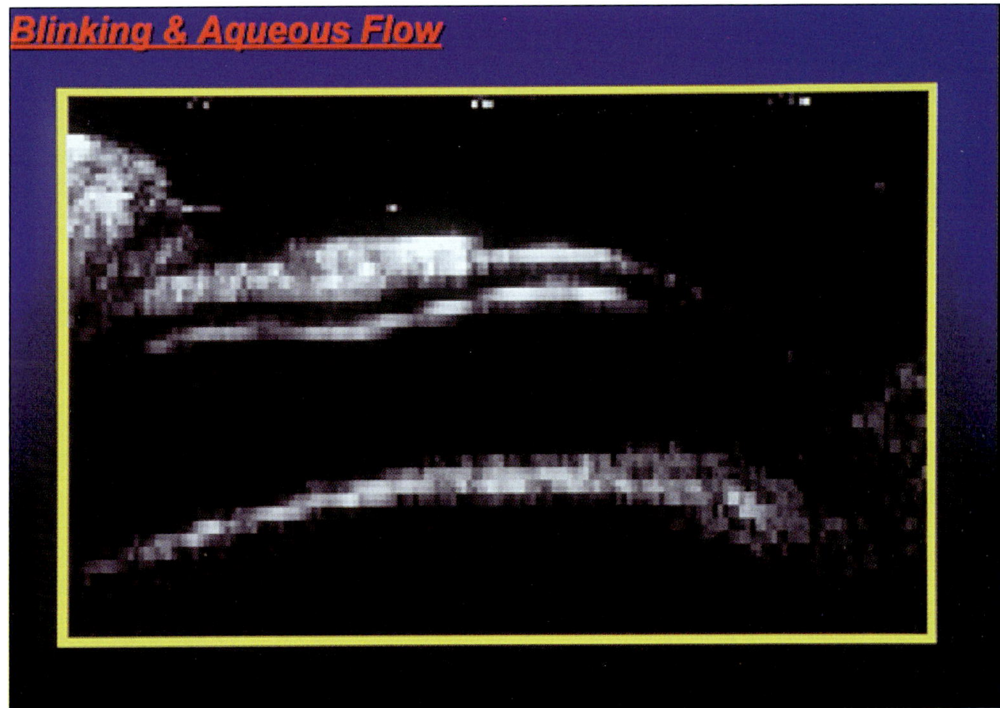



**Figure 10-8b.** During the blink, the cornea indents. Reprinted with permission from Ritch R. A unification hypothesis of pigment dispersion syndrome. *Trans Am Ophthalmol Soc.* In press.

chamber and produces a planar iris configuration (Figure 10-10). Iridectomy appears to prevent the accentuation of the iris concavity that accompanies accommodation.[58] Pilocarpine completely inhibits exercise-induced pigment release and IOP elevation, while iridectomy does so incompletely.[49,59]

## Implications for Treatment

The development of relative pupillary block from age-related increase in lens thickness and loss of accommodation with presbyopia presumably lead to the cessation of pigment liberation in middle age. By eliminating the iris concavity and iridozonular contact, miotic therapy may prevent progression of the disease and the development of glaucoma by immobilizing the pupil and may allow previously existing damage to reverse more readily. Since most PDS patients are young and cannot tolerate pilocarpine drops because of

**Figure 10-9a.** Normal myopic eye prior to accommodation. Reprinted with permission from Ritch R. A unification hypothesis of pigment dispersion syndrome. *Trans Am Ophthalmol Soc.* In press.

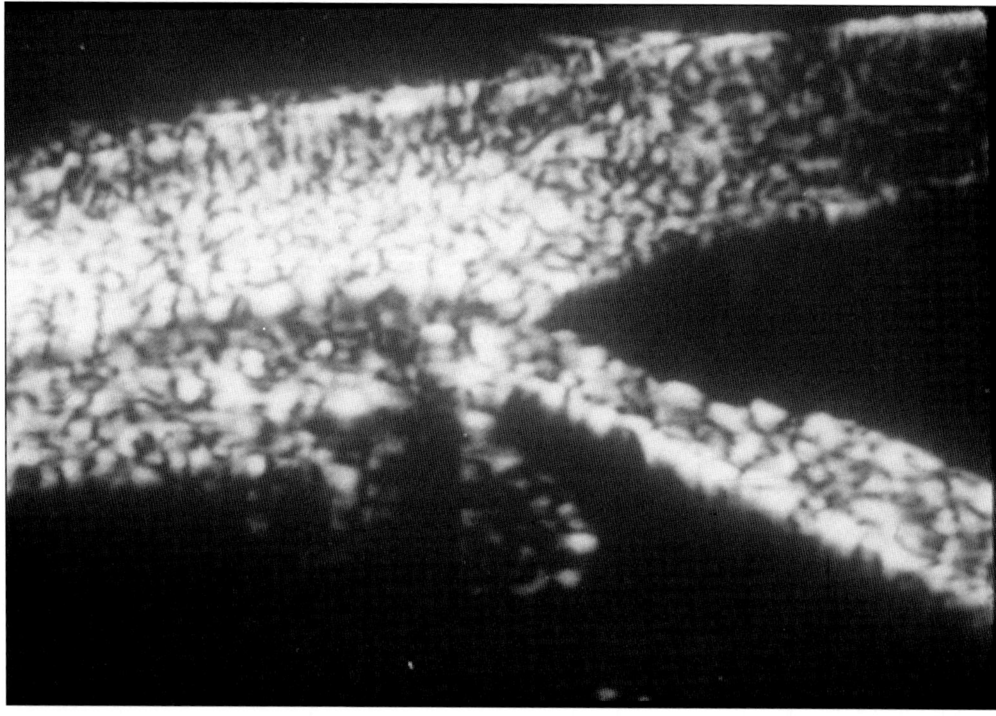

**Figure 10-9b.** Accommodation produces a midperipheral iris concavity mimicking that seen in PDS. Reprinted with permission from Ritch R. A unification hypothesis of pigment dispersion syndrome. *Trans Am Ophthalmol Soc.* In press.

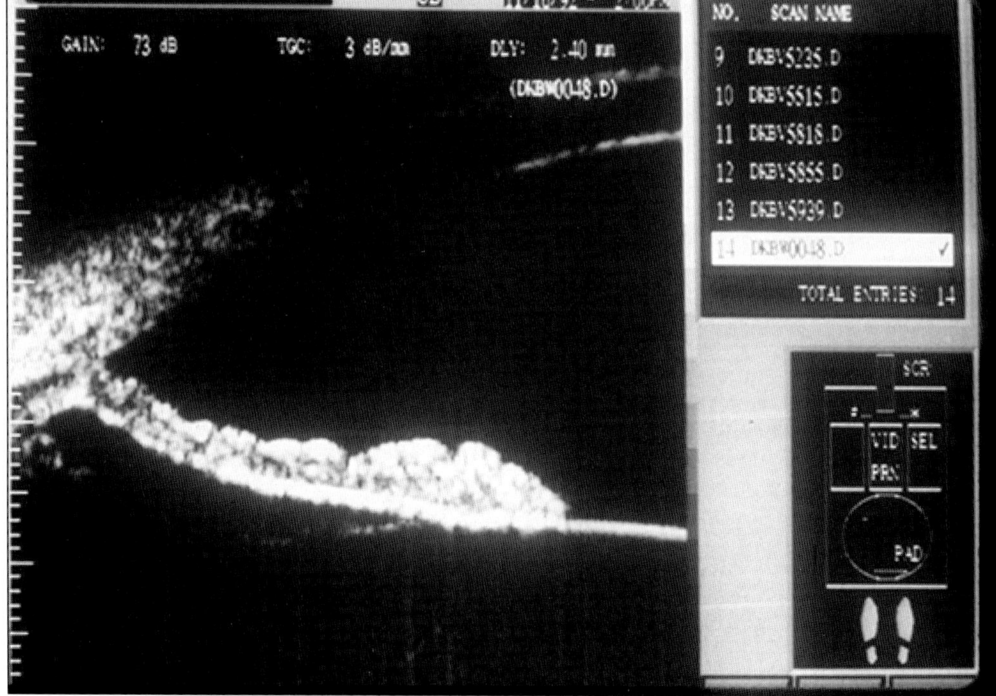

induced myopia and accommodative spasm, pilocarpine Ocuserts have proven to be the best available form of miotic therapy.

Argon laser trabeculoplasty (ALT) is more successful in younger patients with PG than in older ones.[60-62] Pigment in younger patients is largely in the uveoscleral and corneoscleral meshworks, whereas in older ones, it is mainly in the juxtacanalicular meshwork and the inner wall of Schlemm's canal.[61] Patients in the pigment liberation stage who undergo ALT should be maintained on miotics or undergo laser iridectomy after ALT to prevent further contact between the iris and zonules.

Treatment should begin early in order to prevent the development of glaucomatous damage and should be designed to prevent progression of the disease rather than merely lower IOP. Miotic treatment produces a convex iris

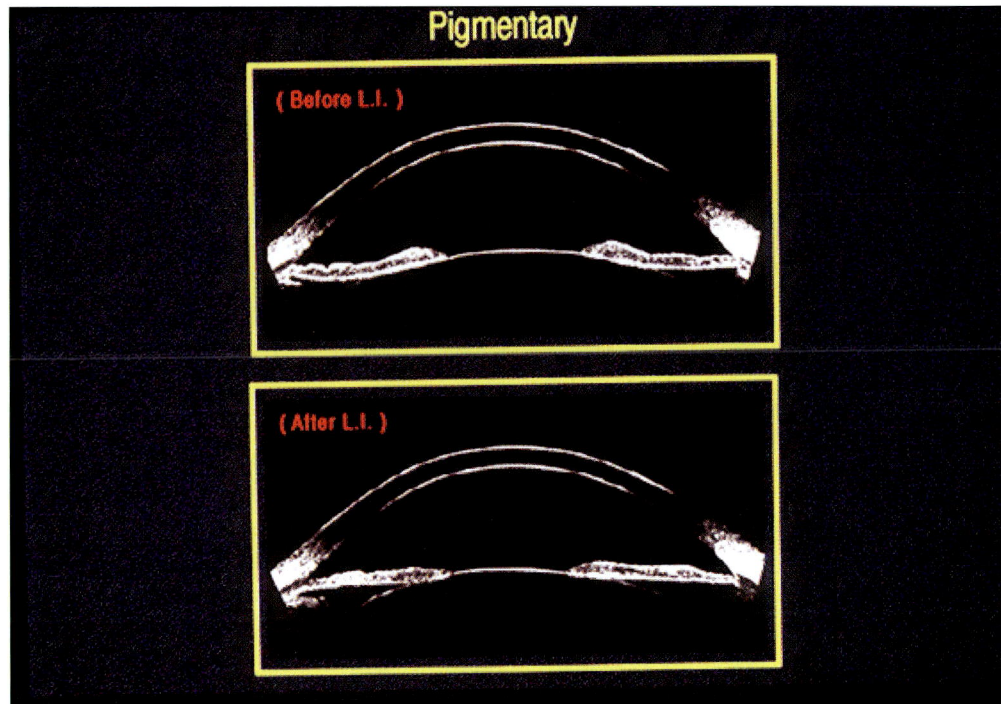


**Figure 10-10.** Laser iridectomy produces a planar iris configuration. Reprinted with permission from Ritch R. A unification hypothesis of pigment dispersion syndrome. *Trans Am Ophthalmol Soc.* In press.

configuration, completely inhibiting pigment liberation, while laser iridectomy produces a planar configuration and may not completely inhibit pigment liberation. Aqueous suppressants theoretically may negatively impact the course of the disease.

Who should undergo laser iridectomy? Iridectomy eliminates active pigment dispersion. Therefore, patients should still be in the pigment liberation stage. If pigment is liberated into the anterior chamber with pupillary dilation, it is suggestive that the patient is still in this stage. Patients who have uncontrolled glaucoma and are facing surgery are also poor candidates for laser iridectomy, since perhaps years are required to achieve functional reconstitution of the trabecular meshwork. We restrict iridectomy to patients under 45 years of age who have elevated IOP with no damage or early glaucomatous damage. Clinical trials are needed to determine whether Ocuserts or iridectomy can normalize IOP in eyes with glaucomatous damage, prevent glaucomatous damage in eyes with elevated IOP, and prevent elevated IOP in normotensive eyes. Since not all patients with PDS go on to develop elevated IOP, and since the iridectomy procedure itself results in significant pigment liberation, we do not advocate treating normotensive eyes at the present time.

## ANGLE-CLOSURE GLAUCOMA

In order to approach treatment of angle-closure glaucoma most effectively, we must understand the differences between the different disorders that cause it and the anatomic and pathophysiologic mechanisms by which they develop.

Just as open-angle glaucoma consists of disorders of diverse etiology related by a final common pathway, angle-closure glaucoma needs to be appreciated within a similar framework. It is a number of different disorders related by a final common pathway, the first step of which is iris apposition to the trabecular meshwork. They are characterized by disordered relationships of anterior segment structures due to changes in size, shape, or position.

Angle-closure can be caused by one or a combination of the following:

- Abnormalities in the relative sizes or positions of anterior segment structures
- Abnormalities in the absolute sizes or positions of anterior segment structures
- Abnormal forces in the posterior segment that alter the anatomy of the anterior segment.

Because the terminology for many of these disorders was developed years ago and has been used inconsistently, it is not ideal for describing angle-closure as we are beginning to understand it today. It remains easier to classify the angle-closure glaucomas in terms of the underlying "mechanism" causing the angle-closure.[63,64]

Relative pupillary block underlies approximately 90% of angle-closure. Laser iridectomy is definitive. The other 10% have either an additional mechanism or combination of mechanisms, which have become well recognized only in recent years. Some of these patients can be made worse by routine treatment for angle-closure, particularly those with intumescent or anteriorly subluxed lenses or malignant glaucoma treated with miotics, who respond paradoxically. Recognition of these other causes of angle-closure in clinical situations is crucial. Understanding the anatomic and pathophysiologic mechanisms involved assists in diagnosis and in optimizing treatment. Until recently, the development of an encompassing schema has been hindered by our inability to visualize the entire anterior segment, limiting our understanding of the underlying anatomic abnormalities. Although slit lamp biomicroscopy and gonioscopy allow us to view the anterior chamber, the posterior chamber, iris-lens relationship, and ciliary body have remained hidden for the most part. Indentation gonioscopy provides accurate information as to the extent of angle-closure and presence of synechiae, but only permits inferential data regarding the structures posterior to the iris.

UBM is ideally suited to study of angle-closure because it can image the angle structures, ciliary body, posterior chamber, and iris-lens relationship simultaneously. In this chapter, we will illustrate how UBM has improved our understanding of angle-closure glaucoma and is helping to elucidate new approaches to therapy.

## Relative Pupillary Block

Relative pupillary block is an impedance to aqueous humor flow between the lens and iris from the posterior chamber to the anterior chamber. The reduced flow causes pressure in the posterior chamber to become higher than that in the anterior chamber. This then causes anterior iris convexity, narrowing of the angle, and, depending on the presence or absence of other incompletely understood factors, acute or chronic angle-closure glaucoma.

Relative pupillary block typically occurs in hyperopic eyes, which have a shorter than average axial length, shallower anterior chamber, thicker lens, more anterior lens position, and smaller radius of corneal curvature.[65-69] Aside from crowding, the anterior segment structures and their anatomic relationships appear normal (Figures 10-11a and 10-11b). Laser iridectomy provides definitive treatment for pupillary block angle-closure glaucoma, providing an alternative pathway for aqueous from the posterior chamber to reach the anterior chamber, eliminating the pressure gradient between the two chambers and allowing the iris to assume a planar configuration. Plugging of the iridectomy by pigment or regrowth of iris pigment epithelium can once again produce pupillary block.

When assessing a patient with a narrow angle for occludability, it is important to perform gonioscopy in a completely darkened room, using the smallest square of slit-beam light in order to avoid stimulating the pupillary light reflex. The narrowest quadrant, usually the superior angle (inferior mirror) is the one that should be observed. At least 2 minutes in total darkness should be allowed for the angle to close before assuming that it is not spontaneously occludable. Indentation

forces the entire iris posteriorly, opening the angle. If synechiae are absent, the angle opens widely. UBM is extremely useful in explaining the situation to the patient. The eye is scanned in both light and dark conditions, and the resultant appearances of the angle can be shown to the patient and graphic explanations given.

## Plateau Iris

Plateau iris configuration refers to an angle appearance in which the iris root angulates forward and then centrally.[70] The iris root is often short and is inserted anteriorly on the ciliary face, so that the angle is shallow and narrow, with a sharp peripheral iris drop-off. The iris surface is relatively flat and the anterior chamber is of relatively normal depth. Plateau iris syndrome refers to the development of angle-closure, either spontaneously or after pupillary dilation, in an eye with plateau iris configuration in the presence of a patent iridectomy.[71-74]

Plateau iris is caused by an anteriorly positioned ciliary body, which narrows the angle by physically supporting the iris root in proximity to the trabecular meshwork (Figures 10-12a and 10-12b).[5,75] The level of the iris with respect to the angle structures, or the "height" to which the plateau rises, determines whether or not the angle will close completely up to the level of Schwalbe's line or only partially, leaving the upper meshwork free of obstruction and leading to chronic angle-closure, a much more common situation in these patients than acute angle-closure (Figure 10-13).[76]

Patients with plateau iris tend to be women in their 30s to 50s and are less hyperopic overall than those with relative pupillary block. On indentation gonioscopy, the ciliary processes prevent posterior movement of the peripheral iris, resulting in the "double-hump sign," in which the iris follows the curvature of the lens, reaches its deepest point at the lens equator, then rises again over the ciliary processes before dropping peripherally. Much more force is needed during gonioscopy to open the angle than in pupillary block because the ciliary processes must be displaced, and the angle does not open as widely (Figures 10-14a and 10-14b).

Some element of pupillary block is often present. As a general rule, the older the patient, the less prominent the angulation of the peripheral iris and the greater the element of pupillary block. Iridectomy is successful at opening the angle when a component of pupillary block is present, but periodic gonioscopy remains indicated, as the angle can narrow further with age due to enlargement of the lens. Continued appositional angle-closure in the presence of a patent iridectomy is an indication for laser iridoplasty.[77-82]

## Iris and Ciliary Body Cysts

Iris and/or ciliary body cysts can produce either acute or chronic angle-closure glaucoma.[83] These are usually easily

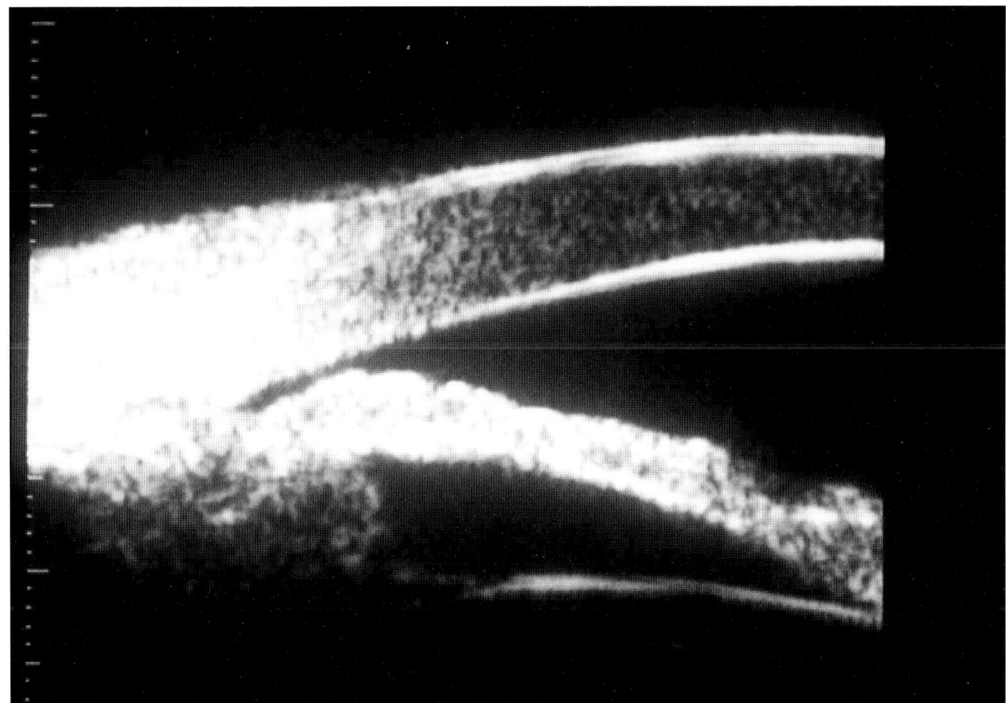

**Figure 10-11a.** The effect of illumination on angle configuration in an eye with pupillary block. Bright illumination. The angle is open. Reprinted with permission from Ritch R, Liebmann J, Tello C. A construct for understanding angle-closure glaucoma: the role of ultrasound biomicroscopy. *Ophthalmol Clin N Amer.* 1995;8:281-293.

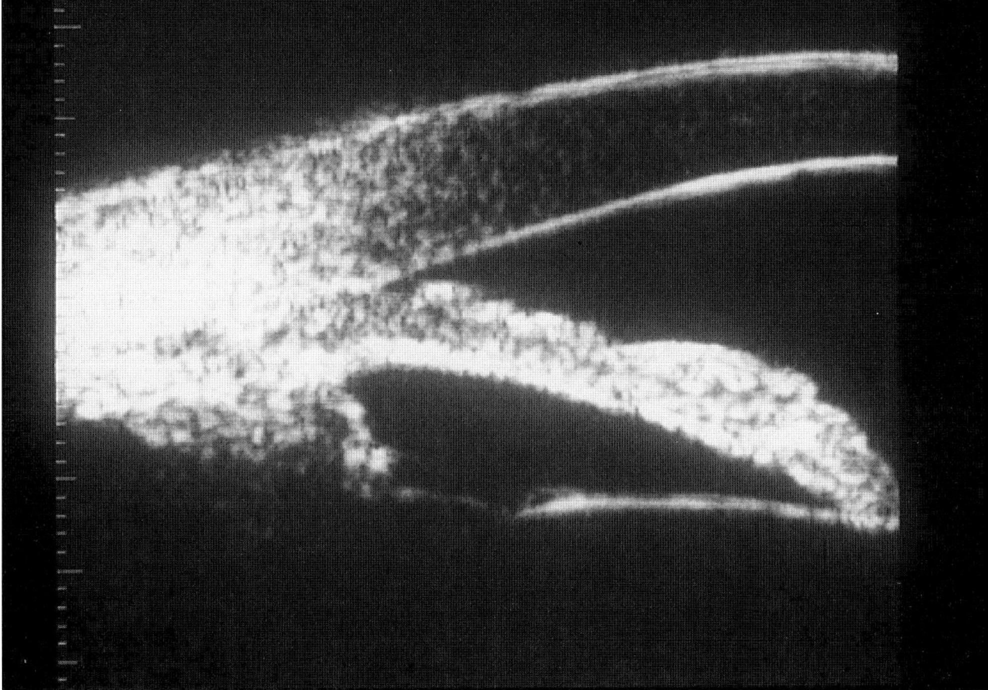

**Figure 10-11b.** Pupillary dilation in a darkened room results in appositional closure. Reprinted with permission from Ritch R, Liebmann J, Tello C. A construct for understanding angle-closure glaucoma: the role of ultrasound biomicroscopy. *Ophthalmol Clin N Amer.* 1995;8:281-293.

**Figure 10-12a.** An eye with plateau iris after laser iridectomy (not shown in this photograph) scanned with room lights on. The anterior chamber is moderately deep, the iris and iris root are comparatively thick, and the iris surface is planar. The ciliary processes are positioned anteriorly and the ciliary sulcus, although present, is minimally defined. The approach to the angle is relatively wide until the point at which the iris root angulates posteriorly, where the angle suddenly becomes extremely narrow. Reprinted with permission from Ritch R, Liebmann JM. Argon laser peripheral iridoplasty: a review. *Ophthalmic Surg Lasers*. 1996;27:289-300.

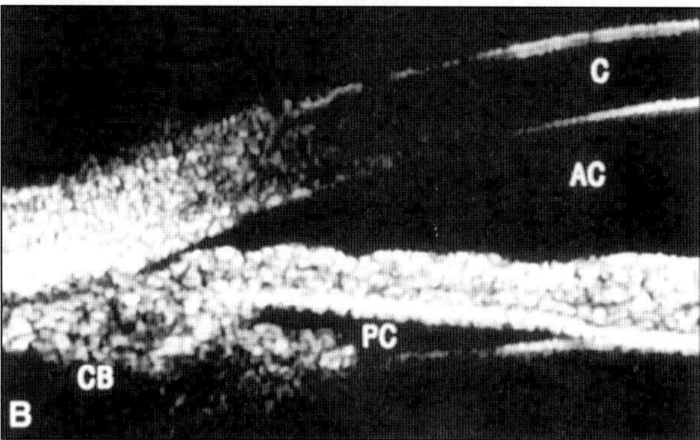


**Figure 10-12b.** The same eye scanned with room lights out. The pupil has dilated and the angle has closed. Laser iridoplasty can open the angle in such an eye by compressing and thinning the peripheral iris stroma. Reprinted with permission from Ritch R, Liebmann JM. Argon laser peripheral iridoplasty: a review. *Ophthalmic Surg Lasers*. 1996;27:289-300.

**Figure 10-13.** Schematic representation of plateau iris. The angle is occludable when the pupil is dilated, but it is the height of the plateau (the extent to which the iris stroma protrudes anteriorly), which determines the level of lateral iridocorneal angle wall that will be occluded, and thus whether IOP will rise. a) Complete plateau iris syndrome. The iris will occlude the meshwork up to Schwalbe's line and IOP will rise. b and c) Incomplete plateau iris syndrome. The iris will occlude the angle to the level of the midmeshwork. The lower on the meshwork that the iris reaches, the less likely a rise in IOP. d) Low plateau. The angle will close only to the top of the scleral spur.

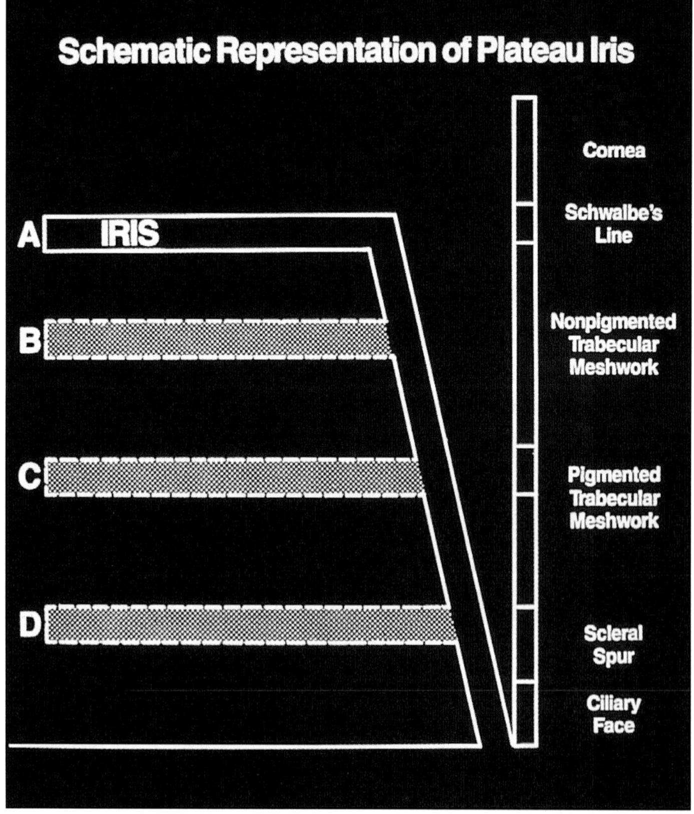

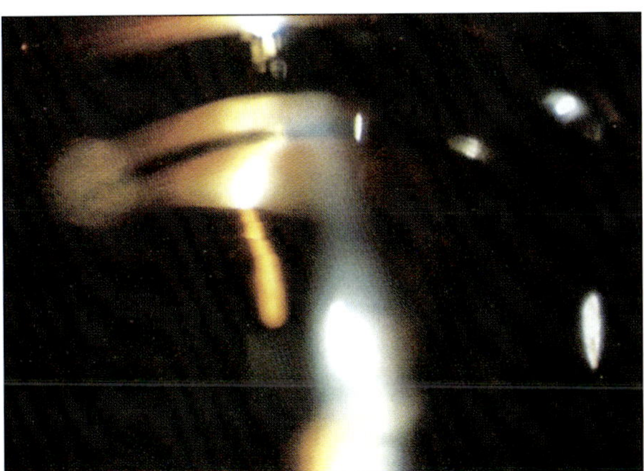

**Figure 10-14a.** Typical gonioscopic appearance of plateau iris. Before indentation, the angle is closed to the mid-trabecular meshwork. The iris assumes a characteristically flat approach to the angle. Reprinted with permission from Ritch R. Plateau iris is caused by abnormally positioned ciliary processes. *J Glaucoma.* 1992;1:23-26.

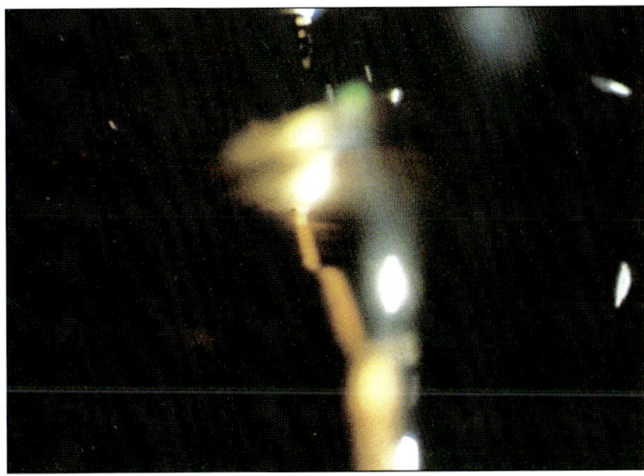

**Figure 10-14b.** With indentation, the deepest displacement of the iris occurs at the lens equator. Reprinted with permission from Ritch R. Plateau iris is caused by abnormally positioned ciliary processes. *J Glaucoma.* 1992;1:23-26.

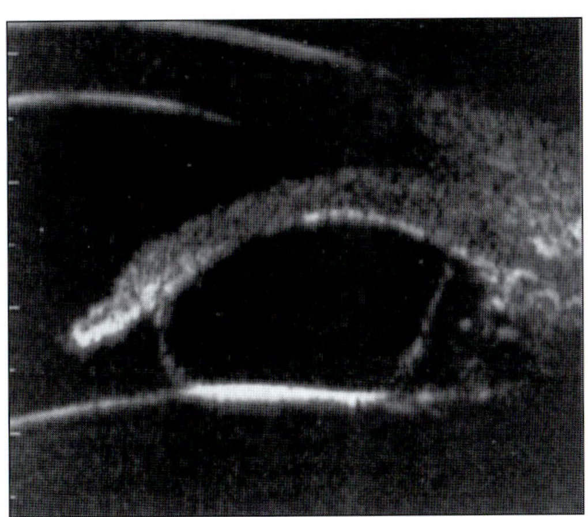

**Figure 10-15a.** A large intraepithelial iris cyst causing angle-closure. Reprinted with permission from Ritch R, Liebmann J, Tello C. A construct for understanding angle-closure glaucoma: the role of ultrasound biomicroscopy. *Ophthalmol Clin N Amer.* 1995;8:281-293.

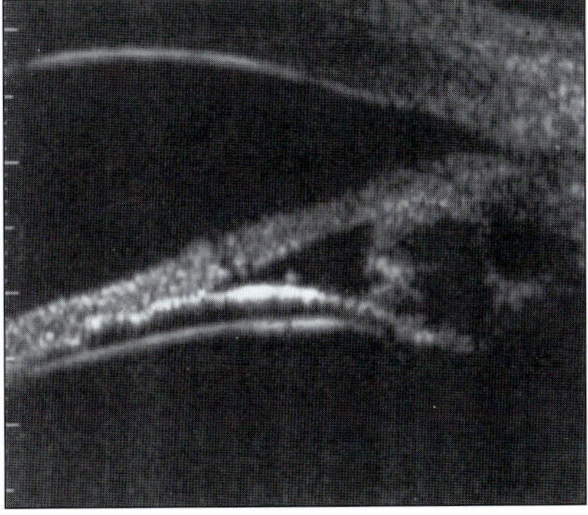

**Figure 10-15b.** The same eye as in Figure 10-15a after laser iridectomy. Smaller, peripheral iris-anterior ciliary epithelial cysts are still present. Reprinted with permission from Ritch R, Liebmann J, Tello C. A construct for understanding angle-closure glaucoma: the role of ultrasound biomicroscopy. *Ophthalmol Clin N Amer.* 1995;8:281-293.

diagnosed, as the angle is closed either in one quadrant or, if cysts are multiple, intermittently. However, when angle-closure mimicking pupillary block occurs, a high index of suspicion and careful gonioscopic evaluation are required.[84] UBM is extremely helpful in making the diagnosis in these patients (Figures 10-15a and 10-15b).

## Abnormalities of the Lens and Zonules

Swelling of the lens may precipitate acute angle-closure glaucoma (phacomorphic glaucoma) (Figures 10-16a and 10-16b). Again, some element of pupillary block may also be present in such patients. This glaucoma is often unresponsive to medical therapy, and paradoxical reactions to pilocarpine are common. Pilocarpine, even in elderly patients, increases axial lens thickness and causes further shallowing of the anterior chamber.[85]

ALPI is effective in breaking attacks of phacomorphic angle-closure.[80] The eye is usually severely inflamed, as these patients usually have been referred after being treated unsuccessfully for a few days. Breaking the attack with iridoplasty allows 2 to 3 weeks for the inflammation and folds in Descemet's to clear, permitting cataract extraction under conditions much closer to ideal. Angle-closure does not recur during this time, since the lens is stationary and

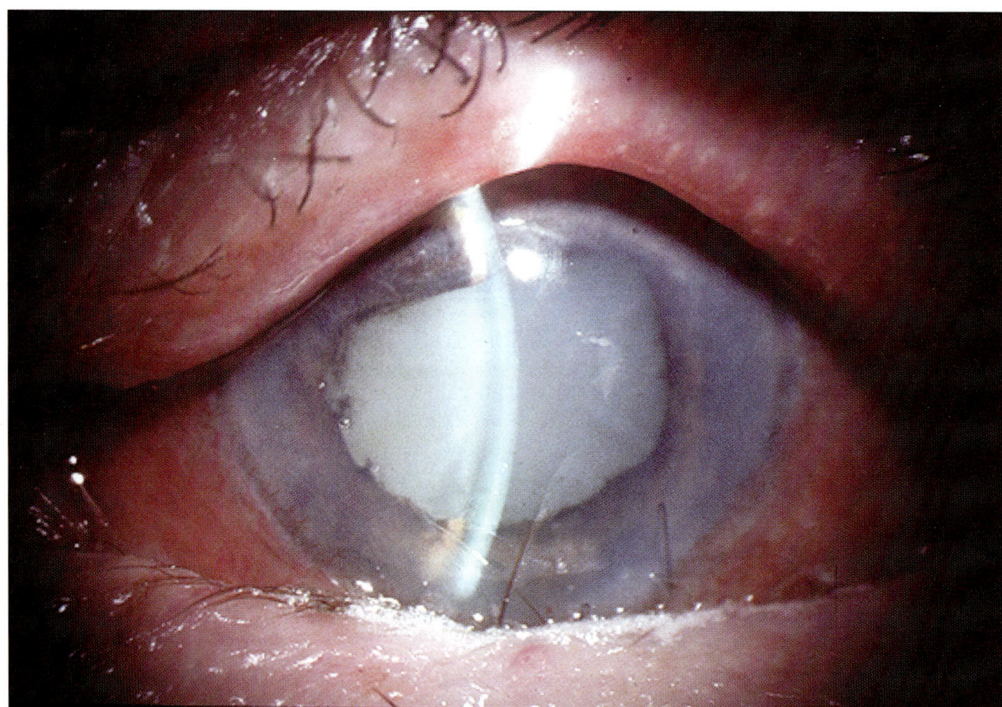

**Figure 10-16a.**
Phacomorphic glaucoma, clinical photograph. Reprinted with permission from Ritch R, Liebmann J, Tello C. A construct for understanding angle-closure glaucoma: the role of ultrasound biomicroscopy. *Ophthalmol Clin N Amer.* 1995;8:281-293.

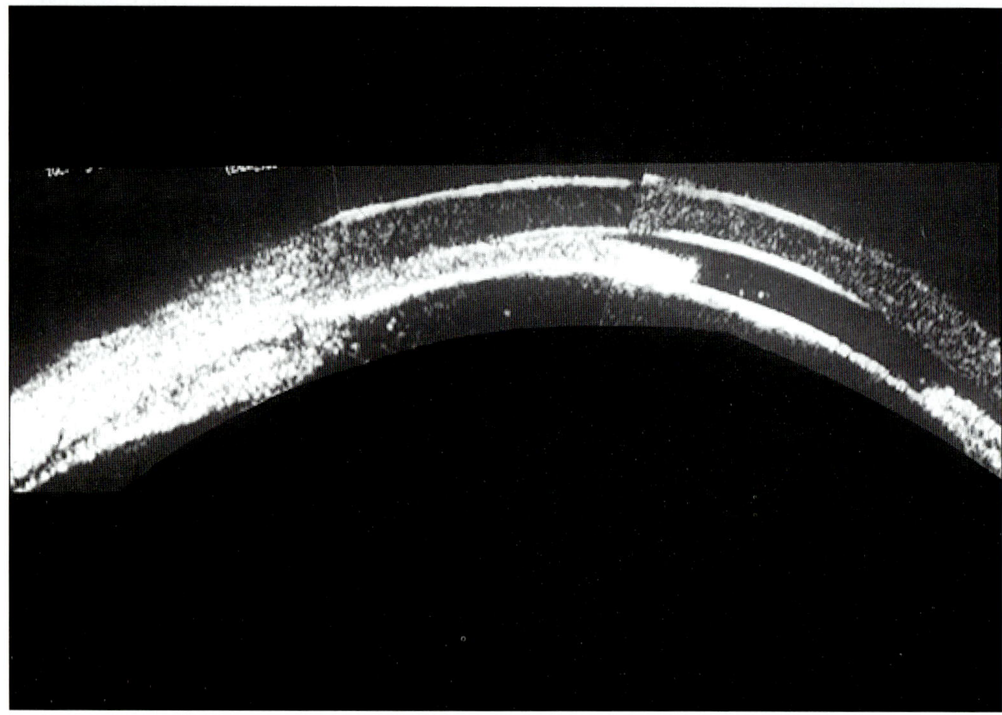

**Figure 10-16b.** Composite UBM of an eye with phacomorphic glaucoma. The anterior chamber is extremely shallow and the lens wedges the iris into the angle and against the cornea. The pars plicata and pars plana can both be seen in this photograph. Reprinted with permission from Ritch R, Liebmann J, Tello C. A construct for understanding angle-closure glaucoma: the role of ultrasound biomicroscopy. *Ophthalmol Clin N Amer.* 1995;8:281-293.

pilocarpine is discontinued at the time of iridoplasty. Any element of pupillary block is treated as soon as possible (usually within 2 to 3 days) after breaking the attack.

In cases of anterior lens subluxation due to trauma or hereditary disorders such as Weill-Marchesani syndrome, iridoplasty is less successful because the pressure of the normal-sized lens against the iris continues, with or without an iridectomy, as long as the underlying cause is present.

Cycloplegics are useful if the zonules are intact, but these may not always be so.[86] If not treated in time, forward lens movement can lead to malignant glaucoma.

## Malignant Glaucoma

Malignant (ciliary block) glaucoma remains a significant challenge to the clinician. It is a multifactorial disease in which the following components may play varying roles:

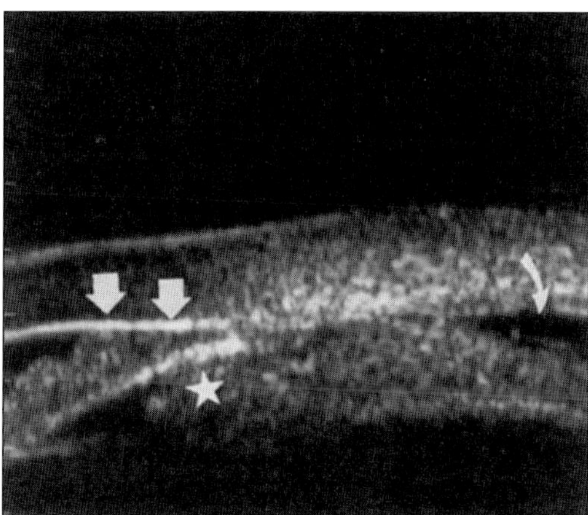

**Figure 10-17.** Anterior rotation of the ciliary processes (star) has forced the peripheral iris against the trabecular meshwork (arrowheads). A shallow retrociliary effusion is present (arrow). Reprinted with permission from Ritch R, Liebmann J, Tello C. A construct for understanding angle-closure glaucoma: the role of ultrasound biomicroscopy. *Ophthalmol Clin N Amer.* 1995;8:281-293.

- Previous acute or chronic angle-closure glaucoma
- Shallow anterior chamber
- Forward lens movement
- Pupillary block by the lens or vitreous
- Loose zonules
- Anterior rotation and/or swelling of the ciliary body
- Thickening of the anterior hyaloid membrane
- Expansion of the vitreous
- Posterior aqueous displacement into or behind the vitreous[87-92]

Analogous to pupillary block, in which the angle is occluded by iris because of a pressure differential between the posterior and anterior chambers, in ciliary block, a pressure differential is presumably created posterior to the lens by aqueous diversion into the vitreous. Primary malignant glaucoma has been thought to result from expansion of the vitreous volume by posterior aqueous displacement, and may occur in phakic, pseudophakic, and aphakic eyes. Anterior rotation of the ciliary body may or may not be present.

Swelling or anterior movement of the ciliary body with forward rotation of the lens-iris diaphragm and relaxation of the zonular apparatus causes anterior lens displacement favoring direct angle-closure (Figure 10-17).[93] Accurate diagnosis and treatment are often more difficult when the initiating event is posterior to the lens-iris diaphragm. Secondary malignant glaucoma occurs when expansion of other posterior segment structures pushes the vitreous and the lens anteriorly, as may happen with intraocular tumors. A syndrome resembling malignant glaucoma can also occur when a wound leak or overfiltration leads to a shallow anterior chamber with forward lens movement, blocking aqueous access to the anterior chamber.

In predisposed eyes, miotic therapy can affect lens position and trigger malignant glaucoma.[87,94-96] Unequal anterior chamber depths, a progressive increase in myopia, or progressive shallowing of the anterior chamber are clues to the correct diagnosis. Malignant glaucoma may occur following cataract surgery with posterior chamber intraocular lens implantation (Figures 10-18a through 10-18g).[12,97-102] Shallowing of the central anterior chamber occurs in pseudophakic malignant glaucoma, but not in pupillary block. Rupture of the anterior hyaloid face is usually curative and allows aqueous to move into the anterior segment.[98]

UBM images are consistent with accepted concepts regarding the posterior diversion of aqueous into the vitreous. Anterior rotation of the ciliary body is present and is compatible with an abnormality of the vitreociliary anatomic relationship leading to aqueous misdirection. The marked forward displacement of the posterior chamber lens and ciliary body reflects enlargement of the vitreous cavity due to a mixture of aqueous and vitreous. Nd:YAG laser hyaloidectomy eliminates the blockage of access of aqueous to the anterior chamber, allowing the structures to move posteriorly, deepen the anterior chamber, and open the angle.[98]

## Synechial Angle Closure

Closure of the angle by peripheral anterior synechiae can be easily imaged by the UBM and both the position and the extent of the synechiae determined (Figure 10-19).

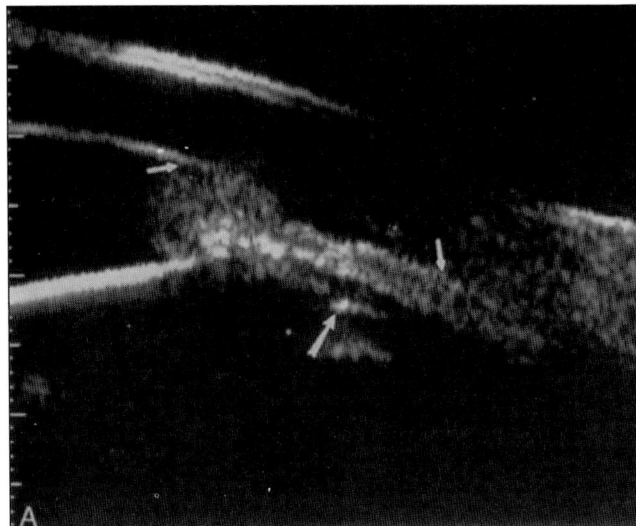

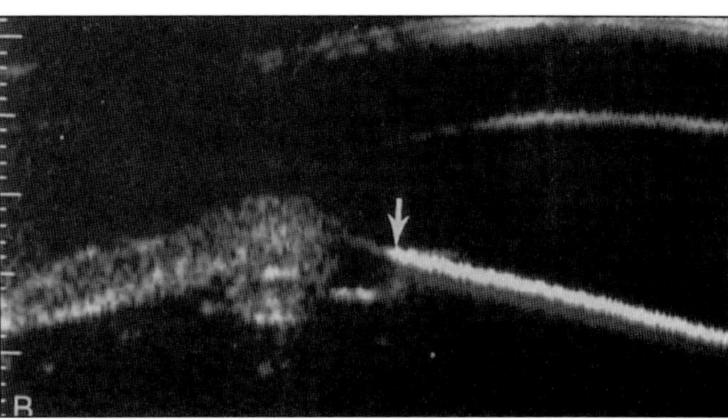

**Figure 10-18b.** The nasal portion of the optic (arrow) is anterior to the iris. Reprinted with permission from Tello C, Chi T, Shepps G, et al. Ultrasound biomicroscopy in pseudophakic malignant glaucoma. Published courtesy of *Ophthalmology* (100:1330-1334, 1993).

**Figure 10-18a.** Pseudophakic malignant glaucoma in an eye with a posterior chamber intraocular lens. In the temporal angle, peripheral iridocorneal apposition is present (small arrows). The haptic is visible beneath the iris (large arrow). Reprinted with permission from Tello C, Chi T, Shepps G, et al. Ultrasound biomicroscopy in pseudophakic malignant glaucoma. Published courtesy of *Ophthalmology* (100:1330-1334, 1993).

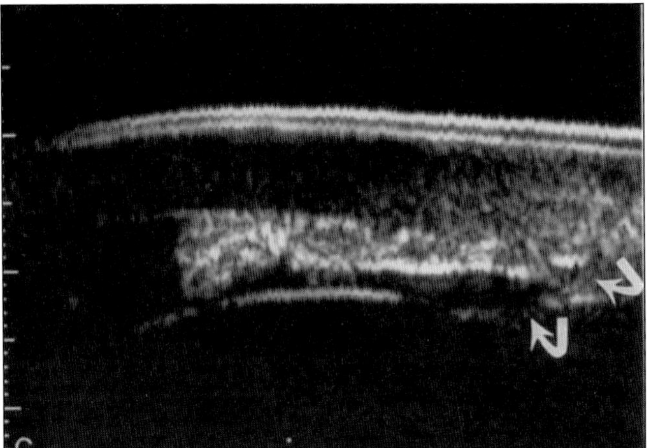

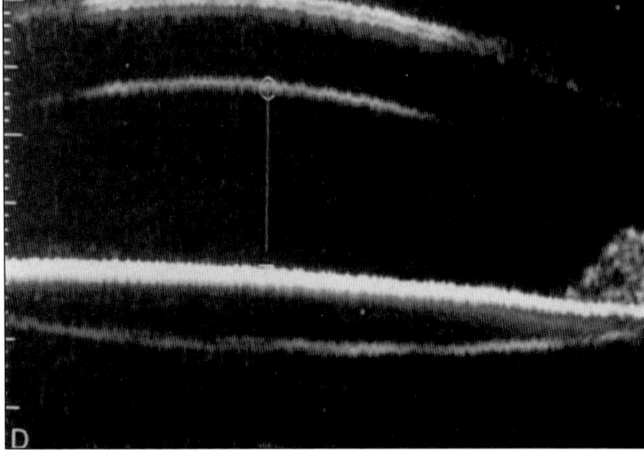

**Figure 10-18c.** Anterior rotation of the ciliary body (arrows) in apposition to the peripheral iris. Reprinted with permission from Tello C, Chi T, Shepps G, et al. Ultrasound biomicroscopy in pseudophakic malignant glaucoma. Published courtesy of *Ophthalmology* (100:1330-1334, 1993).

**Figure 10-18d.** The central anterior chamber is shallow. Reprinted with permission from Tello C, Chi T, Shepps G, et al. Ultrasound biomicroscopy in pseudophakic malignant glaucoma. Published courtesy of *Ophthalmology* (100:1330-1334, 1993).

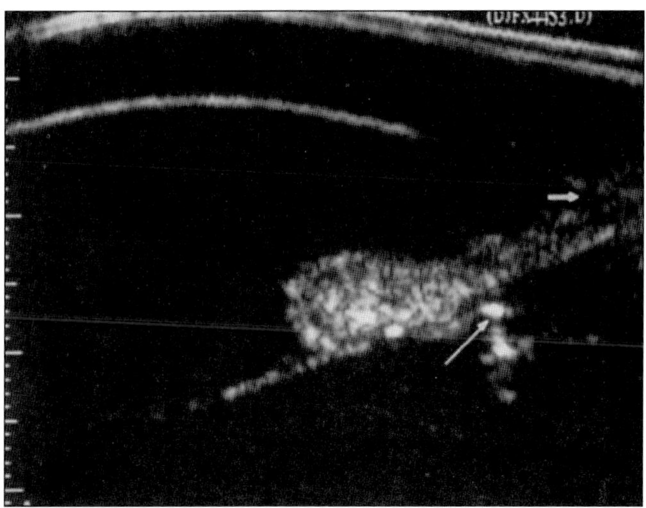

**Figure 10-18e.** After Nd:YAG laser anterior hyaloidectomy, the angle is open (small arrow) and the haptic has moved posteriorly (large arrow). Reprinted with permission from Tello C, Chi T, Shepps G, et al. Ultrasound biomicroscopy in pseudophakic malignant glaucoma. Published courtesy of *Ophthalmology* (100:1330-1334, 1993).

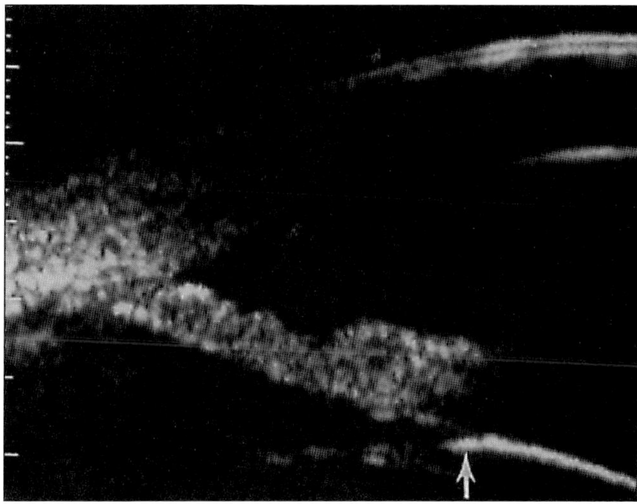

**Figure 10-18f.** The nasal portion of the optic (arrow) is posterior to the iris. Reprinted with permission from Tello C, Chi T, Shepps G, et al. Ultrasound biomicroscopy in pseudophakic malignant glaucoma. Published courtesy of *Ophthalmology* (100:1330-1334, 1993).

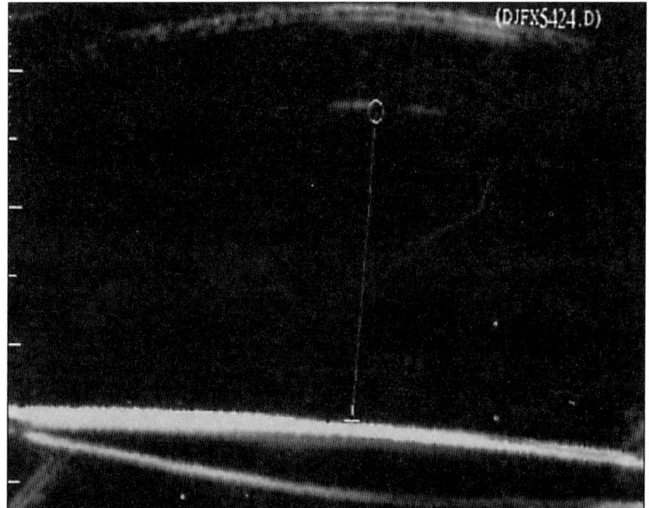

**Figure 10-18g.** The central anterior chamber is deep. Reprinted with permission from Tello C, Chi T, Shepps G, et al. Ultrasound biomicroscopy in pseudophakic malignant glaucoma. Published courtesy of *Ophthalmology* (100:1330-1334, 1993).

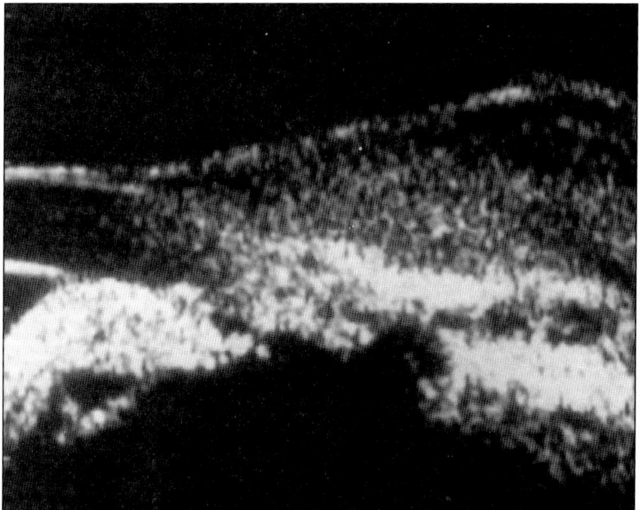

**Figure 10-19.** An eye which had undergoine trabeculectomy and which, on gonioscopy, appeared to have the ostium occluded by iris. UBM, however, shows the iris to be synechially apposed to the anterior meshwork, while the ostium posterior to it is open and leads into a channel created by the scleral flap. The bleb is diffusely edematous without cyst formation. Reprinted with permission from Ritch R, Liebmann J, Tello C. A construct for understanding angle-closure glaucoma: the role of ultrasound biomicroscopy. *Ophthalmol Clin N Amer.* 1995;8:281-293.

# REFERENCES

1. Pavlin CJ, Sherar MD, Foster FS. Subsurface ultrasound microscopic imaging of the intact eye. *Ophthalmology.* 1990;97:244-250.
2. Pavlin CJ, Harasiewicz K, Sherar MD, Foster FS. Clinical use of ultrasound biomicroscopy. *Ophthalmology.* 1991;98:287-295.
3. Pavlin CJ, McWhae JA, McGowan HD, Foster S. Ultrasound biomicroscopy of anterior segment tumors. *Ophthalmology.* 1992;99:1220-1228.
4. Katz NR, Finger PT, McCormick SA, et al. Ultrasound biomicroscopy in the management of malignant melanoma of the iris. *Arch Ophthalmol.* 1995;113:1462-1463.
5. Pavlin CJ, Ritch R, Foster FS. Ultrasound biomicroscopy in plateau iris syndrome. *Am J Ophthalmol.* 1992;113:390-395.
6. Ritch R, Liebmann J, Stegman Z. Mapstone's hypothesis confirmed. *Br J Ophthalmol.* 1995;79:300.
7. Ritch R, Liebmann J, Tello C. A construct for understanding angle-closure glaucoma: the role of ultrasound biomicroscopy. *Ophthalmol Clin N Amer.* 1995;8:281-293.
8. Aslanides IM, Libre PE, Silverman RH, et al. High frequency ultrasound imaging in pupillary block glaucoma. *Br J Ophthalmol.* 1995;79:972-976.
9. Azuara-Blanco A, Spaeth GL, Araujo SV, et al. Plateau iris syndrome associated with multiple ciliary body cysts. Report of 3 cases. *Arch Ophthalmol.* 1996;114:666-668.
10. Kawano Y-I, et al. Ultrasound biomicroscopic analysis of transient shallow anterior chamber in Vogt-Koyanagi-Harada syndrome. *Am J Ophthalmol.* 1996;121:721-723.
11. Pavlin CJ, Easterbrook M, Harasiewicz K, et al. An ultrasound biomicroscopic analysis of angle-closure glaucoma secondary to ciliochoroidal effusion in IgA nephropathy. *Am J Ophthalmol.* 1993;116:341-345.
12. Tello C, Chi T, Shepps G, et al. Ultrasound biomicroscopy in pseudophakic malignant glaucoma. *Ophthalmology.* 1993;100:1330-1334.
13. Potash SD, Tello C, Liebmann J, Ritch R. Ultrasound biomicroscopy in pigment dispersion syndrome. *Ophthalmology.* 1994;101:332-339.
14. Liebmann JM, Tello C, Chew S-J, et al. Prevention of blinking alters iris configuration in pigment dispersion syndrome and in normal eyes. *Ophthalmology.* 1995;102:446-455.
15. Gentile RC, Pavlin CJ, Liebmann JM, et al. Accurate diagnosis of traumatic cyclodialysis clefts by ultrasound biomicroscopy. *Ophthalmic Surg.* 1996;27:97-105.
16. Pavlin CJ, Easterbrook M, Hurwitz JJ, et al. Ultrasound biomicroscopy in the assessment of anterior scleral disease. *Am J Ophthalmol.* 1993;116:628-635.
17. Garcia-Feijoo J, Martin-Cabajo M, Benitez del Castillo JM, Garcia-Canchez J. Ultrasound biomicroscopy in pars planitis. *Am J Ophthalmol.* 1996;121:214-215.
18. Gentile RC, Tello C, Liebmann JM, et al. Ciliary body edema and cyst formation in uveitis. *Br J Ophthalmol.* In press.
19. Yamamoto T, Sakuma T, Kitazawa Y. An ultrasound biomicroscopic study of filtering blebs after mitomycin C trabeculectomy. *Ophthalmology.* 1995;102:1770-1776.
20. Pavlin CJ, Rootman D, Arshinoff S, et al. Determination of haptic position of transsclerally fixated posterior chamber intraocular lenses by ultrasound biomicroscopy. *J Cataract Refract Surg.* 1993;19:573-577.
21. McWhae J, Willerscheidt A, Gimbel H, Freese M. Ultrasound biomicroscopy in refractive surgery. *J Cataract Refract Surg.* 1994;20:493-497.
22. Milner MS, Liebmann JM, Tello C, et al. High-resolution ultrasound biomicroscopy of the anterior segment in patients with dense corneal scars. *Ophthalmic Surg.* 1994;25:284-287.
23. Morinelli EN, Najac RD, Speaker MG, et al. Repair of Descemet's detachments with the assistance of intraoperative ultrasound biomicroscopy. *Am J Ophthalmol.* 1996;121:718-720.
24. Nouby-Mahmoud G, Silverman RH, Coleman DJ. Using high frequency ultrasound to characterize intraocular foreign bodies. *Ophthalmic Surg.* 1993;24:94-99.
25. Coleman KJ, Woods S, Rondeau MJ, Silverman RH. Ophthalmic ultrasonography. *Radiol Clin N Amer.* 1992;30:1105-1114.
26. Iezzi R, Rosen RB, Tello C, et al. Personal computer-based three-dimensional ultrasound biomicroscopy of the anterior segment. *Arch Ophthalmol.* 1996;114:520-524.
27. Sugar HS, Barbour FA. PG: a rare clinical entity. *Am J Ophthalmol.* 1949;32:90-92.
28. Sugar HS. PG: a 25-year review. *Am J Ophthalmol.* 1966;62:499-507.
29. Campbell DG. Pigmentary dispersion and glaucoma: a new theory. *Arch Ophthalmol.* 1979;97:1667-1672.
30. Davidson JA, Brubaker RF, Ilstrup DM. Dimensions of the anterior chamber in pigment dispersion syndrome. *Arch Ophthalmol.* 1983;101:81-83.
31. Lichter PR. PG: current concepts. *Trans Am Acad Ophthalmol Otol.* 1974;78:OP309-313.
32. Zentmayer W. Association of an annular band of pigment on the posterior capsule of the lens with a Krukenberg spindle. *Arch Ophthalmol.* 1938;20:52-57.
33. Scheie HG, Fleischhauer HW. Idiopathic atrophy of the epithelial layers of the iris and ciliary body. A clinical study. *Arch Ophthalmol.* 1958;59:216-228.
34. Brachet A, Chermet M. Association glaucoma pigmentaire et decollement de retine. *Ann D'Oculist.* 1974;207:452-457.
35. Scheie HG, Cameron JD. pigment dispersion syndrome: a clinical study. *Br J Ophthalmol.* 1981;65:264-269.
36. Delaney WVJ. Equatorial lens pigmentation, myopia, and retinal detachment. *Am J Ophthalmol.* 1975;79:194-196.
37. Weseley P, Liebmann J, Walsh JB, Ritch R. Lattice degeneration of the retina and the pigment dispersion syndrome. *Am J Ophthalmol.* 1992;114:539-543.
38. Byer NE. Clinical study of lattice degeneration of the retina. *Trans Am Acad Ophthalmol Otol.* 1965;69:1065-1081.
39. Lichter PR, Shaffer RM. Diagnostic and prognostic signs in PG. *Trans Am Acad Ophthalmol Otol.* 1970;74:984-998.
40. Epstein DL. Pigment dispersion and PG. In: Chandler PA, Grant WM, eds. *Glaucoma.* Philadelphia, Pa: Lea & Febiger; 1979:122.
41. Speakman JS. Pigmentary dispersion. *Br J Ophthalmol.* 1981;65:249.
42. Yanoff M, Fine BS. *Ocular Pathology: A Text and Atlas.* New York: Harper & Row; 1975.
43. Campbell DG. Improvement of PG and healing of transillumination defects with miotic therapy. *Invest Ophthalmol Vis Sci.* 1983;23(Suppl):173.
44. Ritch R. Nonprogressive low-tension glaucoma with pigmentary dispersion. *Am J Ophthalmol.* 1982;94:190-196.
45. Ritch R, Manusow D, Podos SM. Remission of PG in a patient with subluxed lenses. *Am J Ophthalmol.* 1982;94:812-813.
46. Pavlin CJ, Harasiewicz K, Foster FS. Posterior iris bowing in pigmentary dispersion syndrome caused by accommodation. *Am J*

*Ophthalmol.* 1994;118:114-116.

47. Pavlin CJ, Macken P, Trope G, et al. Ultrasound biomicroscopic features of PG. *Can J Ophthalmol.* 1994;29:187-192.

48. Liebmann JM, Tello C, Ritch R. Pigment dispersion syndrome, iris configuration, and blinking. *Invest Ophthalmol Vis Sci.* 1994;35(Suppl):1558.

49. Haynes WL, Alward WLM, Tello C, et al. Incomplete elimination of exercise-induced pigment dispersion by laser iridectomy in pigment dispersion syndrome. *Ophthalmic Surg Lasers.* 1995;26:484-486.

50. Liebmann JM, Langlieb A, Stegman Z, et al. Anterior chamber anatomy in asymmetric pigment dispersion syndrome. *Invest Ophthalmol Vis Sci.* 1995;36(Suppl):S562.

51. Sokol J, Stegman Z, Liebmann JM, Ritch R. Location of the iris insertion in pigment dispersion syndrome. *Ophthalmology.* 1996;103:289-293.

52. Ritch R, Liebmann J, Tello C, Chew SJ. Ultrasound biomicroscopic findings in pigment dispersion syndrome. In: Krieglstein GK, ed. *Glaucoma Update V.* Heidelberg: Kaden Verlag; 1995:290-298.

53. Campbell DG. Iridectomy, blinking and PG. *Invest Ophthalmol Vis Sci.* 1993;34(Suppl).

54. Chew SJ, Tello C, Wallman J, Ritch R. Blinking indents the cornea and reduces anterior chamber volume as shown by ultrasound biomicroscopy. *Invest Ophthalmol Vis Sci.* 1994;35(Suppl):1573.

55. Ritch R. A unification hypothesis of pigment dispersion syndrome. *Trans Am Ophthalmol Soc.* In press.

56. Karickhoff JR. Reverse pupillary block in PG: follow up and new developments. *Ophthalmic Surg.* 1993;24:562-563.

57. McWhae J, Crichton A. Presentation at the International Society for Ophthalmic Ultrasound. Cortina, Italy; 1994.

58. Pavlin CJ, Macken P, Trope G, et al. Accommodation and iridectomy in the pigment dispersion syndrome. *Ophthalmic Surg Lasers.* 1996;27:113-120.

59. Haynes WL, Johnson AT, Alward WLM. Inibition of exercise-induced pigment dispersion in a patient with the pigment dispersion syndrome. *Am J Ophthalmol.* 1990;109:599-601.

60. Lunde MW. Argon laser trabeculoplasty in pigmentary dispersion syndrome with glaucoma. *Am J Ophthalmol.* 1983;96:721-725.

61. Ritch R, Liebmann JM, Robin AL, et al. Argon laser trabeculoplasty in PG. *Ophthalmology.* 1993;100:909-913.

62. Lieberman MF, Hoskins HD Jr, Hetherington J Jr. Laser trabeculoplasty and the glaucomas. *Ophthalmology.* 1983;90:790-795.

63. Shields MD, Ritch R, Krupin TK. Classifications and mechanisms of the glaucomas. In: Ritch R, Shields MB, Krupin T, eds. *The Glaucomas.* St. Louis, Mo: CV Mosby; 1989:751-755.

64. Shields MD, Ritch R. Classifications and mechanisms of the glaucomas. In: Ritch R, Shields MB, eds. *The Secondary Glaucomas.* St. Louis, Mo: CV Mosby; 1982.

65. Lowe RF. Primary angle-closure glaucoma: a review of ocular biometry. *Austral J Ophthalmol.* 1977;5:9-17.

66. Delmarcelle Y, François J, Goes F, et al. Biometrie oculaire clinique (oculometrie). *Bull Soc Ophthalmol Belge.* 1976;1:172.

67. Tomlinson A, Leighton DA. Ocular dimensions in the heredity of angle-closure glaucoma. *Br J Ophthalmol.* 1973;57:475-486.

68. Lowe RF, Clark BAJ. Posterior corneal curvature: correlations in normal eyes and in eyes involved with primary angle-closure glaucoma. *Br J Ophthalmol.* 1973;57:475.

69. Lee DA, Brubaker RF, Illstrup DM. Anterior chamber dimensions in patients with narrow angles and angle-closure glaucoma. *Arch Ophthalmol.* 1984;102:46-50.

70. Tornquist R. Angle-closure glaucoma in an eye with a plateau type of iris. *Acta Ophthalmol.* 1958;36:413.

71. Godel V, Stein R, Feiler-Ofry V. Angle-closure glaucoma following peripheral iridectomy and mydriasis. *Am J Ophthalmol.* 1968;65:555-560.

72. Lowe RF. Primary angle-closure glaucoma: postoperative acute glaucoma after phenylephrine eye-drops. *Am J Ophthalmol.* 1968;65:552.

73. Lowe RF. Plateau iris. *Austral J Ophthalmol.* 1981;9:71.

74. Wand M, Grant WM, Simmons RJ, Hutchinson BT. Plateau iris syndrome. *Trans Am Acad Ophthalmol Otol.* 1977;83:122.

75. Ritch R. Plateau iris is caused by abnormally positioned ciliary processes. *J Glaucoma.* 1992;1:23-26.

76. Lowe RF, Ritch R. Angle-closure glaucoma. Clinical types. In: Ritch R, Shields MB, Krupin T, eds. *The Glaucomas.* St. Louis, Mo: CV Mosby; 1989:839-853.

77. Ritch R. *Techniques of Argon Laser Iridectomy and Iridoplasty.* Palo Alto, Calif: Coherent Medical Press; 1983.

78. York K, Ritch R, Szmyd LJ. Argon laser peripheral iridoplasty: indications, techniques and results. *Invest Ophthalmol Vis Sci.* 1984;25(Suppl):94.

79. Ritch R, Lowe RF, Reyes A. Angle-closure glaucoma—therapeutic overview. In: Ritch R, Shields MB, Krupin T, eds. *The Glaucomas.* St. Louis, Mo: CV Mosby; 1989.

80. Ritch R. Argon laser treatment for medically unresponsive attacks of angle-closure glaucoma. *Am J Ophthalmol.* 1982;94:197.

81. Ritch R, Solomon IS. Glaucoma surgery. In: L'Esperance FA, ed. *Ophthalmic Lasers.* 3rd ed. St. Louis, Mo: CV Mosby; 1989.

82. Ritch R. Argon laser peripheral iridoplasty: an overview. *J Glaucoma.* 1992;1:206-213.

83. Chandler PA, Braconier HE. Spontaneous intra-epithelial cysts of iris and ciliary body with glaucoma. *Am J Ophthalmol.* 1958;45:64.

84. Vela A, Rieser JC, Campbell DG. The heredity and treatment of angle-closure glaucoma secondary to iris and ciliary body cysts. *Ophthalmology.* 1984;91:332-337.

85. Abramson DH, Franzen LA, Coleman DJ. Pilocarpine in the presbyope: demonstration of an effect on the anterior chamber and lens thickness. *Arch Ophthalmol.* 1973;89:100-102.

86. Ritch R, Solomon LD. Argon laser peripheral iridoplasty for angle-closure glaucoma in siblings with Weill-Marchesani syndrome. *J Glaucoma.* 1992;1:243-247.

87. Levene RZ. A new concept of malignant glaucoma. *Arch Ophthalmol.* 1972;87:497.

88. Shaffer RN, Hoskins HD Jr. Ciliary block (malignant) glaucoma. *Trans Am Acad Ophthalmol Otol.* 1978;85:215.

89. Simmons RJ. Malignant glaucoma. *Br J Ophthalmol.* 1972;56:273.

90. Weiss DI, Shaffer RN. Ciliary block (malignant) glaucoma. *Trans Am Acad Ophthalmol Otol.* 1972;76:450.

91. Simmons RJ, Thomas JV, Yaqub MK. Malignant glaucoma. In: Ritch R, Shields MB, Krupin T, eds. *The Glaucomas.* St. Louis, Mo: CV Mosby; 1989.

92. Dueker D. Ciliary-block glaucoma—differential diagnosis and management. *J Glaucoma.* 1994;3:167-170.

93. Phelps CD. Angle-closure glaucoma secondary to ciliary body swelling. *Arch Ophthalmol.* 1974;92:287.

94. Gorin G. Angle-closure glaucoma induced by miotics. *Am J Ophthalmol.* 1966;62:1063.

95. Merritt JC. Malignant glaucoma induced by miotics postoperatively in open-angle glaucoma. *Arch Ophthalmol.* 1977;95:1988.

96. Rieser JC, Schwartz B. Miotic induced malignant glaucoma. *Arch*

*Ophthalmol.* 1972;87:706.

97. Brown RH, Lynch MG, Tearse JE, Nunn RD. Neodymium-YAG vitreous surgery for phakic and pseudophakic malignant glaucoma. *Arch Ophthalmol.* 1986;104:1464-1466.

98. Epstein DL, Steinert RF, Puliafito CA. Neodymium-YAG laser therapy to the anterior hyaloid in aphakic malignant glaucoma. *Am J Ophthalmol.* 1984;98:137.

99. Lynch MG, Brown RH, Michels RG, et al. Surgical vitrectomy for pseudophakic malignant glaucoma. *Am J Ophthalmol.* 1986;102:149-153.

100. Duy TP, Wollensak J. Ciliary block (malignant) glaucoma following posterior chamber lens implantation. *Ophthalmic Surg.* 1987;18:741-744.

101. Reed JE, Thomas JV, Lytle RA, Simmons RJ. Malignant glaucoma induced by an intraocular lens. *Ophthalmic Surg.* 1990;21:177-180.

102. Vajpayee RB, et al. Pseudophakic pupillary-block glaucoma in children. *Am J Ophthalmol.* 1991;111:715.

103. Ritch R, Liebmann JM. Argon laser peripheral iridoplasty: a review. *Ophthalmic Surg Lasers.* 1996;27:289-300.

# CONCLUSIONS

*Joel S. Schuman, MD*

Several questions were posed in the Preface:

- Which, if any, technology for optic nerve head or nerve fiber layer analysis should I buy?
- Which devices can I use to determine blood flow in glaucoma, and what do the results mean?
- What tests should I order on my patients, and what can I expect the tests to tell me?

This text has provided the reader with the accumulated knowledge of individuals with considerable experience as to each of the technologies discussed, and has hopefully equipped the reader with the wisdom to answer each of the questions asked above.

Each of the devices for ONH and NFL imaging appear to do what they set out to do, but each does this in a different way. With many of these technologies the buyer "gets what is paid for." Certain technologies, particularly OCT, offer applications in multiple areas of ophthalmology. CSLO may be used for the examination of macular holes using coronal sections, for focal electroretinography, and for angiography. OCT has utility in retinal diseases, the anterior segment, and lens evaluation, as well as in glaucoma; these are only the uses within ophthalmology. We are currently at a stage with OCT similar to the introduction stage of MRI, when beautiful images of sagitally sectioned brain could be seen in living humans for the first time. The actual utility of MRI grew over time, and like MRI at its introduction, the potential of OCT is still largely untapped.

Ocular blood flow is more complex. Current technologies hint at what might be possible in the future: actual measurement of blood flow in the optic nerve. The work of Harris, Cantor, and Kagemann and of Melamed, Krupsky, and Treister provide major steps in that direction.

Ultrasound biomicroscopy enables clinicians to see immediately posterior to the iris, nearly to the ora serratta. It can provide a dynamic view of the angle structures, allowing the clinician to actually observe angle closure in susceptible individuals. As Ritch, Liebmann, Iezzi, and Tello showed, the UBM is a useful tool both for clinical diagnosis and elucidation of glaucoma mechanisms.

## SUMMARY

"Which, if any, technology for optic nerve head or nerve fiber layer analysis should I buy?" The answer to this question really depends upon the clinician's needs and finances. All clinicians need a slit lamp and an indirect lens (60, 78, or 90 D) with which to examine the ONH and NFL. Any clinician seeing a large volume of glaucoma patients should have the capability for stereoscopic ONH and NFL photography. Most would like the ability to objectively and quantitatively assess the eye as well, which is possible only with an imaging system.

"Which devices can I use to determine blood flow in glaucoma, and what do the results mean?" At the present time, no commercial device has conclusively been shown to demonstrate blood flow. This is still not only an area fertile for investigation, but a hotbed of controversy. The chapters on this topic help to explain the current state-of-the-art, and to allow clinicians to decide whether blood flow analysis is appropriate for selected patients (eg, suspected ocular ischemia, normal tension glaucoma, etc.).

"What tests should I order on my patients, and what can I expect the tests to tell me?" This question requires one to know the degree of uncertainty in the diagnosis of a given patient. If there is little or no doubt as to the presence or absence of glaucoma or its progression, no additional testing is required. Would that this were routinely the case! A more typical patient, for instance, is an individual with suspected glaucoma with large cups and intact neuroretinal rims, an

IOP in the mid-20s, and normal visual fields. In this patient, a test of NFL thickness or using CSLO might either raise or lower the clinician's suspicion level. If, for example, OCT or the NFA showed the NFL to be relatively thick, with no areas of focal thinning, or if the CSLO demonstrated a good neuroretinal rim area, then the patient might be considered a glaucoma suspect, but with low suspicion, or maybe not even a suspect at all.

These devices can be used to support or refute a glaucoma diagnosis, or to detect the presence of change over time; however, more investigation is required to actually use these technologies to make the diagnosis, or to unconditionally demonstrate progression of disease.

All pieces of the glaucoma puzzle must be put together in order to care appropriately for the patient. The clinician must use the clinical patient examination, IOP, ONH, and NFL appearance, visual field data, as well as quantitative data contributed by technology, to detect glaucoma or its progression.

# INDEX